Emotions in the Human Voice

Volume 2: Clinical Evidence

Emotions in the Human Voice

Volume 2: Clinical Evidence

Edited by
Krzysztof Izdebski

PLURAL PUBLISHING
INC.
SAN DIEGO
OXFORD
BRISBANE

PLURAL PUBLISHING
INC.

5521 Ruffin Road
San Diego, CA 92123

e-mail: info@pluralpublishing.com
Web site: http://www.pluralpublishing.com

49 Bath Street
Abingdon, Oxfordshire OX14 1EA
United Kingdom

Typeset in 10.5/13 Garamond by Flanagan's Publishing Services, Inc.
Printed in the United States of America by McNaughton and Gunn

Library of Congress Cataloging-in-Publication Data:

Emotions in the human voice / [edited by] Krzysztof Izdebski.
p. ; cm.
Includes bibliographical references and index.
ISBN-13: 978-1-59756-073-3 (v. 1 : alk. paper)
ISBN-10: 1-59756-073-1 (v. 1 : alk. paper)
ISBN-13: 978-1-59756-118-1 (v. 2 : alk. paper)
ISBN-10: 1-59756-118-5 (v. 2 : alk. paper)
[etc.]
1. Voice—Psychological aspects. 2. Emotions. I. Izdebski, Krzystof.
[DNLM: 1. Affect. 2. Verbal Behavior. 3. Auditory Perception. 4. Emotions.
5. Phonation. 6. Voice Quality. BF 582 E545 2007]
BF592.V64E44 2007
153.6—dc22

2007043352

CONTENTS

FOREWORD

The human voice—what a masterpiece of creation! We laugh with it, we cry with it, we sing with it, we pray with it, we scream with it, we whisper with it—yet, how little do we know about its effect upon the listener. The voice represents our ultimate means of communication from birth to death, yet how little do we know about its impact on human culture and society. While our voice connects us to our fellow humans and other species, we know but little about the mechanics of this transaction.

Even in antiquity, Greek and Roman philosophers were aware that the voice is the mirror of the soul. But it was not until the 20th century and the age of communication that serious investigations were initiated into the relations between the human voice and emotions. Recent research has revealed that the effect of the mother's voice creates a bond with the fetus in utero during the second trimester of pregnancy. With each year of our physical development, the voice and emotions play a more complex role in our adjustment to an ever-more complex world.

The recent Pacific Voice and Speech Foundation Annual Voice Conference on Voice and Emotion held at the Pixar Animation Studios in California represented the first serious attempt to study the complex relations between voice and emotions on a multidisciplinary level. The success of this meeting sparked a global fire of interest to bring together the vast knowledge from various cultures and various specialties, which has not been readily available to interested individuals.

This search extended to academicians and to clinicians, to scientists and to practitioners, to teachers and to writers. In Europe, contributors hail from Scandinavia and Finland in the north; from Italy and Spain in the south; from the United Kingdom, the Netherlands, Belgium, and France in the west; from Russia in the east; and from Germany, Austria, Poland and Switzerland in Central Europe. In the western hemisphere, chapters arrived from the United States, Canada, and Brazil; in the Far East from Japan, and Singapore, and Viet Nam; in the Pacific region from Australia and the Philippines; and in the Middle East from Israel.

The authors represent an equally diverse group of authorities: psychologists, linguists, speech and voice pathologists, physicians, phoniatricians, acousticians, vocal artists and performers, voice coaches, and experts from the fields of radio, computer science, commerce, television, and motion pictures. Over the past several weeks, I have had the opportunity to review this amazing collection of manuscripts, and I am amazed by the wealth and diversity of the submitted information. While the human voice is always one part of the equation, the emotions vary from joy to pain, from sorrow to happiness; from adults to children; from men to women; from spontaneity to stability; from pleasantness to roughness; from health to disease; from the brain to the organs of phonation; from neurology to psychophysiology; from development to recognition; from actor to anime, and—from laughter to love. The information is here and the choice is yours.

All of us share a sincere debt of thanks to the Editor, Dr. Krzysztof Izdebski, an enthusiastic and indefatigable champion of the field of voice, and a dear friend to many of the participating authors. Dr. Izdebski spearheaded the meeting held at the Pixar Studios and has done the lion's share of preparing this book. While all readers will benefit by their study of *Emotions in the Human Voice*, Dr. Izdebski deserves our respect, our admiration, and, above all, our gratitude.

Hans von Leden
Professor of Biocommunications (Emeritus)
University of Southern California
Los Angeles, California

PREFACE

When my long-standing friend and colleague, Tom Murry of New York City, asked me in April of 2004, while we were munching on some tiny canapés during a coffee break at a voice course in Paris, France, to put into a *book* the experiences of the XV Annual Pacific Voice Conference entitled *Emotions and Voice* held at the Pixar Animation Studio in Emeryville, California, in March of that year, I was not sure if he was still my long-standing friend, had had an episode of hypoglycemia, or suddenly became my newest tormentor. As his then semi-casual request is now coming to a semi-completion, I can truly state that Tom had a vision, which he expressed in that Parisian April milieu with a straight, professorial, but somewhat emotive statement, that simply meant, "KI, you can do it! And I count on you." I am not sure that at the time I heard his voice as a challenge or just a friendly call for a potentially interesting volume collecting conference-related papers. Soon, however, I was to find out.

Upon my return to northern California, I started to reconstruct the taste of the canapés, Tom's voice, and the events of the XV Annual Pacific Voice Conference. My recollections were positive, so I began to look optimistically for the missing links and started to compile a list of potential contributors, who for whatever reasons were absent from our March 2005 happening, but who knew a lot. As soon as I began to put all the materials together and outlined a book, I realized the challenge placed on me by Tom.

This challenge came to me as a big surprise, as I am accustomed to writing, to publishing, to presenting, and to creating year after year new and narrowly focused scientific-clinical content that has made the Annual Pacific Voice Conferences (PVC). PVC is more or less an annual educational activity of the San Francisco based Pacific Voice and Speech Foundation that I chair—a hit among the international crowd of working voice clinicians. What struck me, when I really sat down to chart out this endeavor, was not the vastness of the material on human emotions, but how circumscribed the information was relating to *voice and emotions*. Yes, Diane Bless of Madison, Wisconsin, USA, was correct when we first discussed the program of the conference in the fall of 2004 (no, there was no food involved then, just a phone and her ever-friendly voice and loyal support) in saying that the topic of voice and emotions is "*terrific and right on time*."

Luckily, the faculty of the XV PVC responded, and soon I was able to locate and enjoy the enthusiasm of other emotion researchers who for many reasons were unable to be present at the Emeryville happening, and who agreed to contribute to this volume. Specifically, I felt that I am on the right track after connecting with and experiencing the enthusiasm and dedicated intellectual help on this project of Branka Zei Pollermann of Emotion Research Group in Geneva, Switzerland and a Director of Vox, also in Switzerland. Her contribution to the entire concept was pivotal and fundamental, and I hence dare to nominate Branka for the Honorary Editor. "Hvala, Danke, Mercie and Thank you Branka"

Looking for further support, I recruited Hans von Leden. Hans is originally from Silesia (a place where I too lived as a child, though long after his departure), and now he is my fellow Californian, though, alas, of southern part, the City of Angels, Los Angeles (where I also lived for a while when attending UCLA). Hans, a cross-cultural erudite, a clinical and scientific father of voice problems in the USA, and so aware of our peculiar way of living life, simply told me as he always does, using his measured yet so emotive voice, "*Krzysztof, I know you can do it; congratulations, good luck and God bless you.*"

More of the wonderful encouragement came from such professionals as Anne-Maria Laukannen of Tampere, Finland, Isabel Guimaraes and Manuel Pais-Clemente of Portugal, Raul Cruz of Oakland CA, USA, and Lilla Theresa Sadowski of Graz, Austria. Now I was sure that this challenge would eventually come to fruition, and after chatting with all the other researchers who so generously embraced the project and promised to deliver in the most collegial and unselfish way, I knew that the book, or the books, would be a reality.

So there was apparently no way for me to retract. With this generous encouragement and upon Tom Murry's continuous insistence, I called Sadanand Singh at Plural Publishing (again, no fancy food around to distract) and presented to him this project as a matter of fact, and after hearing what was cooking, he simply asked, "*Krys, do you think anybody will buy the book?*" He then passed me to a Lauren Duffy of Plural, who proclaimed, "Oh, I love the whole idea, and I am so excited about this book; when can I have it?" It felt safe, as if we found somebody really, really nice to blame if the book fails to sell.

Really, there have been no books or collections on the subject of emotions of the human voice or on emotions in the human voice, and ours was to be first. The book was to be based on the first-ever truly focused international two-day conference on this topic, namely, the XV Annual Pacific Voice Conference commingled with Pixar Studios' interest in voice and cartoon characters. Was this conference instructional enough to the digital art industry on how to make the voices of the brilliant cartoon characters created by Pixar more emotional, more believable, and more scientifically correct, or are they smart enough on their own? When I contacted Pixar with the idea of a joint meeting on voice and emotions, I was placed in the hands of Randy Nelson, Dean of Pixar University, who embraced the project and went with it blindly, as if a gathering of hundreds of people interested in the emotions of the human voice naturally belonged to the studio. Randy, I do feel guilty for all the flack you may have gotten as a result of this conference, but we had a great time, we learned from your faculty and your environment, and you are a generous host who is greatly missed. And just to let you know, the participants ask for a repeat.

The theme of the conference caught the attention of a Pixar activity tracker, a smart local newspaper writer (you do know that Pixar is a big, big business, and big businesses are carefully watched, and I assume you may know that Pixar was just bought by Disney, and this is also big news), who politely accused the organization of "*going emotional*." Emotions are cardinal no-nos of any big business. And the "accusation" was right on, as in addition to all the fantastic scientific sessions and presentations by Pixar faculty we had an unprecedented opportunity to experience on-line, in real life and in virtual reality, not only a special presentation of the Oscar winning Pixar production of *The Incredibles*, but also to enjoy a 6-hour-long parade of professional voice users (artists) demonstrating vocally coded emotions. This group comprised public speakers, voice-over artists, improvisational actors, stage actors, singers from pop, blues, jazz, country, cabaret, opera, and chorus, storytellers, other performers, cartoon character creators, puppeteers, voice coaches, animators, movie sound creators, and others, all of whom showed their vocally coded emotions in a most remarkable way. Thank you guys, thank you indeed. Pity, then, that the content of these incredible artistic renditions, all focused on highlighting the emotional voice, is missing from this volume.

So what is this book all about? First, it is a *thank you note* to all the contributors, as we all are the editors of equal weight. Next, it is a compilation of the most up-to-date knowledge of what constitutes emotive vocalization *vis-á-vis* currently accepted models of emotions. Obviously, some material is missing and some ideas or results are underrepresented, and obviously, there is room to expand and to improve. Nonetheless, these volumes stand alone and provide a solid reference source on the emotions of the human voice in the most comprehensive way presented so far; the collection also unifies all of us into a cross-cultural family of people who believe in the power of vocal emotions.

The choice of the title for the book was a challenge as well, and many versions were possible. I tossed the two words, *emotions* and *voice*, around in my head for many weeks, and I finally came up with some combinations that meant something to me. So, I asked others to evaluate the power of the final choice of the title. Eventually, *The Emotions in the Human Voice* was selected as the title. Nothing fancy, but these words give a straightforward message and fit among the titles of other publications on the subject of human emotions, e.g., Paul Ekman's 1982 publication entitled, *The Emotions in the Human Face*. Though the outline of the March 2005 XV Annual Pacific Voice Conference on Emotions and Voice was organized to flow thematically as if it were a theatrical production, I found myself in a conflict when trying to organize the chapters in a clustered and seemingly logical or sequential fashion. After an honest discussion with Lauren Duffy of Plural (again during a break between our mutual responsibilities while attending a meeting, this time on Coronado Island near San Diego in Southern California, and enjoying ice tea this time rather than French cuisine), we decided on arranging the chapters essentially in alphabetical order by the author's last name. The reasoning was based on the idea that these volumes represent an anthology of interrelated topics, that as such they can be read in any order, and that only upon consuming them all will a reader be ready to utter an emotive vocalization reflective of his or her personal view of the value of this work or specific criticism.

One more thing shall be mentioned that made my efforts in putting this collection together a real pleasure. This was the willingness of Plural to allow me to design the cover and to include nonscientific illustrations. The acceptance by Plural of this idea placed me on a path to search for illustrators and graphic artists who would be willing to produce a cover and the graphic vignettes to be placed on the left page in front of selected chapters.

I admit that I enjoyed the search very, very much. This search took me into the world of art and graphic design that I deeply respect and admire, and it provided me with an emotional break from thinking about the words and the text only. Once I found the artists that I was looking for, it took very little pressure to persuade both of them to contribute on pro-bono bases. Hence, my special thank-you goes to Daniele Coscone of Italy and to Marta Semkowicz of Poland for agreeing to participate. Honestly, it took some emotional work on my part to make this deal, but that is completely another story.

So here we are, ready to indulge in the text placed in front of us. As you come to read these superb contributions, please note that we do vocalize often, in fact daily or nightly, often really freely and spontaneously, and that at times we vocalize on command, and that our vocalizations do carry plenty of emotive content, content that can be truly revealing, even if we do not realize it.

Krzysztof Izdebski

ACKNOWLEDGMENTS

The following people listed here (not in alphabetical order) contributed significantly to my curiosity, understanding, and studies of vocally transmitted emotions, hence made this book possible, and for that I am profoundly thankful to all them. Because all of you transcend all kinds of boundaries, professions, systems, religions, age, and all else, I simply ask you to accept a humble "thank you" in your native or emotional language and with chosen prosody. If I missed something, or somebody, please yell at me.

Heather Antonissen, Asa Abelin, Jean Abitbol, Albert Bandura, Magda Goldberger, Zdenek Hufnagel, Beata Woytowicz, Mara Behlau, Brasil, Brad Bird, Diane M. Bless, Sylvie Brajtman, Janina Casper, Manuel Pais Clemente, Piero Cosi, Raul M. Cruz, Danielle Coscone, Peter Docter, Maria Dietrich, Carlo Drioli, Steffi Frigo, Anna Paczynska-Izdebski, Grzegorz A W Izdebski, the Singh Family, Piotr Sokolowski Enskoog, Siri Elliason, Karamindan Ghuman, Isabel Guimaraes, Rozalina Gutman, Ioulia Grichkovtsova, Lorrie Grifee, the Seshadri Family, the Asenov Family, Anastasia Vavilova, Venislava Georgieva Georgieva, Hristina Djambazova, Brindis Gudmunsdottir, Lucinda Halstead,

Sabine Hoffmann, Josef Schlomicher-Their, Anna Maria Hortis-Dzierzbicka, the Deutchman Family, Ellen van der Honert, Mirja Ilves, Julian Konrad Matheus Izdebski, Alexandra Michalina Catherina Izdebski, Kazuhiko Kakehi, Arvid Kapas, Gwen Korovin, Jody Kreiman, Marika Kuzma, Anne Maria Laukkanen, Petri Laukka, Heather Lauren, Inneke Mennen, Marilyn C. Izdebski, Norman Boone and the Boones Family, Marilee Monnot, Luiza Renata Motter, Dominique Morsomme, John W. Mullennix, Thomas Murry, Clifford Nass, Randy Nelson (special thanks for being so PIXAR), Marcos de Sarvat Family, Susana Naidich Family, Kevin Pelphrey, Robert Peterson, Daniela Powsner, Anna Petrini, Jeff Pigeon, Beata Ptaszynski, Raquel M. Ramsey, Ruth Rainero, Lorraine Ramig,

Joe Rauft, Kevin Reher, Brian Rosen, Gary Rydstrom, Lilla-Theresa Sadowski, Annett Schirmer, Marta Semkowicz, Tapio Seppänen, Sumi Shigeno, Julia A. Sidorova, Jennifer Spielman, Andrew Stenton, Claude Steinberg, Kimberly M. Steinhauer, Victoria Stevens, Fantisek Sram, The Juergen Wendler Family, Uyi Thompson Stewart, Rebeca Stockley, Brad Story, Dave Stroud, Veikko Surakka, Marc Swerts, Mihoko Teshigawara, Juhani Toivanen, Miriam van Mersbergen, Ingrid Verduyckt, Jerry Weissman, Willy Wellens, Magda van Opstal.

Britta Yilitalo, Hans von Leden, Herbert H. and Sigrid Dedo, Michael Chcial, Edward Damrose, Jeanelle Mifsud, the Thomas Shipp Family, the PIXAR staff, the Bay Area Italian American Community, the Tonnela Family, Gary Pratt, the Monty Upshaw Family, M.T. Sylvia, Maria Pignato, Timothy Willcutts.

Fred Harris, Kito Gamble, Molly Holm, Michael Grossman, Lydia Hyde, Kathleen Antonia, Joel Ben Izzy, Lisa Jenai Hernandez, Lucy Beck, Pam Fry, Karen Mellander-Magoon, Franc D'Ambrosio, Sylvie Sandy Cressman, Heather Lauren, Kathy Kennedy, Dorota Rózanska, Faye Carol, Carolyn Bloom, Martin Stirling, Facing New York. Renata Jaworski, Marianne van Zeeland, Mette Fog Pedersen, Stella Rubin Cognome, Claudia Packman, Annabell Castaldo, Ruth Ann Swenson, Misha Didyk, Oksana, Cairo Cocalis, Kevin Beaty.

Agata Zubel, Cezary Duchnowski, Michala Pedersen, Lisa Popeil, Alfonso Gianluca Gucciaro, Fonta Hadley, Bozena Hammerlink, Luciana Castro, Betty Horwitz, Donald and Angela Bell, Belinda Lew, Tracy Baldwin, Gerald Berke, Jean Zaludek, Florence Blager, Maria Pignati, Branko Stark, Michal Broniatowski Family, Roger Crumley Family, Chantal Bianda

Eugenia Chavez, Steven and Hillary Homs, Adidi Mandpe, Daniel Hartman, Jacob Johnson, Sharon Greenlin, Wendler Family, Viggo Pedersen, Sin-Yong Phua, Lisa van der Ploeg, Per Ake Lindestad, Philippe Dejonkere, Wojtek Chodzko-Zajko, Baska Oksztel-Matoszek, Malgorzata Gorecka-Kumek, "Babcia" Michasia Szymanska, "Babcia" Ebska, Halina Heliodora Izdebski, Julian W. Izdebski, Maryon Meyreson.

Jacob Johnson, the Schindler Family, the E. David Manace Family, the James E. Kline Family, Trinh Green, Gabriela Heimensen, Kirstem Mott, Rick Sklader, Mieczyslaw Dzierzbicki, Krzysztof and Natalia Izdebscy, Faculty, staff and management of Pixar and Ex'Pressions,

I also want to thank all my voice patients residing all over the world, representing so many different countries, culture, languages and ethnic roots, and all the people I met in my life with feminine or masculine names and voices, who came to see me because their voice was suffering, and all those other fine people I met in my life, that remain emotional about the way they talk.

CONTRIBUTORS

Luigi Anolli, Ph.D., Professor
Dipartimento di Scienze Umane per la Formazione
Universita' di Milano-Bicocca
Milano, Italy
Chapter 13

Mara Behlau, Ph.D.
Centro de Estudos da Voz—CEV
São Paulo, SP, Brazil
Chapter 19

Jürg Bernhard, Ph.D.
International Breast Cancer Study Group Coordinating Center
Bern, Switzerland
Chapter 14

Elizabeth J. Carter, Ph.D.
Research Fellow
Laboratory for Developmental Cognitive Neuroscience
Department of Psychology
Carnegie Mellon University
Pittsburgh, Pennsylvania
Chapter 2

Raul M. Cruz, M.D.
Kaiser Permanente Medical Center
Otolaryngology, Head and Neck Surgery
Oakland, California
Chapter 17

Maria Dietrich, Diplom-Heilpädagogin, M.A. CCC-SLP
Communication Science and Disorders
University of Pittsburgh
Pittsburgh, Pennsylvania
Chapter 11

Philip C. Doyle, Ph.D., CCC-SLP
Professor
Voice Production and Perception Laboratory
Department of Otolaryngology-Head, Neck, and Reconstructive Surgery
Schulich School of Medicine and Dentistry
University of Western Ontario
London, Ontario, Canada
Chapter 4

Jo Estill, M.A.
Pittsburgh, Pennsylvania
Chapter 6

Gordon G. Gallup, Jr., Ph.D.
Department of Psychology
State University of New York at Albany
Albany, New York
Chapter 15

Gisele Gasparini, M.Sc.
Centro de Estudos da Voz - CEV
São Paulo, Brazil
Chapter 19

Ioulia Grichkovtsova, Ph.D.
Queen Margaret University College, Edinburgh
Speech and Hearing Sciences
Musselburgh, East Lothian
Chapter 3

Kurt Hammerschmidt, Ph.D.
Research Group Cognitive Ethology,
German Primate Center GmbH—
Leibniz Institute for Primate Research
Göttingen, Germany
Chapter 12

Sabine Hofmann, Dottoressa Logopedista
Studio Logopedico "Mindworks",
Narni, Italy
and Servizio di Audologia e Foniatria
Chapter 16

Maria A. Hortis-Dzierzbicka, M.D.
Center for Craniofacial Disorders
Institute of Mother and Child
Warsaw, Poland
and
Specialized Freestanding Clinical Unit for Speech Treatment and Rehabilitation
Otwock, Poland
Chapter 5

Susan Hughes, Ph.D.
Psychology Department
Albright College
Reading, Pennsylvania
Chapter 15

Krzysztof Izdebski, F.K., M.A., Ph.D., CCC-SLP, FASHA
Chairman: Pacific Voice and Speech Foundation
San Francisco, California
and
Clinical Associate Professor
Voice and Swallowing Center
Department of Otolaryngology-Head and Neck Surgery
Stanford University, School of Medicine
Palo Alto, California
Chapters 5, 8, 14, 16, 17

Alois Mauerhoffer, Professor
Kunst Unversitet, Graz,
Österreich, Steiermark
Chapter 17

Ineke Mennen, Ph.D.
Bilingualish Research Centre
University of Bangor Gwynnedd, Wales
Chapter 3

Marilee Monnot, Ph.D.
Clinical Associate Professor
Department of Neurology, College of Medicine
University of Oklahoma Health Sciences Center
and Center for Alzheimer's and Neurodegenerative Disorders
Veterans Affairs Medical Center
Oklahoma City, Oklahoma
Chapter 7

Dominique Morsomme, Ph.D.
Université Catholique de Louvain
Centre d'Audiophonologie Saint Luc
Bruxelles, Belgium
Chapter 9

Diana Orbelo, Ph.D.
Mayo Clinic
Speech Pathology Department
Rochester, Minnesota
Chapter 7

Kevin A. Pelphrey, Ph.D.
Associate Professor
Laboratory for Developmental Cognitive Neuroscience
Department of Psychology
Carnegie Mellon University
Pittsburgh, Pennsylvania
Chapter 2

Branka Zei Pollermann, Ph.D.
Director, Vox Institute

Geneva, Switzerland
Chapter 1

Elliott Ross, MD, Professor
Department of Neurology, College of Medicine
University of Oklahoma Health Sciences Center
and Center for Alzheimer's and Neurodegenerative Disorders
Veterans Affairs Medical Center
Oklahoma City, Oklahoma
Chapter 7

Lilla-Teresa Sadowski, Mag. Phyl.
Logopädie, Psycho-Sensolinguistik,
Logopädie Austria, Austrian Voice Institute
Institut "Medtrain"
Graz, Österreich
Chapter 16

Elisabeth Scheiner, Ph.D
Department of Neurobiology
German Primate Center GmbH—Leibniz Institute for Primate Research
Göttingen, Germany
Chapter 12

Kimberly M. Steinhauer, Ph.D.
VA Pittsburgh Healthcare System
Think Voice International, LLC
Pittsburgh, Pennsylvania
Chapter 6

Victoria Stevens, Ph.D.
California Institute of the Arts, School of Critical Studies; Psychoanalytic Centre of California; Santa Barbara Graduate Institute for Infant and Child Development.
Los Angeles, California
Chapter 10

Julie Testa, Ph.D.
Mayo Clinic
Psychiatry and Psychology Department
Rochester, Minnesota
Chapter 7

Magda J. M. C. van Opstal
Leuven, Belgium
Chapter 18

Katherine Verdolini Abbott, Ph.D., CCC-SLP
Communication Science and Disorders
University of Pittsburgh
University of Pittsburgh Voice Center
Department of Otolaryngology
University of Pittsburgh Medical Center
Pittsburgh, Pennsylvania
Chapter 11

Ingrid Verduyckt, M.A.
Université Catholique de Louvain
Centre d'audiophonologie Saint Luc
Bruxelles, Belgium
Chapter 9

Hans von Leden, M.D.
Professor of Biocommunications (Emeritus)
University of Southern California
Los Angeles, California
Prologue

Willy A. R. Wellens, Ph.D.
Phoniatrics
ENT, Head and Neck Surgery
University Clinics KULeuven
Leuven, Belgium
Chapter 18

INTRODUCTION

This is one of the shortest introductions the reader of any scientific volume will ever experience. The reason for this brevity is obvious; namely, as the editor of these volumes, I am extremely proud to have been charged with the task of creating this book, yet I clearly recognize that it is not my book, and that it was created by all of us, all of us who are concerned with the topic of emotions expressed, conveyed, produced, perceived, or generated in the context of the human voice.

The concept that the voice is a carrier of emotions is not a new one. In fact voice, emotions, sexuality, guilt, etc., have been discussed in the Talmud, in the Bible, in Hinduism, in Buddhism, in the Koran, and in many other writings on philosophy or on religious doctrines. Many of the contemporary scholars credited with the development of modern thought and scientific truth about life, or about the evolution of life and of the psychological correlates of life (e.g., Darwin, Freud, Fromm, Jung, etc.), have addressed voice and emotions. So, is there anything we can say about this topic that has not been said before?

These volumes provide the *answer*. We are clearly aware that emotional information is and can be conveyed by a variety of means of human communication. Communication involves content, prosody, gesture, facial expressions, paralinguistic aspects, and cultural know-how. We now know that cross-modality inputs affect the production and perception of another modality. We also know that not all aspects are universal, and that it is OK to be restricted by cultural constraints. With respect to voice and emotions, these modalities are, however, still unclear.

Voice is today a fully acknowledged tool of labor, as so much of our interactions are conducted in the absence or the presence of another person, namely, on the phone or over Internet voice transmission, with the voice signals alone carrying all the clues of our well-being or about our emotional state. Hence, it is not a perplexing question, why we are then ready to make assumptions, judgments, choices, firing and hiring, judicial opinions, criminal recommendations, or purchase choices and other crucial decisions about life based on the emotions we experience regardless of this vocal information?

This *second volume* addresses some clinical topics of vocally coded emotions and certainly neglects many pertinent questions, specifically those pertaining to the evidence based treatment of emotionally based voice disorders, the urgent issue, that will be addressed in the future volumes planned for 2009. This specific area has been requested to be placed in focus in the future volumes by Mette F. Pedersen of Denmark, a champion of evidence based clinical research.

This Volume II, if not the entire collection, is not a final word in the quest of understanding what constitutes clinical issues in vocally conveyed emotions, but in my opinion, it is a darn good approximation of the current (2008) state of the art on this subject. Nonetheless, much remains to be discovered and learned. One thing that will become obvious when these volumes are consumed by the reader is the fact that, during the act of acoustically conducted communication, emotional information may be coded and expressed both by the content and by modulation of speech. And although it is almost given that the left brain is in charge of language, emotions are shown to be lateralized to the right part of the brain, and much more is to be learned about cross-brain integration of vocal emotions.

Moreover, similarities in acoustic profiles, intonation, and emotion flow now permit us to assess the extent of how hemispheric lateralization of speech prosody depends on functional instead of acoustical properties. This brings at least one fundamental question into focus; namely, are there acoustical properties of emotions, and if there are, what are they and how do they differ or influence the functional concepts of emotions? The other fundamental question is that of the discovery of what constitutes an emotion in itself. To trivialize this entire concept, I dare to paraphrase Chomsky and Halle who in the epilogue to their then most fundamental work on English phonology (*The Sound Pattern of English*, 1968) proclaimed that the work they had just published suffers from "fundamental scientific inadequacy." Is this volume destined to suffer a similar course? So as not to make this an excuse, I will also dare to quote a Latin doctrine, "*Per risum multum debes cognoscere stultum*," rightly or wrongly stating that the perception of voice cues in the laughter of the emotionally disturbed can point to the source of the type of emotional disturbance that produced such a sound. So then, to cover up my own ignorance, I dare to say, "*Nulla aetas ad discendum sera*" or "It is never too late to learn." With this hope I turn the rest to the reader, and I plea for forgiveness of our ignorance of the scope of the subject we so do love.

Krzysztof Izdebski
Oakland/San Francisco, California,
February 1, 2008

To my two special children,
Alexandra Michalina Catherina
and
Julian Konrad Matheus,
whose voices over
their combined 29 years of life
have never failed
to express their emotions,
emotions and voices
I had so many chances
to misinterpret.

Oakland, San Francisco, California, USA,
and all the many places all over the world,
I found myself working on these volumes

CHAPTER 1

Autonomic Determinants of Vocal Expression of Emotions

Branka Zei Pollermann

Summary

Although the autonomic component of emotional reactions is clinically important, there are little data about its precise role in the communication of emotion. This study investigated the impact of autonomic lesions on the vocal expression of emotions. A group of diabetics was chosen as a cohort because diabetic insulin-dependent patients can suffer diffuse neuropathy capable of producing profound changes affecting normal body reactions. Outcome measures were autonomic function tests, acoustic analyses of vocal emotional expression, and subjective feeling ratings. Standard autonomic function tests were performed to assess the sympathetic and parasympathetic tone (that is, prevailing base levels of sympathetic and parasympathetic activity) in 39 gender-mixed diabetic patients. For both measures subgroups were formed with scores above and below the median. Feelings of joy, anger, and sadness were induced through verbal recall of emotional experiences. The patients rated the intensity of the emotion felt during the recall. Their voices were acoustically analyzed, yielding a number of acoustic parameters related to emotions (Zei & Archinard, 2002).

Indices of global vocal activation, and vocal differentiation of emotions were computed for anger-sadness, joy-sadness, and anger-joy comparisons. The patients' self-reported subjective feeling related to each emotion was coded as well as the intensity of weeping. For each dependent variable, two-factor analysis of variance was applied with the independent variables "sympathetic tone" (high vs. low) and "parasympathetic tone" (high vs. low).

The analyses of variance (ANOVAs) yielded significant effects for vocal variables and the subjective feeling scores. Patients with low parasympathetic tone showed diminished *vocal arousal* in anger and joy and heightened *vocal arousal* in sadness. They had less intense subjective feelings of both sadness and anger. Patients with low sympathetic tone had less pronounced spectral differentiation between anger and joy conditions.

Our findings indicate that diminished autonomic control of cardiovascular reactions is associated with lower intensity of the subjective feelings of sadness and anger, and blunting of vocal signaling of both positively and negatively valenced emotional states.

Theoretical Background

Diabetic neuropathy is the most common complication of diabetes mellitus, both type 1 and type 2. Autonomic diabetic neuropathy is a form of diffuse neuropathy that affects the nerves that serve the heart and internal organs and produce changes in many processes and systems. Damage to the nerves in the cardiovascular system interferes with the body's ability to adjust blood pressure and heart rate in response to normal body reactions, exercise, stress, and emotional challenges. This means that the heart rate can stay unchanged, instead of rising and falling in response to the psycho-physiological demands. It then follows that emotional reactions, as mechanisms of the organism's adaptive functioning, are likely to be affected by impaired or diminished autonomic response.

Autonomic reactions are central to most emotion theories. The James-Lange theory (James, 1894) states that emotional feelings are consequences of peripheral physiological changes supported by the autonomic nervous system (ANS). The Cannon-Bard theory suggests that emotion occurs when the thalamus sends signals simultaneously to the cortex and the ANS, and that different emotions are associated with different patterns of autonomic arousal (Cannon, 1927). Schachter & Singer (1962) proposed a theory holding that discrete emotional experiences derive from cognitive appraisals initiated by the perception of undifferentiated autonomic arousal. As their experiment was concerned with the arousal induced by epinephrine (whose effects are almost a perfect mimicry of a discharge of the sympathetic nervous system such as increase of blood pressure, heart rate, respiration rate, etc.), their results contributed to the understanding of the importance of the sympathetic branch of the ANS and did not allow inferences as to the role of the parasympathetic division of the ANS.

Considering the fact that vagal response is very fast (in the order of 400 milliseconds compared with 20–30 seconds' latency in sympathetic stimulation), studying its role in the regulation of emotion in subjects with parasympathetic lesions appeared meaningful. Berntson and colleagues suggested a model of autonomic regulation based on the concept of "autonomic space" with orthogonal sympathetic and parasympathetic axes, such that stress-induced heart rate increase, for example, could result from an increase of the sympathetic stimulation or a decrease in the parasympathetic stimulation (Berntson, Cacioppo, & Quigley, 1991; 1993a).

In Scherer's component process theory of emotions (Scherer, 1984a; 1984b; Scherer & Scherer, 2001), ANS reactions are one of five components (cognitive appraisal, physiological arousal, expressive reaction, action tendency, and the subjective feeling). It then follows that the presence of impairment in one component should lead to a major change in emotionality. An example is emotional disorders in patients with unilateral brain lesions (Gainotti, 1991). More recently, Damasio's model assigns a major role to the emotional sensations related to the state of the smooth muscles, which in turn are under autonomic control.

It thus appears meaningful to assume that impairment of the autonomic response should lead to a major change in emotionality (Damasio, 1999).

Emotions are usually characterized along two basic dimensions (Lang, 1995; Russel, 2003):

- Arousal (aroused vs. calm), which mainly refers to the physiological arousal involved in the preparation of the organism for an appropriate reaction.
- Valence (pleasant/positive vs. unpleasant/negative), which mainly refers to the overall subjective hedonic feeling.

Our aim was to determine which dimension of an emotional experience is affected by diminished cardiovascular response: arousal, valence, or both. More specifically, the goal was to explore whether the emotions that are characterized by ergotropic arousal (e.g., anger and intense joy) are differentially affected compared with those characterized by trophotropic arousal (e.g., sadness) (Scherer, 1989a, 1989b).

Hypotheses

1. In subjects with low parasympathetic tone, sadness will be expressed and felt to a lesser degree than normally expected for emotions dominated by trophotropic arousal. This hypothesis is based on the assumption that low parasympathetic tone reflects long-term vagal withdrawal, which in turn can result in the overactivity of the counter-regulatory system, that is, the sympathetic system.
2. In subjects with low sympathetic tone, the intensity of the subjective feeling of anger and joy as well as their verbal expression will be lower than expected for emotions dominated by ergotropic arousal. This hypothesis is based on the assumption that low sympathetic tone may prevent full deployment of the states of anger or joy/elation.
3. In subjects with diminished autonomic response, the emotional expression of emotions as well as the corresponding subjective feeling states will be flattened.

Hypotheses 1 and 2 are based on the classical reciprocal model of autonomic regulation, which follows a unidimensional vector or a continuum that extends from dominant sympathetic activation on one end to dominant parasympathetic activation on the other extreme. The state of autonomic control at any given time is characterized by a point on this continuum.

Hypothesis 3 is based on an alternative model of autonomic control (Berntson, Cacioppo, & Quigley, 1991; 1993a) whereby autonomic regulation evolves in a two-dimensional space defined by orthogonal parasympathetic and sympathetic axes. According to this model autonomic control can vary independently within a bivariate "autonomic space" with reciprocal, coactive, or independent changes in the sympathetic and parasympathetic branches of the ANS. The heart being a dually and antagonistically innervated organ, the neural changes and the organ's response may be patterned in terms of coactivation of the sympathetic and parasympathetic systems. The consequent heart rate response could thus be acceleratory, deceleratory, or unchanged from prestimulus levels depending upon which activational input was greater (Berntson et al., 1991; 1993b).

Studying the relationship between diminished cardiovascular response and emotional reactions furthers our understanding of more general psychological consequences of diabetic autonomic lesions. This chapter presents the results of our study.

Methods

Subjects

Thirty-nine French-speaking diabetic patients (17 female and 22 male) varying in age (range = 31-73, mean = 56; SD = 9) and duration of illness (range = 1-36; mean =15; SD = 11) participated in the investigation. None suffered from depression or any somatic disease affecting respiration, phonation, or articulation.

Physiological Measures

Three standard autonomic function tests (Ewing, Campbell, Burt, & Clarke, 1973; Vita et al., 1986) were used to assess each patient's base level autonomic response:

1. Heart rate variability (HRV) during deep breathing at six breaths per minute, expressed as the mean heart rate difference (based on maximum minus minimum heart rate measured during three successive breathing cycles).
2. Immediate heart rate response to standing up expressed as the "30:15 ratio," i.e., the ratio of the largest R-R interval around the 30th beat after starting to stand up to the shortest R-R interval around the 15th beat. The R-R interval is defined as the time duration between two consecutive R waves of the ECG. Both tests quantify the parasympathetic control of the heart with a small sympathetic component (Valensi et al., 1997). They were done by means of Autocaft software (BBC Master, Edinburgh, UK).

Data of both of the above tests were adjusted for age (Valensi et al., 1997) and a cumulative average score (Ewing, Martyn, Young, & Clarke, 1985) was computed into a variable "parasympathetic tone."

The third test involved isometric handgrip exercise as indicator of sympathetic function. It measured the diastolic blood pressure rise during sustained handgrip for 5 minutes. The data were adjusted for gender, and the derived variable was named "sympathetic tone."

Induction of Emotions

The emotions of were self-induced by asking the subjects to verbally recall the situations in their lives which arouse joy, sadness, and anger. This self-recall method has been shown to effectively induce emotional states (McCraty, Atkinson, Tiller, Rein, & Watkins, 1995). At the end of each narrative (lasting on the average about 6 minutes), the subject immediately read aloud a standard sentence on the emotion congruent tone. The sentence read: "ALORS TU ACCEPTES CETTE AFFAIRE." It was presented in block letters without punctuation so as not to suggest any tone of voice.

According to the conceptual and empirical work of Mendolia and Kleck (Mendolia & Kleck, 1993), talking about one's emotional experience directs one's attention to the affect relevant properties of the event. Thoughts brought into awareness from such talk are emotion focused. Verbal description of an emotional experience cues mental images as well as expressive reactions that influence felt emotion (Tesser & Clary, 1978). It is thus " . . . possible to turn a recollection of an event from the past into an emotional experience in the present" (Strack, Schwarz, & Gschneidinger, 1985, p. 219). This is in agreement with Damasio's model of emotional memory retrieval (Damasio, 1989). He suggests that a unique spatiotemporal patterning of the brain activity is retroactivated during the recall of emotion episodes including specific patterns of appraisal and the peripheral somatic and autonomic reactions. According to LeDoux, emotional processing of the contents of speaking involves an integration of cortical sensory inputs to the amygdala (LeDoux, Iwata, Cicchetti, & Reis, 1988). As the central nucleus of the amygdala provides a link with efferent motor systems controlling autonomic and behavioral emotional responses, it is hypothesized that autonomic responses to verbal recall of emotional experiences are similar to those of real-life emotional reactions. Analogous neuropsychological evidence is provided by Farah (1988).

Psychological Measures

In order to control for a possible influence of personality dimensions (Scherer, 1978, 1979; 1981) and anxiety (Scherer, 1986) on voice production mechanisms (including breathing patterns) (Winkworth, 1995), the patients completed Spielberger Anxiety-state scale (Bruchon-Schweitzer, 1993) at the beginning of the interview and prior to the emotion induction. Eysenck Personality Inventory questionnaire (Eysenck, 1970) was administered at the end of the interview. The latter yielded data on extraversion and neuroticism dimensions of personality.

Measures of the Intensity of Felt Emotion, Weeping and Change in Emotionality

Upon each narrative, and after having said the standard sentence, the patient was asked to rate the degree to which he or she felt the just verbally recalled emotion. The intensity of felt emotion was coded on a four-point scale (0–3). Three variables represented the intensity of the subjective feeling related to each condition: FeelA for anger, FeelJ for joy, and FeelS for sadness. As 77% of the subjects wept during the recall of emotional experiences, the intensity of weeping was rated by the experimenter on a four-point scale (0–3), with 0 = absence of weeping; 1 = noticeable tears in the eyes; 2 = abundant tearing; 3 = abundant tearing accompanied by speaking difficulties. At the end of the interview the experimenter asked the subjects whether they thought that their emotional reactions (emotionality) had changed in the last few years. The answers were rated on a four-point scale (0–3).

In summary, the above ratings produced five variables: three related to the intensity of emotions, one to the awareness of change in emotionality, and one to the intensity of weeping.

Measurement of Vocal Expression of Emotions

The subjects' voices were digitally recorded, with the distance of the microphone to the mouth being kept constant. One hundred and seventeen samples of the standard sentence were acoustically analyzed by means of a Macintosh platform software (Keller, 1994), which yielded data on the fundamental frequency (F_0), energy envelopes, long-term average spectra, and the speaking rate.

The relationship between the emotional arousal and vocal expression was first modeled by Williams and Stevens (1972) and has received considerable empirical support (Banse & Scherer, 1996; Scherer, 1981; Simonov, Frolov, & Ivanov, 1980; Williams & Stevens, 1981). Emotional arousal is thus known to be mainly encoded in the fundamental frequency (F_0), in vocal energy, and in the speaking rate. Compared with an emotionally unmarked (neutral) speaking mode, *vocal arousal*[1] of an angry voice would typically be characterized by increased values of some or all of the above parameters, while that of a sad voice would be marked by a decrease in the same parameters. By contrast, the hedonic valence dimension of emotional reactions seems to be mainly reflected in intonation patterns and in spectral characteristics of the speaker's voice.

Drawing on our previous work on acoustic patterns of emotions (Zei & Archinard, 2002), the following vocal parameters were computed: mean F_0, F_0 coefficient of variation, F_0 max/F_0 min ratio, mean voiced energy level, voiced energy range, speaking rate, and long-term average spectra (LTAS). As described by Zei and Archinard (1998), voiced energy range was measured between two midpoint vowel nuclei and it was expressed as the difference in dB between the highest and the lowest peak in voiced energy envelopes. The speaking rate was expressed as the number of syllables uttered per second.

LTAS were computed for each voice sample, yielding 128 data points for a range of 40–5500 Hz. We used a Bark-based strategy of spectral data analysis (Hassal & Zaveri, 1979). The spectrum was divided into 13 bands, each covering a 1.5 Bark interval (Pittam & Gallois, 1986; J. Pittam, B. S. Pittam, Burnstock, & Purves, 1987), and a mean energy value for each band was computed. We thus obtained 13 spectral energy values per emotion and per subject.

Vocal Differentiation of Emotions on the Arousal Dimension

To quantify the degree of vocally expressed emotional arousal, a *vocal-arousal-index* was computed for each emotion. All the vocal variables were normalized by external reference values for healthy

[1]By analogy to the concept of autonomic arousal, we propose the term *vocal arousal* to signify the amount of vocal activation resulting from autonomic arousal.

male and female subjects, (Zei & Archinard, 2002) and a cumulative average score was computed. This procedure yielded three indices: AngerIndx, for *vocal arousal* in anger, JoyIndx for *vocal arousal* in joy, and SadnessIndx for *vocal arousal* in sadness.

To test the hypothesis of flattening of vocal differentiation between high-arousal and low-arousal conditions, an index of vocal differentiation was computed for anger-sadness and joy-sadness comparisons. This was done by calculating the ratio between the value of each vocal parameter (mean F_0, F_0 coefficient of variation, F_0 max/min ratio, voiced energy range, speaking rate) in anger condition and the respective value in sadness condition. The resulting ratios were cumulated into an average score named *vocal-differential index* (VDI). We thus obtained a VDI-anger-sadness and a VDI-joy-sadness.

Vocal Differentiation of Emotions on the Valence Dimension

To assess vocal differentiation of emotions on the valence dimension, we used spectral parameters. The spectral data for anger (a negative emotion with a high level of arousal) were compared with those for joy (a positive emotion with a high level of arousal). The approach was based on previous studies of vocal differentiation of hedonic valence in spectral analyses (Popov, Simonov, Frolov, Khachatur'iants, & Pastushenko, (1971); Zei & Archinard, 2001). The spectral value of each of the 13 bands of the LTAS in anger condition was divided by the respective value in joy condition. The frequency bands found to significantly differentiate the spectra in anger from those in joy covered a range from 600–4370 Hz. A cumulative spectral differential index (Anger/JoySpect) was computed for this range.

In summary, acoustic analyses of the patients' voices yielded 6 indices. Three represented the overall *vocal arousal* in each emotion condition: AngerIndx, JoyIndx, and SadnessIndx; two represented vocal differentiation of a high-arousal vs. a low-arousal emotion: VDI-anger-sadness, VDI-joy-sadness, and one stood for spectral differentiation of a positively valenced vs. a negatively valenced emotion: Anger/JoySpect.

Statistical Analyses

As a first step, covariance tests were applied to check for a possible influence of gender on the dependent variables. The neurological variables (parasympathetic and sympathetic tone) were used as covariates and gender as factor. Gender was significantly associated with three variables: intensity of felt anger ($F = 5.80$; $p = .021$), intensity of felt sadness ($F = 5.83$; $p = .021$), and awareness of change in emotionality ($F = 10.66$; $p = .002$). Female subjects reported higher intensity of felt anger and felt sadness as well as a stronger awareness of change in emotionality. Prior to performing further analyses, the data were adjusted for gender. Partial correlations (with neurological variables being partialed out) were computed to examine the association between dependent variables and the psychological variables (anxiety, extraversion) as well as the subjects' age and duration of illness. The results showed that anxiety score had a significant negative correlation with both AngerIndx

($r = -.41; p < .05$), and VDI-anger-sadness ($r = -.47$; $p < .01$), while extraversion was positively correlated with the awareness of change in emotionality ($r = .33$; $p < .05$) and the intensity of weeping ($r = .45; p < .01$). The latter also displayed a positive correlation with age ($r = .34$; $p < .05$).

As a third step subgroups were formed with scores above and below the median for the independent variables *sympathetic tone* and *parasympathetic tone*. According to the model of autonomic space (Berntson et al., 1991; Cacioppo, Klein, Berntson, & Hatfield, 1993), significant interaction effects between independent variables were expected. We therefore performed two-factor analyses of variance (ANOVA) for each dependent variable with the independent variables parasympathetic tone (high vs. low) and sympathetic tone (high vs. low). Anxiety score was used as a covariate in the ANOVAs for both AngerIndx and VDI-anger-sadness , while extraversion score served as a covariate in the ANOVA for the "awareness of change" and the intensity of weeping. For the latter, age was used as a covariate as well.

Results

Blunting of Feelings of Anger and Sadness

The ANOVAs yielded significant main effects only for the variable *parasympathetic tone*. There was no significant interaction effect between the independent variables. With respect to the main effect, significant differences were found for the intensity of felt anger ($F = 7.21$; $p = .011$), the intensity of felt sadness ($F = 12.59$; $p = .001$), the intensity of weeping ($F = 14.5$; $p = .001$), and for the awareness of change in emotionality ($F = 4.9$; $p = .034$). The subjects with a low parasympathetic tone felt lower intensity of anger and sadness, wept less, and had a higher degree of awareness of change in their emotional reactions. The following examples illustrate qualitative descriptions of change in emotionality as described by the patients with low parasympathetic tone:

> "Before, my emotions were more spontaneous."
>
> "I have fewer negative emotions."
>
> "Unpleasant emotions are better controlled, while pleasant emotions are more freely experienced."
>
> "I feel less anger and more joy."
>
> "My emotions are calmer."
>
> "I am more passive, especially regarding anger."
>
> "My emotional reactions are less spontaneous."
>
> "My emotions used to come automatically; now I don't react quickly."

Blunting of Vocal Expression of Emotional Arousal

The ANOVAs for overall *vocal arousal* indices AngerIndx, JoyIndx, and SadnessIndx as dependent variables yielded significant results only for the parasympathetic tone only. The anxiety score was used as a covariate for AngerIndx.

The individuals with low parasympathetic tone displayed lower *vocal arousal* in both anger ($F = 5.07$; $p = .031$) and joy ($F = 7.35$; $p = .01$) while they had a higher degree of *vocal arousal* in sadness ($F = 15.24$; $p = .000$) (Figure 1-1). There was no significant interaction effect between independent variables.

Diminished Vocal Differentation of Emotions

The ANOVAs for vocal-differential indices yielded highly significant main effects for the parasympathetic tone only: VDI-anger-sadness ($F = 40.85$; $p = .000$) and VDI-joy-sadness ($F = 40.59$; $p = .000$). Vocal differentiation of emotions (anger vs. sadness and joy vs. sadness) was lower in the group with low parasympathetic tone (Figure 1-2). The anxiety score was used as a covariate in the ANOVA for VDI-anger-sadness. There was a significant but weak interaction effect between the independent variables only in the ANOVA for the VDI-joy-sadness ($F = 6.6$; $p = .01$).

Blunting of Vocal Expression of Emotional Valence

The ANOVA with anger/joy spectral differential (Anger/JoySpect) as dependent variable yielded a significant main effect only for the sympathetic tone ($F = 6.82$; $p = 0.01$). The subjects with low sympathetic tone produced smaller spectral differences between anger and joy than did the subjects with high sympathetic tone (Figure 1-3). There was a significant interaction effect between parasympathetic and sympathetic tone ($F = 5.66$; $p = 0.02$).

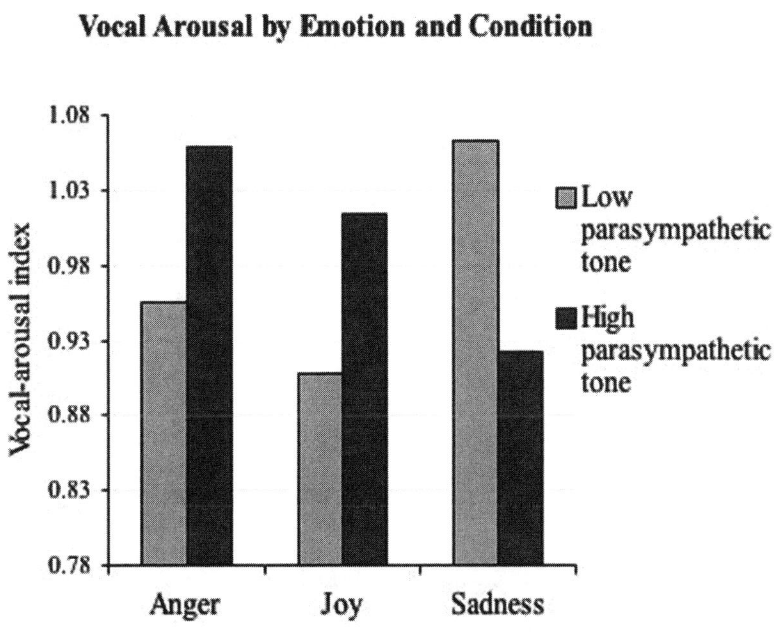

Figure 1–1. Degree of overall *vocal arousal* in anger, joy, and sadness by condition (group with low vs. group with high parasympathetic tone).

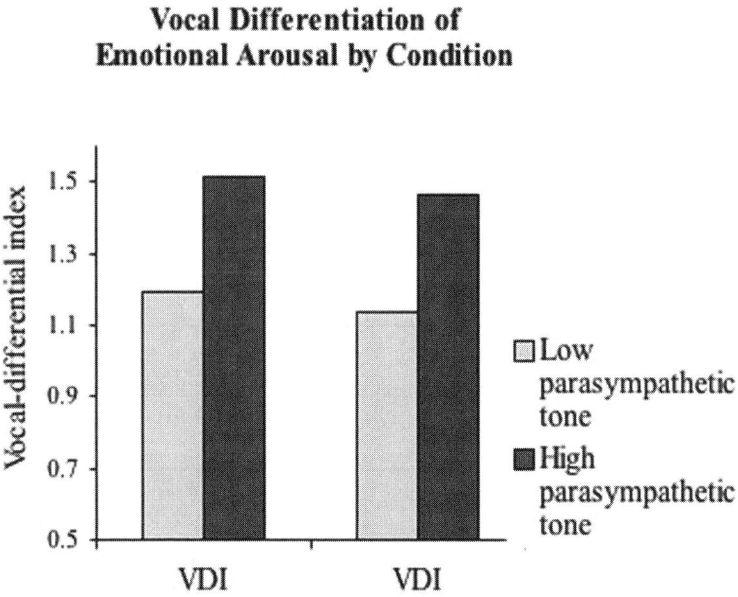

Figure 1–2. VDI = vocal-differential index reflecting the degree of vocal differentiation of emotions on the arousal dimension: anger vs. sadness and joy vs. sadness by condition (group with low vs. group with high parasympathetic tone).

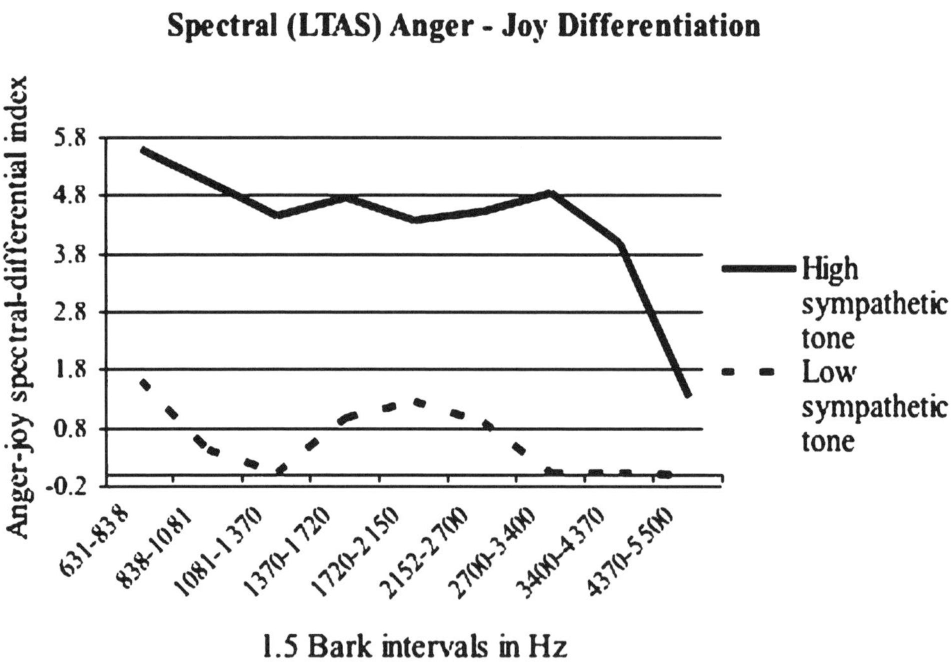

Figure 1–3. Anger-joy spectral-differential index reflecting the degree of spectral differentiation of two high-arousal emotions differing on the dimension of valence (anger vs. joy) displayed by by condition (group with low vs. group with high sympathetic tone).

Discussion

Current literature on emotionally induced autonomic arousal has been characterized by a tendency to focus more on the sympathetic than the parasympathetic system's contribution, neglecting a possible interaction between both branches of the ANS. This study allowed us to explore the relationship between the base-line levels of sympathetic and parasympathetic activity in diabetic patients and their vocally expressed emotional reactions (independent of their prominent personality traits and/or anxiety state).

Diabetics were chosen as a cohort group to test this relationship because, at an advanced stage of the disease, diabetics can exhibit autonomic neuropathy capable of producing profound changes affecting normal body reactions. This study investigated the impact of base-line autonomic tone on the vocal expression of emotions.

Marked group differences in feeling states were observed for the variable *parasympathetic tone*. The subjects with low parasympathetic tone experienced lower intensity of anger and sadness and wept less. Now, the observed diminished weeping may be due to a weaker emotional response, but it can also be related to the fact that the nerve fibers that carry the impulses to the lachrymal gland are part of the parasympathetic nervous system (Frey, 1985), so that destruction of the parasympathetic nerves (as found diabetic autonomic neuropathy) causes diminished tearing, while damage to the sympathetic nerves causes little change (DeJong, 1979).

Furthermore, individuals with low parasympathetic tone exhibited blunting on the level of vocal expression of emotions. Their overall *vocal arousal* in anger and joy was lower, while in sadness it was higher than expected for these conditions. Such a pattern of emotional flattening is congruent with the works of Porges (Porges, Arnold, & Forbes, 1973), who demonstrated that the level of vagal tone (defined as the amount of inhibitory influences on the heart by the parasympathetic nervous system) influences behavioral patterns in children, particularly in the expression and regulation of emotion (Porges, 1995; Porges & Byrne, 1992; Porges, Doussard-Roosevelt, & Maiti, 1994). Porges showed that the measurement of vagal tone could be used as an index of general reactivity predisposing an individual to be hypo- or hyperactive. Other studies relate base-level vagal activity to general expressivity (Stifter, Fox, & Porges, 1989).

Our finding about low parasympathetic tone being associated with an unusually high *vocal arousal* in sadness (emotion usually characterized by high trophotropic activation) could be explained by the fact that a long-term vagal withdrawal permits a relative overactivity of the counter-regulatory sympathetic system. It is therefore not surprising that in individuals with low parasympathetic tone the speech patterns characterizing anger or joy are poorly differentiated from those characterizing sadness. Consistent with the above results is the finding that individuals with disease induced low parasympathetic tone report a stronger feeling of change in emotionality. A different picture emerges for the sympathetic tone. Neither the overall *vocal arousal* nor the subjective feeling states were significantly associated with the sympathetic tone. Our hypothesis 2 was thus not confirmed. However, the group with high sympathetic tone differed significantly from the group with low sympathetic tone only in the spectral differentiation of emotional valence: anger vs. joy (see Figure 1-3). The subjects with high sympathetic tone showed bigger spectral differentiation.

The contribution of the parasympathetic system to emotionality has been especially emphasized within the framework of developmental psychology (Porges, 1983). Porges and colleagues describe the relation between vagal tone and emotional response in the following way (Porges et al., 1994, p. 172):

> Changes in Respiratory Sinus Arrhythmia amplitude in response to sensory, cognitive, and visceral challenges represent a "central command" to regulate vagal efferents originating in the right nucleus ambiguous and terminating in the heart, soft palate, pharynx, larynx, bronchi, and oesophagus. These changes in nucleus ambiguous regulation of peripheral autonomic activity support the expression of emotion, motion, and communication by regulating metabolic output (i.e., shifts in heart rate) and organs involved in the production of vocalisations.

These authors link the vagal control of the sino-atrial node to cardiovascular states facilitating emotion related fight-flight behaviors. Their model emphasizes the bidirectional physiological characteristics of the vagus (efferent + afferent feedback) whereby any dysfunction of the circuit could result in affective disorders. Other studies relate base-level vagal tone to general expressivity (Stifter et al., 1989).

As mentioned earlier, historically, the vagus and other components of the parasympathetic nervous system had not been incorporated in theories of emotion. Porges proposed a model whereby the vagal circuit of emotion regulation incorporates lateral brain function with the regulation of the peripheral autonomic nervous system in the expression of emotion. He convincingly showed that baseline levels of cardiac vagal tone and vagal tone reactivity are associated with behavior, the expression of emotion, and self-regulation skills.

The relation between vocal expression and the vagus is found in studies of neural control of vocalization, which have shown that vocalization is modulated by afferent input from the pulmonary and upper airways, which in turn is mediated by sensory receptors in the vagus nerve. Summation of pulmonary vagal and upper airway afferent discharge with the periaqueductal gray matter (PAG) motor output has the potential to result in a more adaptive and integrated response. Integrations of specific motor patterns for sound production by PAG neurons may offer an explanation for the well-known association between emotional and vocal control where fluctuations in emotional experiences alter the respiratory and laryngeal motor patterns in human speech and song (Davis, Zhang, Winkworth, & Bandler, 1996).

As to the interaction between parasympathetic and sympathetic activation of the ANS, our results only partially support the hypothesis of autonomic control evolving within a bivariate "autonomic space" with conjunct action of both branches. We found rather weak (albeit statistically significant) interactions between parasympathetic and sympathetic tone for both arousal and valence dimensions of emotions. No interaction was observed for the subjective feeling component of emotions. The latter was found to be associated with parasympathetic tone only.

Conclusions

Our results support the main hypothesis that diminished autonomic response is associated with emotional blunting. They also point to a major role played by the parasympathetic branch of the ANS. More specifically, patients with low parasympathetic tone feel lower intensity of anger and sadness, and display blunting of vocally expressed emotional arousal. The sympathetic branch of the ANS played a role only in the spectral differentiation of emotional valence (anger vs. joy).

To the extent that an individual's autonomic tone is inherent to his or her personality, one could expect autonomic lesions to impact some of the prominent personality traits. In a recent study, Schweiger and colleges found that individuals with high vagal tone are less inhibited and do not try to deny feelings (Schweiger, Witling, Genzel, & Block, 1998). It thus appears that our finding relating a disease induced change in the vagal tone to the awareness of change in emotionality, may have psychological consequences for the patients' personality. The assumption is based on the fact that emotion experiences provide continuity in the functioning of personality. Emotional feeling states that remain constant over time link the stability of emotion experience to personality (Barrett & Campos, 1987; Izard, Libero, Putnam, & Haynes, 1993). Caroll Izard and colleagues have convincingly demonstrated how emotions become linked to particular thoughts to form affective-cognitive structures, which in turn combine into cognition-emotion-action patterns that characterize the individual's style of adaptive behavior and contribute to the development of personality.

We can thus expect subjects with impaired cardiovascular reactions to have altered emotional experiences with subsequent consequences for the regulation of the organism's interaction with physical and social environment. Indeed, vocal signaling of emotional states serves an important function of regulating social interactions. It not only provides information about the speaker's attitudes and behavioral tendencies, but it is also informative about the speaker's acceptance of social and cultural demands and expectations (Gregory, Webster, & Huang, 1993; Rosenfeld, 1987). Altered vocal signaling of emotions may therefore impact the person's social functioning.

To conclude, we believe that damage to the nerves in the cardiovascular system not only affects the autonomic responsivity, its flexibility, and its balance, but it also induces a CNS-ANS dysregulation (Friedman & Thayer, 1998) resulting in a dysregulation of the organism's adaptive biological and social response to environmental challenges.

Acknowledgments. I extend special thanks to Professor Krzysztof Izdebski for his constructive remarks in the elaboration of the manuscript, to Dr. Yves Morel for his administration of the autonomic function tests, and to Véronique Ullmann for her work on qualitative assessment of the patients' verbal comments.

References

Banse, R., & Scherer, K. R. (1996). Acoustic profiles in vocal emotion expression. *Journal of Personality & Social Psychology, 70*(3), 614-636.

Barrett, K. C., & Campos, J. J. (1987). Perspectives on emotional development. ii:

A functionalist approach to emotions. In J. D. Osofsky (Ed.), *Handbook of infant development* (2nd ed., pp. 555-578). Oxford, UK: John Wiley and Sons.

Berntson, G. G., Cacioppo, J. T., & Quigley, K. S. (1991). Autonomic determinism: The modes of autonomic control, the doctrine of autonomic space, and the laws of autonomic constraint. *Psychological Review, 98*(4), 459-487.

Berntson, G. G., Cacioppo, J. T., & Quigley, K. S. (1993a). Cardiac psychophysiology and autonomic space in humans: Empirical perspectives and conceptual implications. *Psychological Bulletin, 114*(2), 296-322.

Berntson, G. G., Cacioppo, J. T., & Quigley, K. S. (1993b). Respiratory sinus arrhythmia: Autonomic origins, physiological mechanisms, and psychophysiological implications. *Psychophysiology, 30*(2), 183-196.

Bruchon-Schweitzer, M. (1993). *Spielberger: Inventaire d'anxiété état-trait, forme y*. Paris: Editions du Centre de Psychologie Appliquée.

Cacioppo, J. T., Klein, D. J., Berntson, G. G., & Hatfield, E. (1993). The psychophysiology of emotion. In M. Lewis & J. Haviland (Eds.), *Handbook of emotions* (pp. 119-141). New York: The Guilford Press.

Cannon, W. B. (1927). The James-Lange theory of emotion: A critical examination and an alternative theory. *American Journal of Psychology*, (39), 106-124.

Damasio, A. R. (1989). Time-locked multiregional retroactivation: A systems-level proposal for the neural substrates of recall and recognition. *Cognition, 33*(1-2), 25-62.

Damasio, A. R. (1999). *The feeling of what happens: Body and emotion in the making of consciousness* (1st ed.). New York: Harcourt Brace.

Davis, P. J., Zhang, S. P., Winkworth, A., & Bandler, R. (1996). Neural control of vocalization: Respiratory and emotional influences. *Journal of Voice, 10*(1), 23-38.

DeJong, R. N. (1979). *The neurologic examination: Incorporating the fundamentals of neuroanatomy and neurophysiology.* Hagerstown, MD: Harper & Row.

Ewing, D. J., Campbell, I. W., Burt, A. A., & Clarke, B. F. (1973). Vascular reflexes in diabetic autonomic neuropathy. *Lancet, ii*, 1354-1356.

Ewing, D. J., Martyn, C. N., Young, R. J., & Clarke, B. F. (1985). The value of cardiovascular autonomic function tests: 10 years experience in diabetes. *Diabetes Care, 8*(5), 491-498.

Eysenck, H. J. (1970). *The structure of human personality*. London: Methuen.

Farah, M. J. (1988). Is visual imagery really visual? Overlooked evidence from neuropsychology. *Psychological Review, 95*(3), 307-317.

Frey, W. H., II (1985). *Crying: The mystery of tears*. Minneapolis, MN: Winston Press.

Friedman, B. H., & Thayer, J. F. (1998). Autonomic balance revisited: Panic anxiety and heart rate variability. *Journal of Psychosomatic Research, 44*(1), 133-151.

Gainotti, G. (1991). *Frontal lobe damage and disorders of affect and personality*. Edinburgh, UK: Churchill Livingstone.

Gregory, S. W., Webster, S., & Huang, G. (1993). Voice pitch and amplitude convergence as a metric of quality in dyadic interviews. *Language and Communication, 13*, 195-217.

Hassal, J. H., & Zaveri, K. (1979). *Acoustic noise measurements*. Naerum, Denmark: Büel & Kjaer.

Izard, C. E., Libero, D. Z., Putnam, P., & Haynes, O. M. (1993). Stability of emotion experiences and their relations to traits of personality. *Journal of Personality and Social Psychology, 64*(5), 847-860.

James, W. (1894). The physical basis of emotion. *Psychological Review* (1), 516-529.

Keller, E. (1994). Signalyze 3.0. Lausanne, Switzerland: InfoSignal.

Lang, P. (1995). The emotion probe: Studies of motivation and attention. *American Psychologist, 50*(5), 372-385.

LeDoux, J. E., Iwata, J., Cicchetti, P., & Reis, D. J. (1988). Different projections of the central amygdaloid nucleus mediate autonomic and behavioral correlates of conditioned fear. *Journal of Neuroscience, 8*(7), 2517-2529.

McCraty, R., Atkinson, M., Tiller, W. A., Rein, G., & Watkins, A. D. (1995). The effects of emotions on short-term power spectrum analysis of heart rate variability. *American Journal of Cardiology*, *76*(14), 1089-1093.

Mendolia, M., & Kleck, R. E. (1993). Effects of talking about a stressful event on arousal: Does what we talk about make a difference? *Journal of Personality and Social Psychology*, *64*(2), 283-292.

Pittam, J., & Gallois, C. (1986). Predicting impressions of speakers from voice quality: Acoustic and perceptual measures. *Journal of Language and Social Psychology*, *5*, 233-247.

Pittam, J., Pittam, B. S., Burnstock, G., & Purves, R. D. (1987). Discrimination of five voice qualities and prediction to perceptual ratings. *Phonetica*, *44*(1), 38-49.

Popov, V. A., Simonov, P. V., Frolov, M. V., Khachatur'iants, L. S., & Pastushenko, L. T. (1971). Chastotnyi spektr rechi kak pokazatel' stepeni i kharaktera emotsional'nogo napriazheniia u cheloveka. *Zhurnal Vysshei Nervnoi Deiatelnosti Imeni I. P. Pavlova*, *21*(1), 104-109.

Porges, S. W. (1983). Heart rate patterns in neonates: A potential diagnostic window to the brain. In T. Field & A. Sostek (Eds.), *Infants born at risk: Psychological, perceptual, and cognitive processes* (pp. 3-22). New York: Grune & Stratton.

Porges, S. W. (1995). Cardiac vagal tone: A physiological index of stress. *Psychophysiology*, *32*(4), 301-318.

Porges, S. W., Arnold, W. R., & Forbes, E. J. (1973). Heart rate variability: An index of attentional responsivity in human newborns. *Developmental Psychology*, *8*, 85-92.

Porges, S. W., & Byrne, E. A. (1992). Research methods for measurement of heart rate and respiration. *Biological Psychology*, *34*(2-3), 93-130.

Porges, S. W., Doussard-Roosevelt, J. A., & Maiti, A. K. (1994). Vagal tone and the physiological regulation of emotion. *Monographs of the Society for Research in Childhood Development*, *59*(2-3), 167-186.

Rosenfeld, H. M. (1987). Conversational control functions of nonverbal behavior. In A. W. Siegman & S. Feldstein (Eds.), *Nonverbal behavior and communication* (pp. 563-601). Hillsdale, NJ: Lawrence Erlbaum Associates.

Russell, J. A. (2003). Core affect and the psychological construction of emotion. *Psychological Review*, *110*(1), 145-172.

Schachter, S., & Singer, J. (1962). Cognitive, social, and physiological determinants of emotional state. *Psychological Review* (69), 379-399.

Scherer, K. R. (1978). Personality inference from voice quality. The loud voice of extraversion. *European Journal of Social Psychology*, *8*, 4674-4687.

Scherer, K. R. (1979). Personality markers in speech. In K. R. Scherer & H. Giles (Eds.), *Social markers in speech* (pp. 147-209). Cambridge, UK: Cambridge University Press.

Scherer, K. R. (1981). Vocal indicators of stress. In J. K. Darby (Ed.), *Speech evaluation in psychiatry* (pp. 171-187). New York: Grune & Stratton.

Scherer, K. (1984a). On the nature and function of emotion: A component process approach. In K. Scherer & P. Ekman (Eds.), *Approaches to emotion* (pp. 293-318). Hillsdale, NJ: Lawrence Erlbaum Associates.

Scherer, K. R. (1984b). Emotion as a multicomponent process: A model and some cross cultural data. *Review of Personality and Social Psychology*, *5*, 37-63.

Scherer, K. R. (1986). Dynamics of stress: Physiological, psychological and social perspectives. In M. H. Appley & R. Trumbull (Eds.), *Voice, stress, and emotion* (pp. 157-179). New York: Plenum Press.

Scherer, K. (1989a). Vocal correlates of emotional arousal and affective disturbance. In H. *Wagner* & A. *Manstead* (Eds.), *Handbook of social psychophysiology* (pp. 165-197). Chichester, UK: Wiley.

Scherer, K. R. (1989b). Emotion psychology can contribute to psychiatric work on affect disorders: A review. *Journal of the Royal Society of Medicine*, *82*(9), 545-547.

Scherer, K. R., & Scherer, U. (1981). Speech behavior and personality. In J. K. Darby (Ed.), *Speech evaluation in psychiatry* (pp. 115-135). New York: Grune & Stratton.

Schweiger, E., Witling, W., Genzel, S., & Block, A. (1998). Relationship between sympathovagal tone and personality traits. *Personality and Individual Differences, 25*, 327-337.

Simonov, P. V., Frolov, M. V., & Ivanov, E. A. (1980). Psychophysiological monitoring of operator's emotional stress in aviation and astronautics. *Aviation, Space, and Environmental Medicine, 51*(1), 46-49.

Stifter, C. A., Fox, N. A., & Porges, S. W. (1989). Facial expressivity and vagal tone in five- and ten-month-old infants. *Infant Behavior and Development, 12*, 127-113.

Strack, F., Schwarz, N., & Gschneidinger, E. (1985). Happiness and reminiscing: The role of time perspective, affect, and mode of thinking. *Journal of Personality and Social Psychology, 49*, 1460-1469.

Tesser, A. C. L., & Clary, G. (1978). Affect control: Process constraints versus catharsis. *Cognitive Therapy and Research, 2*(3), 265-274.

Valensi, P., Gautier, J. F., Amarenco, G., Sauvanet, J. P., Leutenegger, M., & Attali, J. R. (1997). Neuropathie autonome chez le diabetique. *Diabetes & Metabolism, 23*(1), 89-99.

Vita, G., Princi, P., Calabro, R., Toscano, A., Manna, L., & Messina, C. (1986). Cardiovascular reflex tests. Assessment of age-adjusted normal range. *Journal of Neurological Science, 75*(3), 263-274.

Williams, C. E., & Stevens, K. N. (1972). Emotions and speech: Some acoustical correlates. *Journal of the Acoustical Society of America, 52*(4), 1238-1250.

Williams, C. E., & Stevens, K. N. (1981). Vocal correlates of emotional states. In J. K. Darby (Ed.), *Speech evaluation in psychiatry* (pp. 221-240). New York: Grune & Stratton.

Winkworth, A. L., Davis, P. J., Adams, R. D., & Ellis, E. (1995). Breathing patterns during spontaneous speech. *Journal of Speech and Hearing Research, 38*(1), 124-144.

Zei, B., & Archinard, M. (1998). La variabilité du rythme cardiaque et la différentiation prosodique des émotions. In (Ed.), *Actes des XXIIèmes Journées d'Etudes sur la Parole* (pp. 167-170). June, Martigny, Switzerland.

Zei, B., & Archinard, M. (2001). Emotional Consequences of Diabetic Neuropathy [abs]. *Psychosomatic Medicine, 63*, 186.

Zei, B., & Archinard, M. (2002). Acoustic patterns of emotions. In E. Keller, G. Bailly, A. Monagham, J. Terken, & M. Huckvale (Eds.), *Improvements in speech synthesis* (pp. 237-245). Chichester, UK: Wiley.

CHAPTER 2

Brain Mechanisms for Social Perception

Elizabeth J. Carter and Kevin A. Pelphrey

Abstract

Social perception consists of the initial stages of evaluating interpersonal interactions using gaze direction, body movement, body language, and other types of biological motion. By using this information to interpret the intentions of others, we choose courses of action. The amygdala, fusiform gyrus, and superior temporal sulcus compose the "social brain": the brain regions involved in social perception analyses. Here we describe the roles of each of these three regions, particularly focusing on the unique contributions of the superior temporal sulcus region to social perception, and discuss how cognitive neuroscience methods including functional magnetic resonance imaging and eye tracking can help elucidate how they work together and separately. Additionally, we illustrate the importance of the social perception system by describing autism, a developmental disorder in which the components of the social brain work in an atypical fashion. Finally, we suggest future directions for this research and implications for our knowledge of typical and atypical development.

Defining Social Perception

Imagine that you are walking home alone late at night from a party in an unfamiliar, slightly dangerous part of your city. As you go quickly down the sidewalk, you see movement out of the corner of your eye. It's a man coming out of the alley! What do you do?

Social perception is a term used to describe the process of analyzing the actions and intentions of other people. You have realized that the movement is a man, but how can you assess whether he's threatening or friendly? First, you can attempt to identify him—if you know who he is, you can more easily decide whether this encounter is potentially problematic. However, say that you don't recognize him. Now you must determine his intentions. To do so, you would use the information that you have readily available: his body language, facial expression, and eye gaze. If he's looking to the ground, does not seem to see you, has a neutral facial expression, and does not directly approach you, he is probably not going to cause you harm. However, if he stares straight at you with an angry face and clenched fists while advancing, you would probably pick up the pace and perhaps hail the next cab that drove by.

These initial stages of evaluating the actions and intentions of others that form social perception are typically covert and automatic: the full assessment of the man coming out of the alley could be done almost instantaneously, even without conscious awareness. Social perception abilities fall within a larger domain of mental processes that also includes social cognition, mentalizing, theory of mind, and social attention. It could be a prequel to some of these more complicated processes, such as theory of mind —the ability to understand that other people hold unique beliefs and desires and that their behavior reflects those (Wellman, 1990).

The Social Brain

A network of interconnected structures in the brain (i.e., the *social brain*) contributes to social perception capabilities (see Figure 2-1). Models of this network typically focus on three interconnected structures, the amygdala, the superior temporal sulcus, and the fusiform gyrus. The amygdala plays a role in making emotional and social judgments about people, such as deciding by a man's facial expression that he is angry or threatening. It was proposed by Brothers (1990) that the amygdala, superior temporal sulcus and gyrus, and the orbitofrontal cortices compose a neural circuit supporting social perception and cognition.

The amygdala is a complex structure composed of a number of nuclei and highly interconnected with other areas of the brain, including the hippocampus, the thalamus, basal forebrain, brainstem, and claustrum (Amaral & Insausti, 1992; Amaral, Veazey, & Cowan , 1982). Animal research implicates the amygdala in fear conditioning in rodents (LeDoux, 1996), as well as judgment of the basic motivational significance and complex social significance of stimuli (e.g., Brothers, Ring, & Kling, 1990; Rolls, 1992), food preferences and sexual behaviors (Brown & Schafer, 1888; Kluver & Bucy, 1938; 1939), and assessing threat and danger in the environment (Emery et al., 2001) in nonhuman primates.

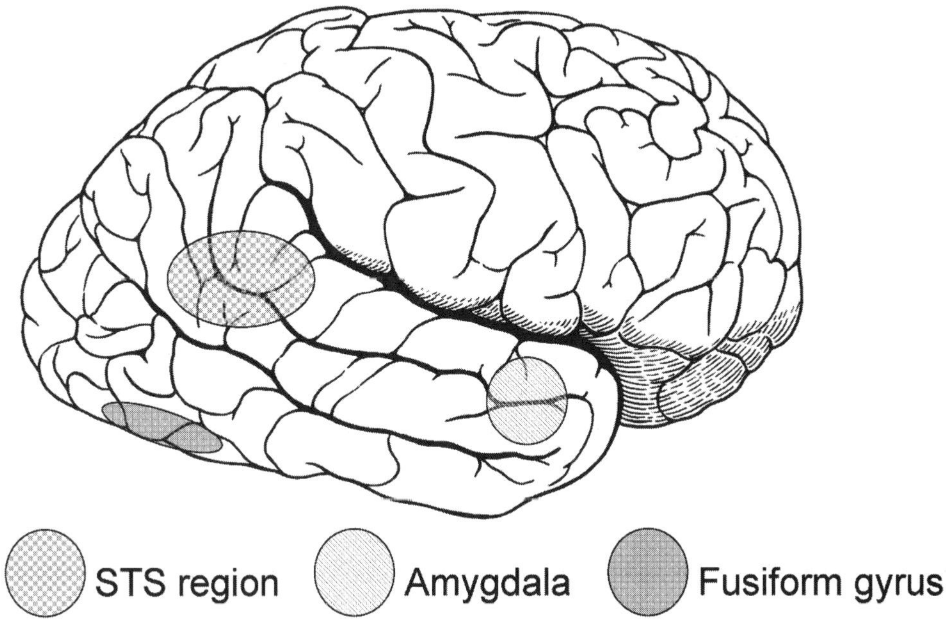

Figure 2–1. Artistic rendering of the components of the "social brain." Note that the location of the amygdala has been projected to the surface of the brain. Figure reproduced with permission from "Neuroanatomical Substrates of Social Cognition Dysfunction in Autism," by K. Pelphrey, Adolphs, and Morris, 2005, *Mental Retardation and Developmental Disabilities Research Reviews*, *10*(4), p. 261.

Lesion and neuroimaging studies have also implicated the amygdala for human social perception. Social information processing deficits have been identified in humans with amygdala lesions, including problems recognizing facial expressions of emotions, especially fear (Adolphs, Tranel, H. Damasio, & A. Damasio, 1994; Anderson & Phelps, 2000; Broks et al., 1998; Sprengelmeyer et al., 1999). Functional neuroimaging studies have shown amygdala activation when typically developing patients view fearful faces, even when performing a task unrelated to emotion (Breiter et al., 1996; Morris et al., 1996). When participants viewed these faces subliminally in a backward-masking paradigm, the amygdala was still consistently activated, indicating that rapid, automatic processing can take place in this region even in the absence of conscious awareness of a face (Whalen et al., 1998). Even with the minimal facial information of only the sclera of the eyes of a fearful face, activation was found in the amygdala (Whalen et al., 2004).

The amygdala is also important for social judgments. Individuals with amygdala lesions consider people in photographs to be more trustworthy and approachable than do individuals without these lesions (Adolphs, Tranel, & A. R. Damasio, 1998). In functional neuroimaging studies of the same task, neurologically normal individuals show activation in the amygdala, superior temporal sulcus, insular cortex, and orbitofrontal cortex (Winston, Strange, O'Doherty, & Dolan, 2002). This supports the animal findings that implicate the amygdala in threat assessment (Adolphs et al., 1999; Adolphs, H. Damasio, Tranel, Cooper, & A. R. Damasio, 2000). Adolphs and colleagues (2005) found that an individual with complete bilateral amygdale lesions, patient S.M., also had abnormal visual scanpaths when viewing emotionally expressive faces, failing to fixate on the eyes and improperly judging the emotions. When she was directly instructed to look at the eyes, her deficit in identifying the emotions disappeared. However, it reappeared as soon as she forgot the instruction. This suggests that the amygdala plays a role in directing the visual system to seek out the eyes as socially important (Adolphs et al., 2005).

An area of the lateral portion of the fusiform gyrus, often referred to as the *fusiform face area*, has been shown to be important for face perception. For example, when presented with faces versus scrambled images or nonface objects in fMRI research, face-evoked activity was found bilaterally (although generally more strongly in the right hemisphere) in this area of the fusiform gyrus (e.g., Kanwisher, McDermott, & Chun, 1997; McCarthy, Puce, Gore, & Allison, 1997; Puce, Allison, Asgari, Gore, & McCarthy, 1996). When electrodes were inserted in the ventral occipitotemporal cortical surface during brain surgery, this area displayed face-specific evoked activity within 200 ms of the stimulus presentation. Also, prosopagnosia resulted from electrical stimulation of this area (Allison, McCarthy, Nobre, Puce, & Belger, 1994). The fusiform gyrus appears to be important for face detection and processing the static aspects of faces used for identification (Haxby et al., 2000; McCarthy, 1999).

The superior temporal sulcus region includes the superior temporal sulcus proper, portions of the superior and middle temporal gyri, and areas of the angular gyrus (Allison, Puce, & McCarthy, 2000). Functional neuroimaging studies have implicated this region for social perception, particularly the posterior superior temporal sulcus region for biological motion perception (for reviews, see Allison et al., 2000; Decety & Grezes, 1999). In this chapter, we will focus on describing a program of research conducted in our laboratory over the past few years that has helped to delineate the role of the posterior superior temporal sulcus region in perceiving and understanding the actions and intentions of others. But first, we will take a step back to describe methods for studying social perception.

Methods for Studying Social Perception

We will focus on the use of two cognitive neuroscience methods throughout this chapter. One commonly used technique is functional magnetic resonance imaging (fMRI), which takes advantage of the brain's property of having different levels of blood oxygenation in regions with varied levels of neural activity. Tracking changes in this blood oxygenation level-dependent (BOLD) contrast can provide an indirect measure of brain activity in a variety of areas. Advantages of this method are that it can be done on large numbers of people repeatedly without ionizing radiation or invasive procedures. This technique can be used to interpret brain response to a variety of stimuli presented in various sensory modalities to participants.

Tracking eye movements provides powerful information about the decisions that a person's brain has made about whether something is important (Rayner, 1998). Typically, people fixate with their eyes areas within a visual scene that they perceive to be important because they get more detailed, higher resolution information by foveating these regions. A number of dependent measures can be provided by tracking eye movements: (a) saccade direction (what direction the eyes move); (b) fixation dwell time (how long the individual looks in a certain location); (c) fixation latency time (how long it takes to move the eyes to a target); and (d) pupil dilation (a measure of autonomic arousal). Long visual fixations on particular areas of the scene can therefore be considered to denote attention and interest and therefore perceived significance of the item at which a person is looking.

In concert with these two cognitive neuroscience techniques, we employ animated, virtual reality stimuli for the participants to observe. These stimuli are convenient and powerful because they strike a balance between being naturalistic and being very easily controlled for different, potentially confounding variables.

A Role for the Superior Temporal Sulcus Region in Action and Intention Understanding

In one of our first studies, we sought to determine whether the superior temporal sulcus region responds selectively to biological motion or more generally to other complex coherent motions. This study was needed because many functional neuroimaging studies of biological motion had used as stimuli point-light displays of walking figures and compared the resulting activations with those evoked by the same display elements moving in a random or noncoherent manner. Although these studies had established that biological motion activates the superior temporal sulcus region, the use of random motion controls had left open the possibility that coordinated and meaningful nonbiological motion might activate these same brain regions and thus called into question their specificity for processing biological motion. We sought to clarify further the role of the superior temporal sulcus in processing biological motion as compared to random motion and coherent, organized, nonbiological motion. We designed an fMRI study with four different motion conditions involving animations of (a) a walking man, (b) a walking robot, (c) a disjointed mechanical figure with the same components as the robot, and (d) a ticking grandfather clock. In this way, we were able to control for whether the figure was biological, whether the motion was biological, and whether the motion was organized. By comparing responses in the superior temporal sulcus for the human and robot figures, we determined that the superior temporal sulcus is sensitive to biological motion itself, not merely to the superficial characteristics of the stimulus. The superior temporal sulcus responded more strongly to biological motion (the human and robot) than to a nonmeaningful but complex nonbiological motion (the mechanical figure) and a complex and meaningful nonbiological motion (the clock). Importantly, not every brain region showed this pattern of effects. We observed a dissociation of function between the superior temporal sulcus region and an area more posterior and inferior to the superior temporal sulcus region corresponding to the more generally motion-sensitive visual area MT+/V5 (e.g., McCarthy et al., 1995). Whereas the superior temporal sulcus region "preferred" biological motion, MT+/V5 responded equally to all four types of motion. From this study, we were able to conclude that the superior temporal sulcus region is involved in social perception by representing perceived actions, but the study left open the question of whether the superior temporal sulcus region is involved in processing the intentions of observed actions.

In our next study, we began to tackle the question of intention understanding by conducting a study to determine whether the superior temporal sulcus region was sensitive to the goal-directedness of observed gaze shifts. During fMRI scanning, our participants watched as a small checkerboard appeared and flickered in an animated character's visual field (Figure 2-2; left panel).

On goal-directed (congruent) trials, the character shifted her gaze towards the checkerboard, acting in accordance with the subject's presumed expectations. On nongoal-directed (incongruent) trials, the character shifted her gaze away from the checkerboard and towards empty

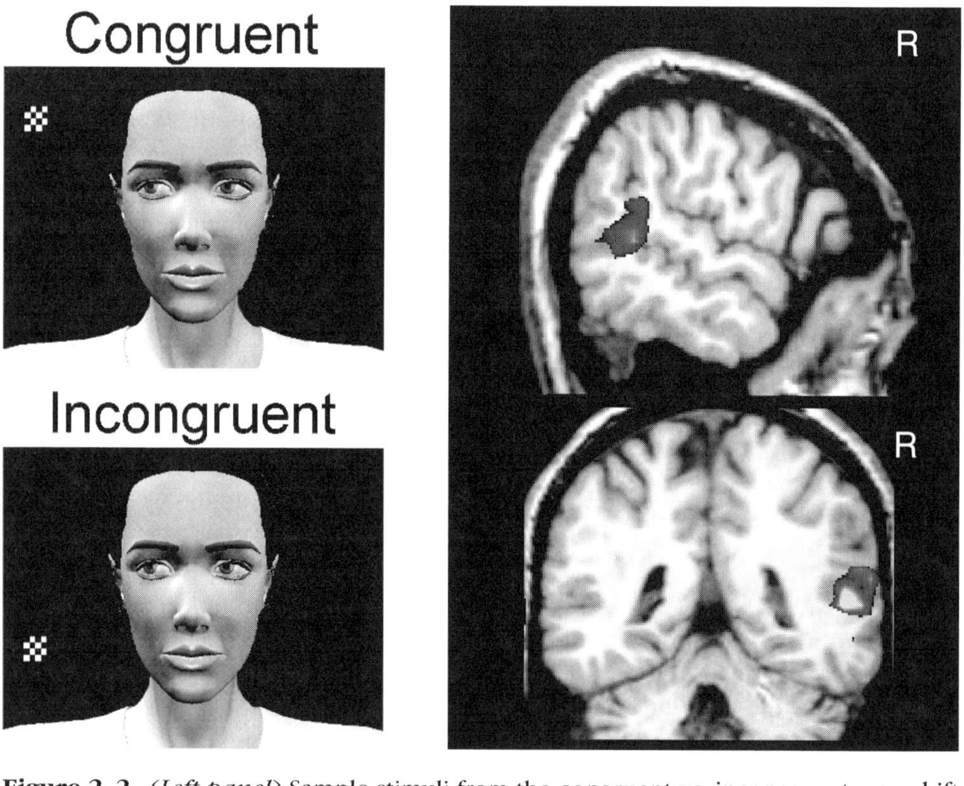

Figure 2–2. (*Left panel*) Sample stimuli from the congruent vs. incongruent gaze shift paradigm. (*Right panel*) Incongruent > congruent activity in the right posterior superior temporal sulcus region. Figure reproduced with permission from "Brain Mechanisms for Interpreting the Actions of Others from Biological-Motion Cues," by K. Pelphrey and Morris, 2006, *Current Directions in Psychological Science*, *15*(3), p.138.

space, violating the participant's likely expectations. We hypothesized that the superior temporal sulcus region would be sensitive to the intentions conveyed by others' actions; therefore, activity evoked in this region would differentiate between congruent and incongruent trials. This differentiation, we reasoned, would reflect an ability to link the perception of the gaze shift with its mentalistic significance. We observed more activity in the right posterior superior temporal sulcus region for incongruent than for congruent gaze shifts (Figure 2-2; right panel), suggesting that additional processing was required when the character violated the participants' expectations. Although this study focused upon the superior temporal sulcus region, similar effects were also observed in the intraparietal sulcus and fusiform gyrus. These initial findings have since been replicated in children, using the same eye-gaze paradigm (Mosconi, Mack, McCarthy, & Pelphrey, 2005). This study allowed us to conclude that the superior temporal sulcus region is sensitive to the goal-directed structure of actions.

We next wondered whether the effects of context observed in our study of gaze processing were unique to the goals and social intentions conveyed by gaze shifts. We designed a study in which participants viewed an animated character making reaching-to-grasp movements either toward (congruent) or away (incongruent) from a blinking dial. Both conditions evoked significant posterior superior temporal sulcus activity that was strongly right lateralized. We again observed a functional dissociation: incongruent trials evoked significantly greater activity in the superior temporal sulcus region than did congruent trials, while an area posterior and inferior to the superior temporal sulcus (likely corresponding to area MT+/V5) responded equally to congruent and incongruent movements. Parietal cortical regions, including the superior parietal lobule and the anterior intraparietal sulcus, also responded equally to congruent and incongruent movements, but they also showed evidence for differential responding based on the hand and arm (left or right) of the animated character used to make the reaching-to-grasp movement. The results of this study further suggested that a region of the posterior superior temporal sulcus is involved in analyzing the intentions of other people's actions and that activity in this region is sensitive to the context of observed biological motions.

Several regions of the brain are organized somatotopically (i.e., of or related to the body) such that different cortical regions contain spatially segregated representations of body parts. We next speculated about whether the superior temporal sulcus region was organized in such a fashion. We conducted an imaging experiment to compare activity elicited by movement of the eyes, mouth, or hand (Figure 2-3; top panel).

Each motion evoked robust activation in the right superior temporal sulcus region. While there was substantial overlap of the activation maps in this region, the spatial distribution of hemodynamic response amplitudes differentiated the movements (Figure 2-3; bottom panel). Mouth movements elicited activity along the mid-posterior superior temporal sulcus, while eye movements elicited activity in more superior and posterior portions of the right posterior superior temporal sulcus region. Hand movements activated more inferior and posterior portions of the superior temporal sulcus

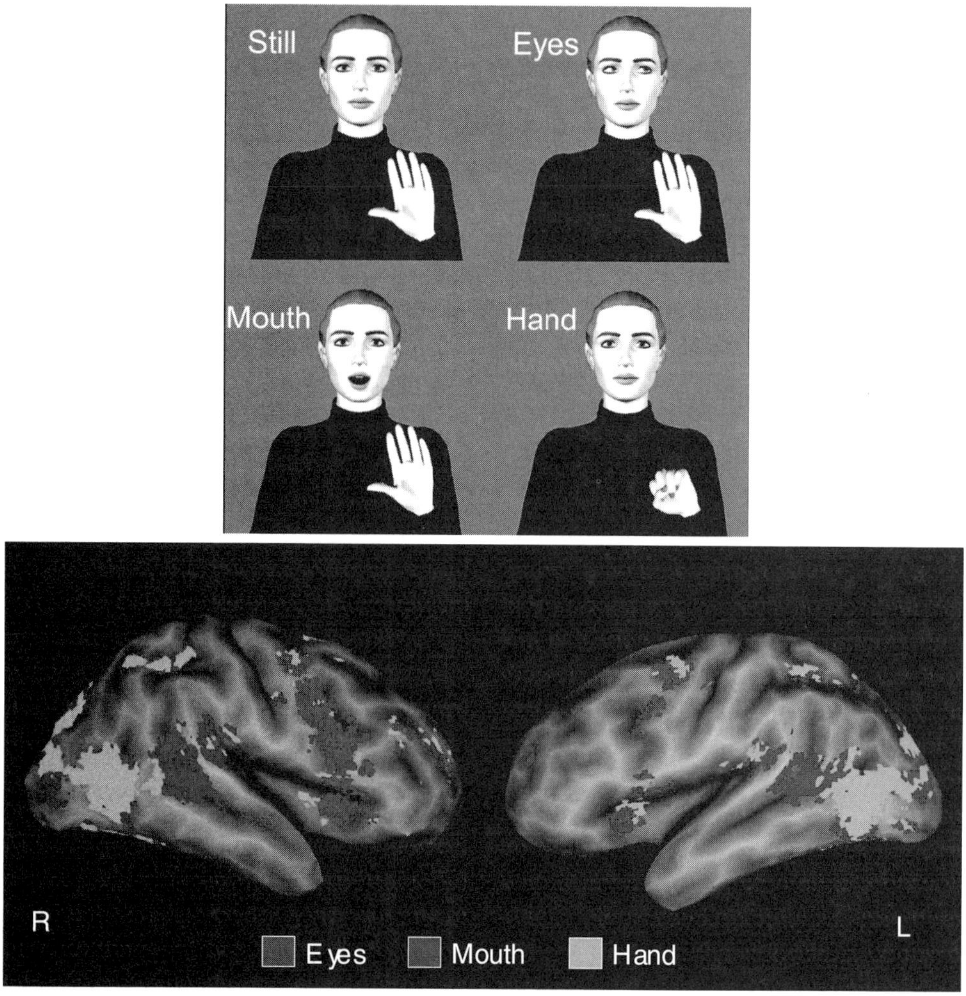

Figure 2–3. (*Top panel*) Sample stimuli for our study comparing brain responses to eye, hand, and mouth movements. (*Bottom panel*) Activation maps showing the distribution of activity in response to the observation of eye, hand, and mouth movements along the lateral surfaces of the left and right cerebral cortices. Figure modified from "Functional Anatomy of Biological Motion Perception in Posterior Temporal Cortex: An fMRI Study of Eye, Mouth, and Hand Movements," by K. Pelphrey, Morris, Michelich, Allison, and McCarthy, 2005, *Cerebral Cortex*, *15*(12) p. 1867–1869.

region within the posterior continuing branch of the superior temporal sulcus. Hand-evoked activity also extended into the inferior temporal, middle occipital, and lingual gyri. This topography may, in part, reflect the role of particular body motions in different functional activities. For example, the area of activity evoked by hand movements was close to an area previously identified as relating to manipulable objects such as tools (Beauchamp, Lee, Haxby, & Martin, 2002). Also, the activation patterns in response to mouth movements were near areas implicated in speech understanding and audiovisual speech integration (Calvert & Campbell, 2003; Wright, Pelphrey, Allison, McKeown, & McCarthy , 2003).

With these findings in hand, we next sought to explore the role of the superior temporal sulcus in processing social intentions in a much more explicitly social encounter similar to the rendezvous with a stranger described in the opening section of this chapter. In a virtual environment consisting of a hallway, an animated, male stranger turned a corner, walked towards the participant, and as he passed shifted his gaze toward (mutual gaze) or away from (averted gaze) the participant while maintaining a neutral facial expression (Figure 2-4; top panel).

The motion of the man walking towards the subject and that of his gaze shift evoked robust activity in the right posterior superior temporal sulcus region and the right fusiform gyrus. Mutual gaze evoked greater activity in the superior temporal sulcus than did averted gaze (Figure 2-4; bottom panel). In contrast, the fusiform gyrus responded equally to mutual and averted gaze, demonstrating a functional dissociation between the two social brain areas. Thus, the fusiform gyrus might have been functioning as a face detector and responding to a looming face, but the superior temporal sulcus region was involved in assessing the stranger's intentions. This study advanced our understanding of the role of the superior temporal sulcus region in social perception by demonstrating its sensitivity to the social context in which a specific biological motion occurs.

Finally, in the most recent study of this series, we investigated the necessity of biological motion for activation of the posterior superior temporal sulcus in circumstances in which the rapid approach of the observer to a virtual human induced the observer to make inferences about the character. We reasoned that a brain system for inferring another's intentions would be strongly engaged as the subject approached the virtual human, therefore allowing us to dissociate activity evoked by a subject's reflexive inference about intentions from that subject's perception of biological motion. Using a virtual reality environment, subjects experienced themselves walking towards a complex scene composed of animate and/or inanimate objects. During social trials, the scene contained a virtual human either making a simple gesture (scratching his face) or standing completely still. During nonsocial trials, the scenes contained items, such as furniture, a face portrait, and a clock, but not the virtual human. We demonstrated strong activity in the posterior superior temporal sulcus while the observer approached the social scene, but only when the virtual human was making gestures. This result emphasizes the importance of biological motion for inferring the intentions of others.

Taken together, our studies demonstrate the important role played by the superior temporal sulcus region in social perception. It is involved in perceiving biological motion, analyzing the goals implicit in movement, and comparing the intentions of others with their performance. Our studies of eye-gaze processing reveal the involvement of the superior temporal sulcus region in understanding that gaze direction might indicate another person's attention, desire, or intentions.

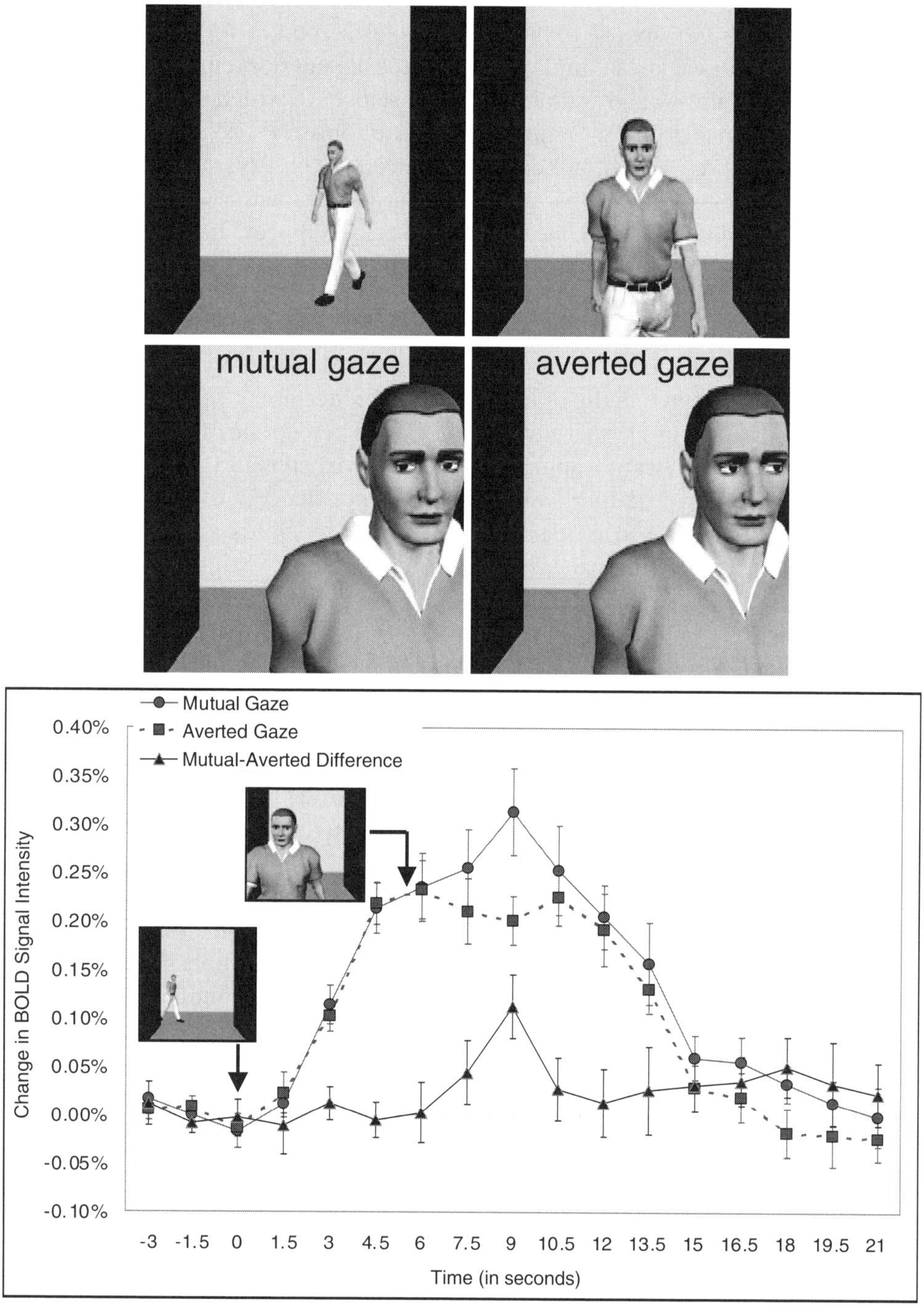

Figure 2–4. (*Top panel*) Mutual vs. averted gaze paradigm. (*Bottom panel*) Responses from the superior temporal sulcus region to mutual and averted gaze (*lines with circles and triangles*) and the difference waveform (*line with squares*). Figure modified from "When strangers pass: Processing of mutual and averted social gaze in the superior temporal sulcus," by K. A. Pelphrey, R. J. Viola, and G. McCarthy, 2004, *Psychological Science*, *15*(9), p. 601.

Autism, Social Perception, and the Superior Temporal Sulcus

Autism is a severe, pervasive developmental disorder characterized by deficits in three domains: (a) social interaction, (b) communication skills, and (c) restricted interests and repetitive, stereotyped behaviors [DSM-IV; American Psychiatric Association (APA), 1994]. There is a wide range of variation in abilities within these domains; however, all three types of deficits are present to some degree in individuals with autism. Additionally, there is a large range of intellectual capacities: although many of these individuals exhibit mental retardation, others have average or even superior abilities.

Social impairment is the primary, unique feature of autism (Kanner, 1943; Wing & Gould, 1979). Early problems in social perception, such as joint attention, are indicators of autism (Baron-Cohen, 1995; Dawson et al., 2002; Lord et al., 1997; Sigman et al., 1999). Also, these children fail to recognize biological motion in point-light displays, where lights are placed on the joints of people in a dark room and can be seen as they move around (Blake, Turner, Smoski, Pozdol, & Stone, 2003; Klin, Jones, Schultz, & Volkmar, 2003). Additionally, individuals with autism have a hard time identifying the emotions portrayed by faces in photographs, particularly fear and anger (Adolphs, Sears, & Piven, 2001; Pelphrey et al., 2002).

In order to explore emotional recognition deficits in individuals with autism, we quantified visual attention to faces (Pelphrey et al., 2002). In an eye-tracking study of adults looking at photographs of faces, we found that the adults with autism spent more time looking at the nonfeature portions of the face (e.g., forehead, cheeks) than did typical adults. Additionally, there was a corresponding decrease in the visual examination of core features (i.e., the eyes, nose, and mouth) by the individuals with autism relative to the individuals without autism. This suggested disorganized face processing and could be related to their overarching social perception problems. Similar results were reported in another study of scanpaths over faces by individuals with autism by Klin and colleagues (2002).

An impaired understanding of the implications of gaze direction is also characteristic of autism. Baron-Cohen (1995) showed pictures of a cartoon face named Charlie looking at one of four types of candy to children with typical development, mental retardation, or autism. When asked, "What is Charlie's favorite candy?" the typically developing children and those with mental retardation correctly responded with the name of the candy at which Charlie was looking. However, the children with autism failed to do this. However, when shown a different set of pictures with faces looking towards or away from them, all of the children could correctly answer the question, "Which one is looking at you?" Together, these results suggest that children with autism can perceive gaze direction, but they do not link it with its social and mental significance.

These deficits, combined with our prior findings on gaze perception in the superior temporal sulcus region, suggested that dysfunction in this area could relate to autism (Pelphrey, Morris, & McCarthy, 2005). In order to test this hypothesis, we used fMRI and our congruent versus incongruent eye-gaze paradigm to determine whether the superior temporal sulcus region of individuals with autism would differentiate between the contexts in which the gaze shifts occurred. The neurotypical individuals showed more evoked activity in this region in response to the unexpected, incongruent gaze shifts than to the congruent shifts. Although the same brain regions were activated in the individuals with autism, the superior temporal sulcus region did not differentiate between the two conditions. Lack of modulation in this area could be a potential mechanism for the gaze processing deficits in this disorder.

We did note that there was a great deal of individual variation in the amount of differentiation in the superior temporal sulcus region for the group of participants with autism. The source of this variation remained unknown. Thus, we decided to do a set of exploratory correlational analyses integrating the fMRI data with diagnostic information from a widely used tool, the Autism Diagnostic Interview—Revised (ADI-R; Lord, Rutter, & Le Couteur, 1994). This assessment includes scoring of reciprocal social interaction, communication (both verbal and nonverbal), and restricted, repetitive, stereotyped behaviors; scores increase with the severity of dysfunction. We found that levels of differentiation in the superior temporal sulcus region highly correlated with scores in the areas of reciprocal social interaction and nonverbal communication such that more severely impaired individuals showed less differentiation in brain activation. This suggests that the neurofunctional impairment in the superior temporal sulcus relates to phenotypic dysfunction in autism, and further research could clarify activity patterns as biomarkers for this disorder.

By combining virtual reality stimuli, fMRI, and eye-tracking techniques, we can learn more about the social deficits seen in autism. Moreover, it could be possible to use virtual reality and eye-tracking information to create more engaging stimuli and help intervene in the course of development. Through creation of more realistic social interactions, it might be possible to teach people with autism how to react and interact more appropriately. In combination with fMRI, more could be learned about the nature and duration of effects of interventions on the brain.

Weaving Together Components of the Social Brain

Though we have emphasized the role of the superior temporal sulcus region, this approach does not fully reflect the interactions of this region with others in the social brain. It is unlikely that this area is acting in isolation; the entire network undoubtedly works together when an individual is first placed in a social situation. For example, let's consider the alley encounter described in the beginning of this chapter. First, the amygdala would be rapidly and automatically engaged in assessing potential threats and determining the distribution of processing resources accordingly. The fusiform face area would be involved in perceptually representing the face in order to attempt to identify the other person. The superior temporal sulcus would analyze body information such as gaze direction, gait, and facial movements, and it would aid in the amygdala's identification of emotional facial expressions. Together, all of the information from these three regions would be integrated quickly in order for you to decide which course of action you wish to take after you notice the stranger.

To learn more about the relationships between these regions, researchers are using functional connectivity while participants watch social scenes from movies. Hasson and colleagues (2004) were able to obtain activations from functional regions of interest, including the amygdala, superior temporal sulcus, and fusiform gyrus, while having participants watch *The Good, the Bad, and the Ugly*. This indicates that more naturalistic viewing paradigms can be used to research the social brain. Additionally, Bartels and Zeki (2005) analyzed activation maps from natural viewing by correlating the activity in different brain regions in order to determine which areas of the cortex most commonly worked together. They found that functional connectivity is highly related to anatomical connectivity (Bartels & Zeki, 2005).

By using emotionally laden movie scenes with auditory and visual components and social interactions among the characters, we can learn more about the social brain. Using fMRI, one could examine virtual reality and photorealistic movies and scenes to see how the patterns of brain activation compare. Additionally, eye tracking could be used in order to see if visual scanpaths change for virtual versus natural stimuli. Virtual reality stimuli are often preferred for research because of the ability to have total control over every item and movement in the scene. Recent improvements in animation techniques have increased the realism of the characters and scenes. On the one hand, the rise in the ability to make highly realistic, animated social interactions that can be used in the scanners has improved our capacity to research the social brain. On the other hand, we could employ fMRI and eye-tracking techniques to investigate the realism and efficacy of these animated stimuli relative to actual film recordings of similar actions.

In Figure 2-5, we show eye-tracking data from two different social scenes in *The Incredibles*.

In the left panels, we show "hot spot" maps of where an adult research participant was looking at two different times at dinner table settings. The right-hand panels show the order and duration of fixations on various areas within the scenes. The data from the top row of images demonstrate that the participant spent the vast majority of her time looking at the faces of the three people present, particularly the young female, who was actually the most prominent in the social interaction depicted. In the bottom row, the data again make evident that the human characters receive more visual attention than the background, especially the two children who unexpectedly find themselves hanging in midair. We can combine this information with fMRI data during viewing of the same movie to analyze the interaction between what the participants look at and find interesting and how their brains react. In this way, parallel advances in the arts and sciences of character animation and functional neuroimaging could lead to important discoveries about how the human brain perceives and processes the emotions, intentions, and actions of other people.

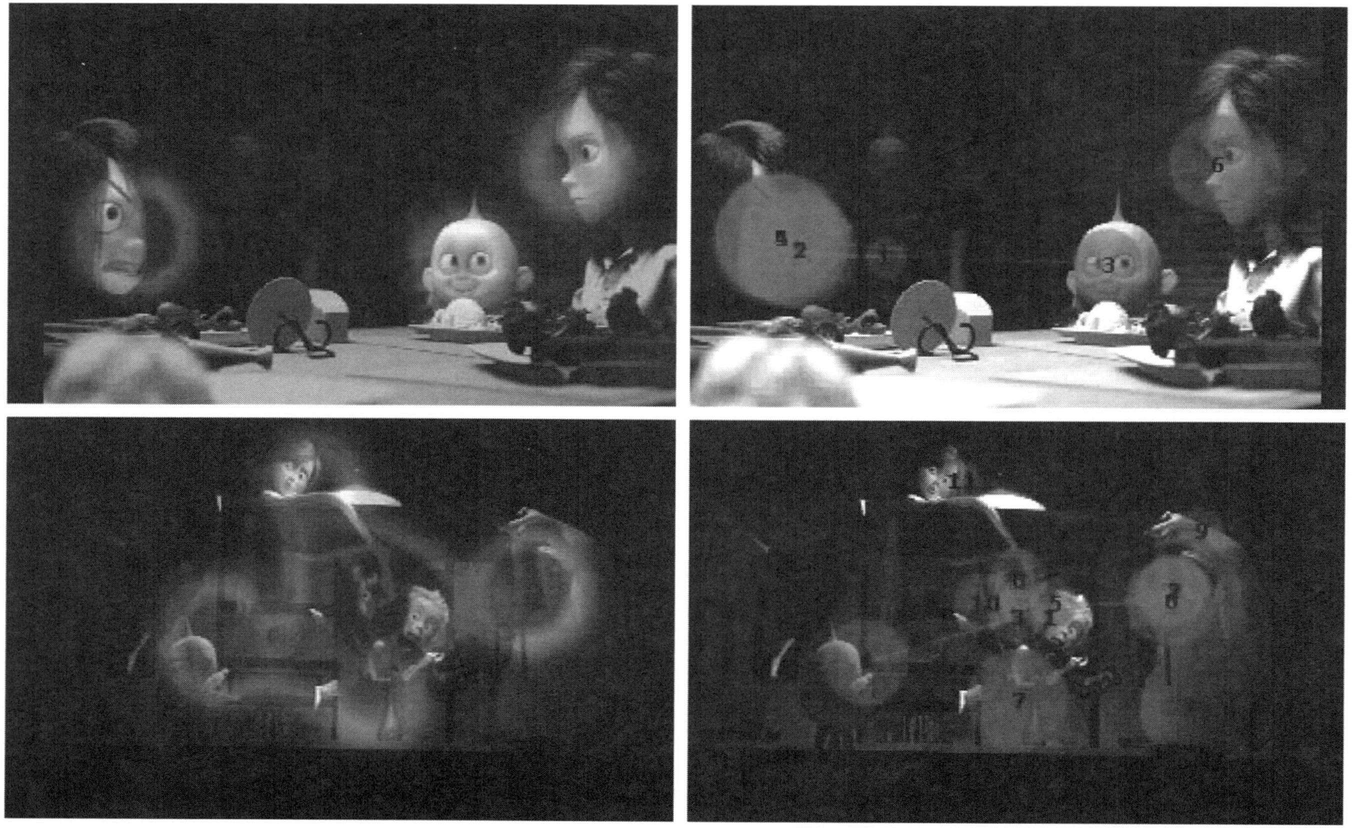

Figure 2–5. (*Left panels*) "Hot spot" maps show how much the participant viewed areas of the scenes. The color gradient is such that red signifies the greatest and blue signifies the least amount of looking time. (*Right panels*) The circles represent fixations with the numbers delineating the order in which those fixations were made and the size of the circles signifying the amount of time spent looking in each place.

Acknowledgments. A Career Development Award from the National Institutes of Health, National Institute of Mental Health grant K01-MH071284, supports Dr. Pelphrey. We gratefully acknowledge our collaborators James Morris, Yvette Peters, Heather Lucas, Gregory McCarthy, and Truett Allison.

References

Adolphs, R., Damasio, H., Tranel, D., Cooper, G., & Damasio, A. R. (2000). A role for somatosensory cortices in the visual recognition of emotion as revealed by three-dimensional lesion mapping. *Journal of Neuroscience, 20*(7), 2683-2690.

Adolphs, R., Gosselin, F., Buchanan, T. W., Tranel, D., Schyns, P., & Damasio, A. R. (2005). A mechanism for impaired fear recognition after amygdala damage. *Nature, 433*(7021), 68-72.

Adolphs, R., Sears, L., & Piven, J. (2001). Abnormal processing of social information from faces in autism. *Journal of Cognitive Neuroscience, 13*(2), 232-240.

Adolphs, R., Tranel, D., & Damasio, A. R. (1998). The human amygdala in social judgment. *Nature, 393*(6684), 470-474.

Adolphs, R., Tranel, D., Damasio, H., & Damasio, A. (1994). Impaired recognition of emotion in facial expressions following bilateral damage to the human amygdala. *Nature, 372*(6507), 669-672.

Adolphs, R., Tranel, D., Hamann, S., Young, A. W., Calder, A. J., Phelps, E. A., et al. (1999). Recognition of facial emotion in nine individuals with bilateral amygdala damage. *Neuropsychologia, 37*(10), 1111-1117.

Allison, T., McCarthy, G., Nobre, A., Puce, A., & Belger, A. (1994). Human extrastriate visual cortex and the perception of faces, words, numbers, and colors. *Cerebral Cortex, 4*(5), 544-554.

Allison, T., Puce, A., & McCarthy, G. (2000). Social perception from visual cues: Role of the STS region. *Trends in Cognitive Science, 4*(7), 267-278.

Allison, T., Puce, A., Spencer, D. D., & McCarthy, G. (1999). Electrophysiological studies of human face perception. I: Potentials generated in occipitotemporal cortex by face and non-face stimuli. *Cerebral Cortex, 9*(5), 415-430.

Amaral, D. G., & Insausti, R. (1992). Retrograde transport of d-[3h]-aspartate injected into the monkey amygdaloid complex. *Experimental Brain Research, 88*(2), 375-388.

Amaral, D. G., Veazey, R. B., & Cowan, W. M. (1982). Some observations on hypothalamo-amygdaloid connections in the monkey. *Brain Research, 252*(1), 13-27.

American Psychiatric Association. (1994). *Diagnostic and statistical manual of mental disorders* (text revision). Washington, DC: American Psychiatric Association.

Anderson, A. K., & Phelps, E. A. (2000). Expression without recognition: Contributions of the human amygdala to emotional communication. *Psychological Science, 11*(2), 106-111.

Baron-Cohen, S. (1995). *Mindblindness: An essay on autism and theory of mind.* Cambridge, MA: MIT Press.

Bartels, A., & Zeki, S. (2005). Brain dynamics during natural viewing conditions—A new guide for mapping connectivity in vivo. *NeuroImage, 24*, 339-349.

Beauchamp, M. S., Lee, K. E., Haxby, J. V., & Martin, A. (2002). Parallel visual motion processing streams for manipulable objects and human movements. *Neuron, 34*, 149-159.

Blake, R., Turner, L. M., Smoski, M. J., Pozdol, S. L., & Stone, W. L. (2003). Visual recognition of biological motion is impaired in children with autism. *Psychological Science, 14*, 51-57.

Breiter, H. C., Etcoff, N. L., Whalen, P. J., Kennedy, W. A., Rauch, S. L., Buckner, R. L., et al. (1996). Response and habituation of the human amygdala during visual processing of facial expression. *Neuron, 17*(5), 875-887.

Broks, P., Young, A. W., Maratos, E. J., Coffey, P. J., Calder, A. J., Isaac, C. L., et al. (1998). Face processing impairments after encephalitis: Amygdala damage and recognition of fear. *Neuropsychologia, 36*(1), 59-70.

Brothers, L. (1990). The social brain: A project for integrating primate behavior and neurophysiology in a new domain. *Concepts in Neuroscience, 1*, 27-51.

Brothers, L., Ring, B., & Kling, A. (1990). Response of neurons in the macaque amygdala to complex social stimuli. *Behavior and Brain Research, 41*, 199-213.

Brown, S., & Schafer, E. A. (1888). An investigation into the functions of the occipital and temporal lobes of the monkey's brain. *Philosophical Transactions of the Royal Society of London, Series B: Biological Science, 179*, 303-327.

Calvert, G. A., & Campbell, R. (2003). Reading speech from still and moving faces: The neural substrates of visible speech. *Journal of Cognitive Neuroscience, 15*, 57-70.

Dawson, G., Munson, J., Estes, A., Osterling, J., McPartland, J., Toth, K., et al. (2002). Neurocognitive function and joint attention ability in young children with autism spectrum disorder versus developmental delay. *Child Development, 73*(2), 345-358.

Decety, J., & Grezes, J. (1999). Neural mechanisms subserving the perception of human actions. *Trends in Cognitive Science, 3*(5), 172-178.

Emery, N. J., Capitanio, J. P., Mason, W. A., Machado, C. J., Mendoza, S. P., & Amaral, D. G. (2001). The effects of bilateral lesions of the amygdala on dyadic social interactions in rhesus monkeys (*macaca mulatta*). *Behavioral Neuroscience, 115*(3), 515-544.

Emery, N. J., Lorincz, E. N., Perrett, D. I., Oram, M. W., & Baker, C. I. (1997). Gaze following and joint attention in rhesus monkeys (*macaca mulatta*). *Journal of Computational Psychology, 111*(3), 286-293.

Hasson, U., Nir, Y., Levy, I., Fuhrmann, G., & Malach, R. (2004). Intersubject synchronization of cortical activity during natural vision. *Science, 303*, 1634-1640.

Haxby, J. V., Hoffman, E. A. & Gobbini, M. I. (2000). The distributed human neural system for face perception. *Trends in Cognitive Sciences, 4*(6), 223-233.

Haxby, J. V., Horwitz, B., Ungerleider, L. G., Maisog, J. M., Pietrini, P., & Grady, C. L. (1994). The functional organization of human extrastriate cortex: A PET-RCBF study of selective attention to faces and locations. *Journal of Neuroscience, 14*(11, Pt. 1), 6336-6353.

Kanner, L. (1943). Autistic disturbances of affective contact. *Nervous Child, 2*, 217-250.

Kanwisher, N., McDermott, J., & Chun, M. M. (1997). The fusiform face area: A module in human extrastriate cortex specialized for face perception. *Journal of Neuroscience, 17*(11), 4302-4311.

Klin, A., Jones, W., Schultz, R., & Volkmar, F. (2003). The enactive mind—from actions to cognition: Lessons from autism. *Philosophical Transactions of the Royal Society of London, Series B, 358*, 345-360.

Klin, A., Jones, W., Schultz, R., Volkmar, F., & Cohen, D. (2002). Visual fixation patterns during viewing of naturalistic social situations as predictors of social competence in individuals with autism. *Archives of General Psychiatry, 59*(9), 809-816.

Kluver, H., & Bucy, P. (1938). An analysis of certain effects of bilateral temporal lobectomy in the rhesus monkey, with special reference to "psychic blindness." *Journal of Psychology, 5*, 33-54.

Kluver, H., & Bucy, P. (1939). Preliminary analyses of the functions of temporal lobes in monkeys. *Archives of Neurology and Psychiatry, 42*, 979-1000.

LeDoux, J. (1996). Emotional networks and motor control: A fearful view. *Progress in Brain Research, 107*, 437-446.

Lord, C., Pickles, A., McLennan, J., Rutter, M., Bregman, J., Folstein, S., et al. (1997). Diagnosing autism: Analyses of data from the

Autism Diagnostic Interview. *Journal of Autism and Developmental Disorders, 27*(5), 501-517.

Lord, C., Rutter, M., & Le Couteur, A. (1994). Autism Diagnostic Interview—Revised: A revised version of a diagnostic interview for caregivers of individuals with possible pervasive developmental disorders. *Journal of Autism and Developmental Disorders, 24*, 659-685.

McCarthy, G. (1999). Physiological studies of face processing in humans. In M. S. Gazzaniga (Ed.), *The new cognitive neurosciences* (2nd ed., pp. 393-410). Cambridge, MA: MIT Press.

McCarthy, G., Puce, A., Gore, J. C., & Allison, T. (1997). Face-specific processing in the human fusiform gyrus. *Journal of Cognitive Neuroscience, 9*(5), 605-610.

McCarthy, G., Spicer, M., Adrignolo, A., Luby, M., Gore, J., & Allison, T. (1995). Brain activation associated with visual motion studied by functional magnetic resonance imaging in humans. *Human Brain Mapping, 2*, 234-243.

Morris, J. S., Frith, C. D., Perrett, D. I., Rowland, D., Young, A. W., Calder, A. J., et al. (1996). A differential neural response in the human amygdala to fearful and happy facial expressions. *Nature, 383*(6603), 812-815.

Mosconi, M. W., Mack, P. B., McCarthy, G., & Pelphrey, K. A. (2005). Taking an "intentional stance" on eye-gaze shifts: A functional neuroimaging study of social perception in children. *NeuroImage, 27*(1), 247-252.

Pelphrey, K. A., Mitchell, T. V., McKeown, M. J., Goldstein, J., Allison, T., & McCarthy, G. (2003). Brain activity evoked by the perception of human walking: Controlling for meaningful coherent motion. *Journal of Neuroscience, 23*(17), 6819-6825.

Pelphrey, K. A., Morris, J., & McCarthy, G. (2004). Grasping the intentions of others: The perceived intention of an action influences activity in the superior temporal sulcus during social perception. *Journal of Cognitive Neuroscience, 16*, 1706-1716.

Pelphrey, K. A., Morris, J., & McCarthy, G. (2005). Neural basis of eye gaze processing deficits in autism. *Brain, 128*(5), 1038-1048.

Pelphrey, K. A., Sasson, N. J., Reznick, J. S., Paul, G., Goldman, B. D., & Piven, J. (2002). Visual scanning of faces in autism. *Journal of Autism and Developmental Disorders, 32*(4), 249-261.

Pelphrey, K. A., Singerman, J. D., Allison, T., & McCarthy, G. (2003). Brain activation evoked by perception of gaze shifts: The influence of context. *Neuropsychologia, 41*(2), 156-170. [Erratum appears in *Neuropsychologia, 41*(11), 1561-1562].

Pelphrey, K. A., Viola, R. J., & McCarthy, G. (2004). When strangers pass: Processing of mutual and averted social gaze in the superior temporal sulcus. *Psychological Science, 15*(9), 598-603.

Puce, A., Allison, T., Asgari, M., Gore, J. C., & McCarthy, G. (1996). Differential sensitivity of human visual cortex to faces, letterstrings, and textures: A functional magnetic resonance imaging study. *Journal of Neuroscience, 16*(16), 5205-5215.

Rayner, K. (1998). Eye movements in reading and information processing: 20 years of research. *Psychological Bulletin, 124*, 372-422.

Rolls, E. T. (1992). Neurophysiological mechanisms underlying face processing within and beyond the temporal cortical visual areas. *Philosophical Transactions of the Royal Society of London, Series B: Biological Science, 335*(1273), 11-20; discussion 20-11.

Sigman, M., Ruskin, E., Arbeile, S., Corona, R., Dissanayake, C., Espinosa, M., et al. (1999). Continuity and change in the social competence of children with autism, down syndrome, and developmental delays. *Monographs of the Society for Research in Child Development, 64*(1), 1-114.

Sprengelmeyer, R., Young, A. W., Schroeder, U., Grossenbacher, P. G., Federlein, J., Buttner, T., et al. (1999). Knowing no fear.

Proceedings of the Royal Society of London, Series B: Biological Sciences, 266(1437), 2451-2456.

Tootell, R. B. H., Reppas, J. B., Kwong, K. K., Malach, R., Born, R. T., Brady, T. J., et al. (1995). Functional analysis of human MT and related visual cortical areas using magnetic resonance imaging. *Journal of Neuroscience, 15*(4), 3215-3230.

Wellman, H. M. (1990). *The child's theory of mind.* Cambridge, MA: The MIT Press.

Whalen, P. J., Kagan, J., Cook, R. G., Davis, F. C., Kim, H., Polis, S., et al. (2004). Human amygdala responsivity to masked fearful eye whites. *Science, 306*(5704), 2061.

Whalen, P. J., Rauch, S. L., Etcoff, N. L., McInerney, S. C., Lee, M. B., & Jenike, M. A. (1998). Masked presentations of emotional facial expressions modulate amygdala activity without explicit knowledge. *Journal of Neuroscience, 18*(1), 411-418.

Wing, L., & Gould, J. (1979). Severe impairments of social interaction and associated abnormalities in children: Epidemiology and classification. *Journal of Autism and Developmental Disorders, 9*(1), 11-29.

Winston, J. S., Strange, B. A., O'Doherty, J., & Dolan, R. J. (2002). Automatic and intentional brain responses during evaluation of trustworthiness of faces. *Nature Neuroscience, 5*(3), 277-283.

Wright, T. M., Pelphrey, K. A., Allison, T., McKeown, M. J., & McCarthy, G. (2003). Polysensory interactions along lateral temporal regions evoked by audiovisual speech. *Cerebral Cortex, 13*(10), 1034-1043.

Zeki, S., Watson, J. D. G., Lueck, C. J., Friston, K. J., Kennard, C., & Frackowiak, R. S. J. (1991). A direct demonstration of functional specialization in human visual cortex. *Journal of Neuroscience, 11*, 641-649.

CHAPTER 3

Child Speech and Emotions: A Cross-Linguistic Perspective

Ioulia Grichkovtsova and Ineke Mennen

Abstract

The main objective of this research is to investigate the production of affective speech by bilingual and monolingual children cross-linguistically. Cross-linguistic differences in affective speech may lead bilingual children to perceive and to express emotions differently in their two different languages. A cross-linguistically comparable corpus of eight bilingual Scottish-French children and 16 monolingual peers, average age 8, was recorded according to the developed methodology. This chapter presents preliminary results on pitch range, peak alignment, and speech rate for bilingual children and their monolingual peers, comparing their emotions and languages.

Introduction

The area of affective speech research has received much attention over the last years. Nevertheless, the effects of individual and cultural differences on affective speech production are still largely neglected. Most cross-linguistic studies concern the perception of vocal emotions (Scherer, Banse, & Wallbott, 2001). They show that humans can recognize vocal emotions with an accuracy percentage well above chance, even in unknown languages, though the level of accuracy is higher in native and close to native languages. The research suggests that vocal realization of emotions is based both on universal mechanisms and cultural conventions. A large number of acoustic parameters were identified as possible means to express emotions in speech: pitch range, intonational patterns, voice quality, rhythm, and so on. At the same time, the usage of these means, their level of importance, and their meaning vary across languages (Abelin & Allwood, 2000; Chen, 2005).

Studies of cross-linguistic production are still quite rare (Boula de Mareuil, Célérier, & Toen, 2002). They usually involve a very small number of speakers per language and disregard a widely observed phenomenon in affective speech —a high interspeaker and intraspeaker variability. Individual speakers have a large number of possible acoustic means to express emotions and a high flexibility of choice and manner of usage that can be considered appropriate in their language and speech community. The existing research is primarily concerned with adults, and studies of child affective speech are very rare and mostly based on perception only (Clément, 1999; Van der Meulen, Janssen, & Den Os, 1997).

The main objective of this research is to investigate the production of affective speech by bilingual (raised in two languages from birth) and monolingual children cross-linguistically in Scottish English and French. Socio-emotional competence is essential for effective communication, and it is one of the priorities in child development. Bilinguals communicate their emotions in two different languages, and they have to use acoustic means related to affective speech appropriately.

Being raised in two different languages and cultures, bilinguals may be competent to express affective states in their two languages. So, our first hypothesis is that bilingual affective productions may fall in the acceptable range in each of their languages. On the other hand, bilinguals produce two languages that differ in some acoustic correlates for affective states. Bilinguals may have a wider range of means and ways to express emotions, and their affective realization may not strictly correspond to those of monolinguals in each of their two languages. This phenomenon has been attested to in bilingual studies of other phonetic aspects (Aoyama, Flege, Guion, Akahane-Yamada, & Yamada, 2004; Mennen, 2004). Thus, our second hypothesis is that bilinguals may represent a particular group of speakers who express vocal emotions in a different manner than monolinguals.

Methodology

The starting point for this study was to develop an appropriate methodology to record child affective speech. Though spontaneous speech is claimed to contain the most authentic emotions, its collection gives rise to numerous difficulties: speakers should be recorded without knowing it, while expressing their emotions naturally, but such a routine is ethically problematic, especially with children. Thus, this study uses only acted speech, which does not suffer the same ethical problems. Moreover, acting of emotions can be presented as a game to children, so that they can be more naturally involved in the expression of emotions. Acting has already been effectively used in the study of child facial expressions of emotions (Field & Walden, 1983). Visual materials were developed in a realistic manner together with a professional illustrator and based on the research of facial expressions. They represent a child expressing four emotions (happiness, sadness, anger, and fear); the child's gender and age are adapted to that of the recorded children. The randomized cards have 16 repetitions for each emotion. One token utterance was selected with a similar sound and prosodic structure for English and French: "*I see a banana there./Je vois une banane, moi.*" The subject is instructed to say the token utterance in the same way as the child in the picture; thus, the child is playing emotions through association with the drawing. Visual materials played a very important part in the recordings: they served as the reference of the expressed emotions, and an affect inducing material, as the subjects associate themselves with the picture.

Neutral state was not represented as a facial expression card; neutral utterances were recorded in a separate test at the very beginning of the recording session. In this test, the child was instructed to say the token utterance (*I see * there./Je vois *, moi.*) with a word from a pile of cards (picture naming); 16 repetitions of the original word (*banana/banane*) were mixed among the others. Later all the utterances with the original token wording were selected for analysis. A small number of utterances was rejected due to noise, hesitation, or incorrect wording. Sixteen monolingual and eight bilingual children were recorded in total. Bilingual children were recorded in two separate sessions (one for each language) by different experimenters in order to control for language mode and code-switching; there was a period of about 2 weeks between the sessions. This methodology allowed us to record a cross-linguistically comparable corpus of 8 bilingual Scottish-French children and 16 monolingual peers, aged between 7 and 10. Socio-economic status of children was matched.

Participants

This paper presents data for four bilingual girls and four monolingual French girls, taken from the recorded corpus. Monolingual children (children labeled 5-8) were recorded in Normandy, France. They are all 8 years old. Bilingual children (children labeled 1-4) were all born in Edinburgh, Scotland, with a French mother and a Scottish father, except child 3 whose parents are French. Child 1 is 10, child 2 is 7, child 3 is 9, and child 4 is 8 years old. They go to mainstream Edinburgh schools, and attend the same French afternoon school twice a week.

Recordings

All children were recorded with a TASCAM DA-P1 portable DAT recorder either in the recording studio or in a quiet schoolroom. The speech was digitized and stored at 44,100 Hz. The analysis was performed on the speech down-sampled to 22,050 Hz.

Measurements

Using WaveSurfer software, acoustic measurements of pitch range variation, peak alignment, and speech rate were taken. All the utterances were manually labeled at the following pitch points: *IF0* (initial value of F_0), *H1* (the peak of the first accented word), *V* (valley, the lowest point between two peaks), *H2* (the peak of the main accented word—main accent), *FL* (final low—the lowest value after the peak). In cases where there was no well-defined peak, an absolute F_0 max value was taken near the accented syllable. Segment duration measurements were taken manually on the whole utterance. F_0 and time values were then extracted automatically to data files with the help of ESPS algorithm, and again checked manually for any pitch perturbation or voice quality errors.

Pitch Range

Following Ladd (1996), we describe pitch range using two partially independent measures of variation: overall level and span. Overall level refers to the "height" of a speaker's voice; span refers to the width of pitch frequencies covered by a speaker (how big the excursions are). We take *FL* point as a measure of the overall level, and the difference of *H2* and *FL* as a measure of the span. These measures have been shown (Patterson, 2000) to give better and perceptually more relevant results than the more commonly used measures, such as statistical moments (mean, standard deviation, difference between maximum and minimum F_0, etc.). All out pitch measures are expressed in semitones. The conversion of frequencies in Hertz into semitones is performed according to:

$$st = \frac{12}{\log_{10}(2)} \times \log_{10}\left(\frac{F_0}{50}\right),$$

where F_0 is the fundamental frequency in Hz, and $\log_{10}$ is the logarithm function to base 10.

As pitch range usage is well known for high individual differences, it was decided to normalize the pitch values. For each measurement, F_0 values were expressed on a speaker-specific normalized scale, which was derived by assigning 100% to the maximum F_0 value and 0% to the minimum F_0 value used by the speaker in our measurements. This approach is based on normalizing models, suggested by Rose (1987). Thus, all F_0 values were normalized according to the following formula:

$$st_{norm} = \frac{st - st_{min}}{st_{max} - st_{min}} \times 100,$$

where *st* is a measured F_0 value for a given speaker in semitones; *stnorm* expresses semitones on a percentage scale of the individual speaker's pitch range; *stmin* and *stmax* are the minimum and maximum F_0 values used by the speaker in our measurements.

Peak Alignment and Speech Rate

Recent research showed that peak alignment is an important measurement for cross-linguistic and second language acquisition studies (Mennen, 2004), and we believe that it might also be relevant for the present study. We present the peak alignment ratio: the ratio of the distance of the main peak from the onset of the main accented vowel as a function of the duration of that vowel. Speech rate was calculated as the number of syllables per second.

Results

This paper presents results on pitch range (overall level and span), peak alignment ratio, and speech rate for four Scottish English-French bilingual and four monolingual French children, comparing their emotions and languages. Separate multivariate ANOVAs were carried out for each child. There were two factors: *emotion* (five levels: anger, fear, sadness, happiness, and neutral) and *language* (two levels: English and French) for bilinguals; and one factor: *emotion* (the same five levels) for monolinguals. The dependent variables were pitch span, pitch level, peak ratio, and speech rate. The significance of factor language varied across the dependent variables. Factor emotion was significant across all the variables with several exceptions for some children, and a post hoc Bonferroni test was carried out to investigate better its significance.

Pitch Range Results

The results for pitch range are shown in Figure 3-1 and Figure 3-2; their statistical significance is shown in Table 3-1. The results show no significant effect of factor language for the dependent variable level of child 1 and child 2, and of factor emotion for the dependent variable span of child 6. In all the other cases, children use pitch range parameters to realize emotions. Bilingual children also use these parameters to differentiate some

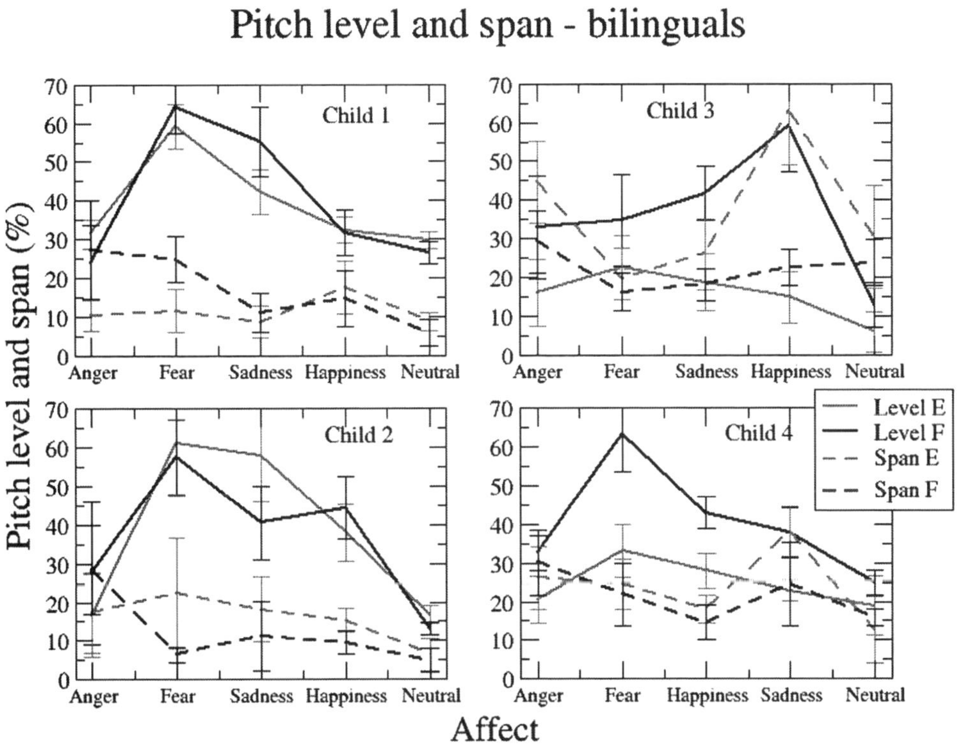

Figure 3–1. Results of pitch level and span for bilingual children. Gray represents English language, black—French language.

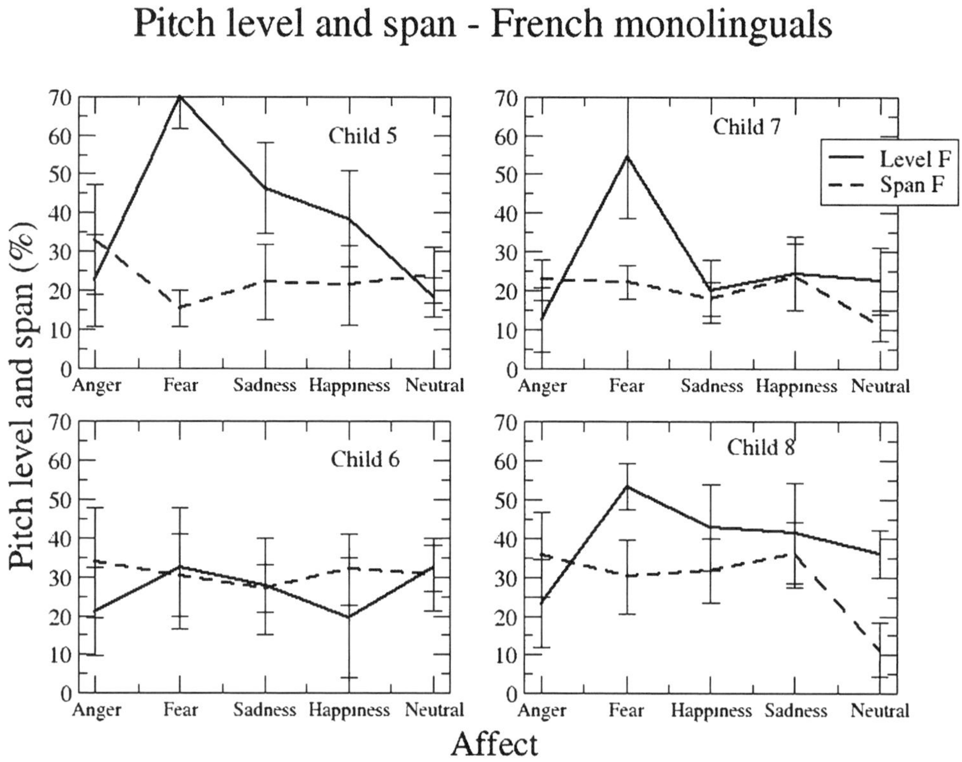

Figure 3–2. Results of pitch level and span for French monolingual children. Gray represents English language, black—French language.

Table 3–1. MANOVA results for dependent variables—pitch span and level. The value is significant at $p < 0.05$

Child	Factor	Span	Level
1	Emotion	$F(4,145)=21$ $p < 0.000$	$F(4,145)=178$ $p < 0.000$
1	Interaction	$F(4,145)=16$ $p < 0.000$	$F(4,145)=13$ $p < 0.000$
2	Language	$F(1,126)=5.9$ $p < 0.017$	$F(1,126)=0.6$ $p < 0.425$
2	Emotion	$F(4,126)=13$ $p < 0.000$	$F(4,126)=71$ $p < 0.000$
2	Interaction	$F(4,126)=8.3$ $p < 0.000$	$F(4,126)=7.1$ $p < 0.000$
3	Language	$F(1,145)=98$ $p < 0.000$	F $(1,145)=190$ $p < 0.000$
3	Emotion	$F(4,145)=39$ $p < 0.000$	$F(4,145)=39$ $p < 0.000$
3	Interaction	$F(4,145)=22$ $p < 0.000$	F $(4,145)=20$ $p < 0.000$
4	Language	$F(1,153)=4.9$ $p < 0.027$	$F(1,153)=264$ $p < 0.000$
4	Emotion	$F(4,153)=33$ $p < 0.000$	$F(4,153)=91$ $p < 0.000$
4	Interaction	$F(4,153)=7.4$ $p < 0.000$	$F(4,153)=18$ $p < 0.000$
5	Emotion	$F(4,75)=7$ $p < 0.000$	$F(4,75)=62$ $p < 0.000$
6	Emotion	$F(4,63)=0.8$ $p < 0.562$	$F(4,63)=2.9$ $p < 0.028$
7	Emotion	$F(4,75)=15$ $p < 0.000$	$F(4,75)=34$ $p < 0.000$
8	Emotion	$F(4,75)=22$ $p < 0.000$	$F(4,75)=18$ $p < 0.000$
9	Emotion	$F(4,63)=3.4$ $p < 0.014$	$F(4,63)=27.1$ $p < 0.000$
10	Emotion	$F(4,71)=29.2$ $p < 0.000$	$F(4,71)=24.6$ $p < 0.000$
11	Emotion	$F(4,75)=11.2$ $p < 0.000$	$F(4,75)=99.2$ $p < 0.000$
12	Emotion	$F(4,78)=92.7$ $p < 0.000$	$F(4,78)=49.5$ $p < 0.000$

emotions in their two languages. Children 2, 3, and 4 separate happiness in their two languages in span, children 1 and 2 separate fear in span, and child 1 separates anger in span. Children 3 and 4 separate sadness and happiness in level. All other emotions overlap in the two languages in their realizations. Post hoc tests were run to study the differences between particular emotions.

Post Hoc Tests for Span

Child 1 realizes happiness with the widest span than the other emotions in English; it is the only emotion that is significantly different. In French, anger and fear have the widest span; they are not significantly different from each other, but are from the other emotions. Sadness and neutral have the narrowest span. Child 2 differs from child 1, as she realizes fear with the widest span in English, which is statistically significant. It is followed by anger, sadness, happiness (not significantly different), and neutral, with the narrowest span. In French span, only anger is significantly different from the rest of the emotions, with the widest span. Child 3 results show that happiness has the widest span in English, as for child 1. Happiness is followed by anger, which is also significantly different from the other emotions. Neutral, sadness, and fear have the narrowest span, and they do not differ. In French, anger has the widest span, but it is not significantly different from neutral; the other emotions have a narrower span than neutral, and they do not differ much from each other. Child 4 has happiness with the widest span in English; it is significantly different from the other emotions. In French, anger has the widest span, but it is not significantly different from happiness. The other emotions have a similar narrower span.

French monolingual child 5 also has anger with the widest span; it is significantly different from the other emotions, except neutral, which overlaps both with anger and the other emotions with the narrower span. Child 6 realizes anger and happiness with a wider span than the rest of emotions, but the difference is not significant. Child 7 separates only neutral from the other emotions with the significantly narrower span; happiness and anger have slightly wider span, but it is not significant. Child 8 follows the same realization pattern as child 7, only neutral is significantly different with the narrowest span.

Post Hoc Tests for Level

Post hoc results for child 1 in English level show that fear has the highest level. It is followed by sadness, which is also significantly different from the other emotions. Finally, happiness, anger, and neutral have the lowest similar level. French has exactly the same pattern. In English, child 2 realizes fear and sadness with the highest level, anger and neutral have the lowest similar level, and happiness is in between these two groups and significantly different. In French, fear, sadness, and happiness have the highest level; they are followed by anger, which overlaps with sadness. Neutral has the lowest level, and it is considerably different from the other emotions. Child 3 realizes only neutral significantly different from the other emotions in English level. In French, happiness has the highest level; it is followed by anger, fear, sadness (not different from each other), and finally neutral with the lowest level, and it is significantly different. Child 4 has fear with the highest level, which is significantly different from the rest of emotions, except sadness. All the other emotions overlap in English. In French, fear has the highest level; it is followed by sadness and happiness (not significantly different) and by anger (not significantly different from happiness); neutral is the lowest.

Child 5 results show that fear has the highest level and is significantly different from the rest of emotions; it is followed by sadness and happiness, then by anger and neutral. Child 6 almost does not separate emotions by level; she has two groups—fear, neutral, and sadness with higher level, and happiness and anger with lower level, but these differences are almost not significant. Child 7 differentiates fear from the rest of emotions with the highest level, the other emotions overlap. Child 8 has fear with the highest level; it is followed by sadness, happiness, and neutral (sadness is not significantly different from fear), and finally, anger has the lowest level; it is significantly different from the other emotions.

Peak Alignment Results

The results for peak alignment are shown in Figure 3-3; their statistical significance is shown in Table 3-2. The results show

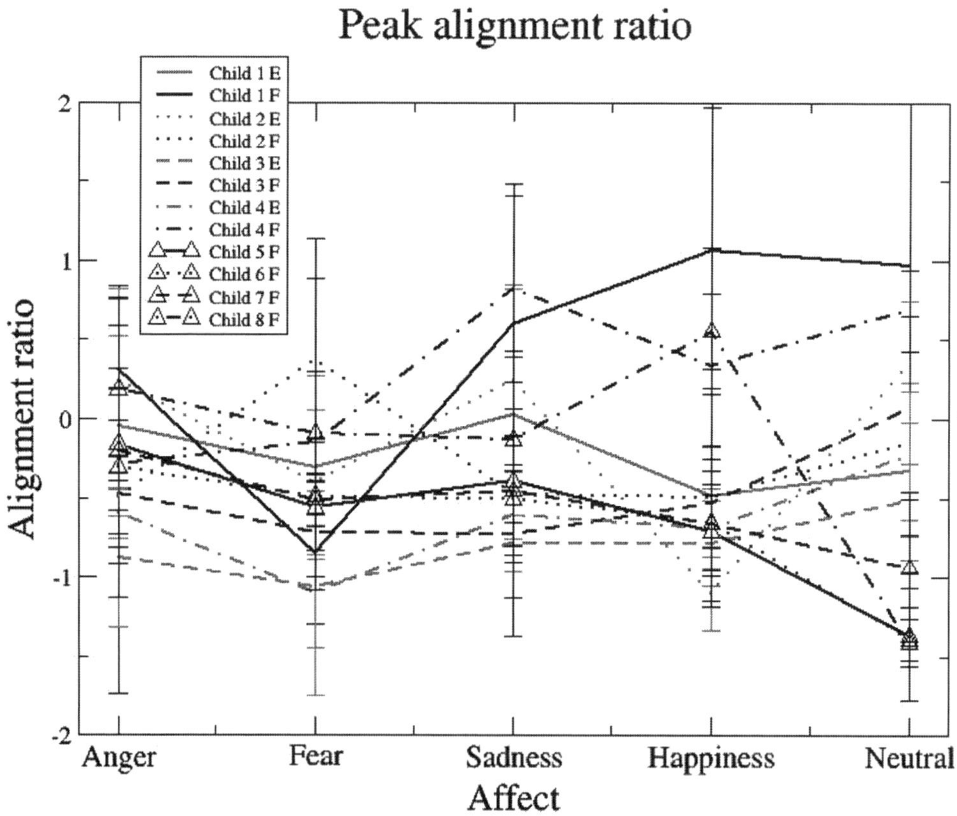

Figure 3–3. Results of peak alignment ratio for bilingual and French monolingual children. Gray represents English language, black—French language.

Table 3–2. MANOVA results for dependent variables—peak alignment and speech rate. The value is significant at $p < 0.05$

Child	Factor	Alignment	Speech Rate
1	Language	$F(1,145)=21$ $p < 0.000$	$F(1,145)=52$ $p < 0.000$
1	Emotion	$F(4,145)=6$ $p < 0.000$	$F(4,145)=11$ $p < 0.000$
1	Interaction	$F(4,145)=7$ $p < 0.000$	$F(4,145)=1.7$ $p < 0.144$
2	Language	$F(1,126)=0.9$ $p < 0.346$	$F(1,126)=33$ $p < 0.000$
2	Emotion	$F(4,126)=6.6$ $p < 0.000$	$F(4,126)=17$ $p < 0.000$
2	Interaction	$F(4,126)=7.1$ $p < 0.000$	$F(4,126)=5.8$ $p < 0.000$
3	Language	$F(1,145)=24$ $p < 0.000$	$F(1,145)=82$ $p < 0.000$
3	Emotion	$F(4,145)=11$ $p < 0.000$	$F(4,145)=39$ $p < 0.000$
3	Interaction	$F(4,145)=1.7$ $p < 0.152$	$F(4,145)=29$ $p < 0.000$
4	Language	$F(1,153)=172$ $p < 0.000$	$F(1,153)=18$ $p < 0.000$
4	Emotion	$F(4,153)=22$ $p < 0.000$	$F(4,153)=52$ $p < 0.000$
4	Interaction	$F(4,153)=6.4$ $p < 0.000$	$F(4,153)=7.9$ $p < 0.000$
5	Emotion	$F(4,75)=14$ $p < 0.000$	$F(4,75)=6.6$ $p < 0.000$
6	Emotion	$F(4,63)=14$ $p < 0.000$	$F(4,63)=9$ $p < 0.000$
7	Emotion	$F(4,75)=7.5$ $p < 0.000$	$F(4,75)=7.5$ $p < 0.000$
8	Emotion	$F(4,75)=29$ $p < 0.000$	$F(4,75)=1.4$ $p < 0.256$
9	Emotion	$F(4,63)=3.5$ $p < 0.012$	$F(4,63)=32.6$ $p < 0.000$
10	Emotion	$F(4,71)=5.6$ $p < 0.001$	$F(4,71)=12.6$ $p < 0.000$
11	Emotion	$F(4,75)=12.5$ $p < 0.000$	$F(4,75)=33.6$ $p < 0.000$
12	Emotion	$F(4,78)=16.6$ $p < 0.000$	$F(4,78)=27$ $p < 0.000$

no significant effect of factor language for child 2, and of interaction between the two factors for child 3. Some bilingual children differentiate emotions in their two languages: child 1 separates happiness in her two languages, and child 4 separates sadness, happiness, and neutral by peak alignment. For all the children, peak alignment realization is influenced by some affective states. Post hoc tests show differences between particular emotions. In English child 1 differentiates happiness from the other emotions, except neutral; it has the peak set farthest before the accented vowel. In French, fear has the peak before the accented vowel and is separated from the other emotions, which have the peak on the accented vowel, and do not differ. In English, child 2 realizes happiness as significantly different from the other emotions; it is the furthest away from the onset of the accented vowel. It is followed by fear, which is also significantly different and set before the vowel. The other emotions are realized after the vowel onset and do not differ. In French, fear is significantly different from the others; it is the only one to be after the vowel onset. In English, child 3 separates only neutral from the other emotions. In all the emotions, the peak occurs before the vowel onset. In French, it is again the neutral that is significantly different, and it is the only one to be after the vowel onset. The results for child 4 show that only fear is significantly different. All the peaks are realized before the vowel onset. In French, fear and anger are realized after the vowel onset; anger does not differ only from fear, but fear does not differ also from happiness. The three monolingual French children 5, 6, and 7 have the same realization pattern: the peaks are realized before the vowel onset, and neutral is significantly different from the other emotions. Child 8 also differentiates neutral from the others; the peak is realized after the vowel onset in all the emotions except neutral.

Speech Rate Results

The results for speech rate are shown in Figure 3-4; their statistical significance is shown in Table 3-2. The results show no significant effect of factor emotion for child 8, and of interaction between the two factors for child 1. Bilingual children differentiate some emotions in their two languages: child 1 separates anger in her two languages, child 2 separates happiness, and children 3 and 4 separate neutral. Post hoc tests were run to study differences between particular emotions. Child 1 has fear with the lowest speech rate in both languages, while anger has the highest speech rate in English (though it is significantly different only from fear). In French, anger is not significantly different from fear, which has the lowest speech rate and which is separated from the other emotions. Child 2 has fear with the highest speech rate in both languages: in English, fear is significantly different from anger and sadness, which have similar lowest rate; in French, it dif-

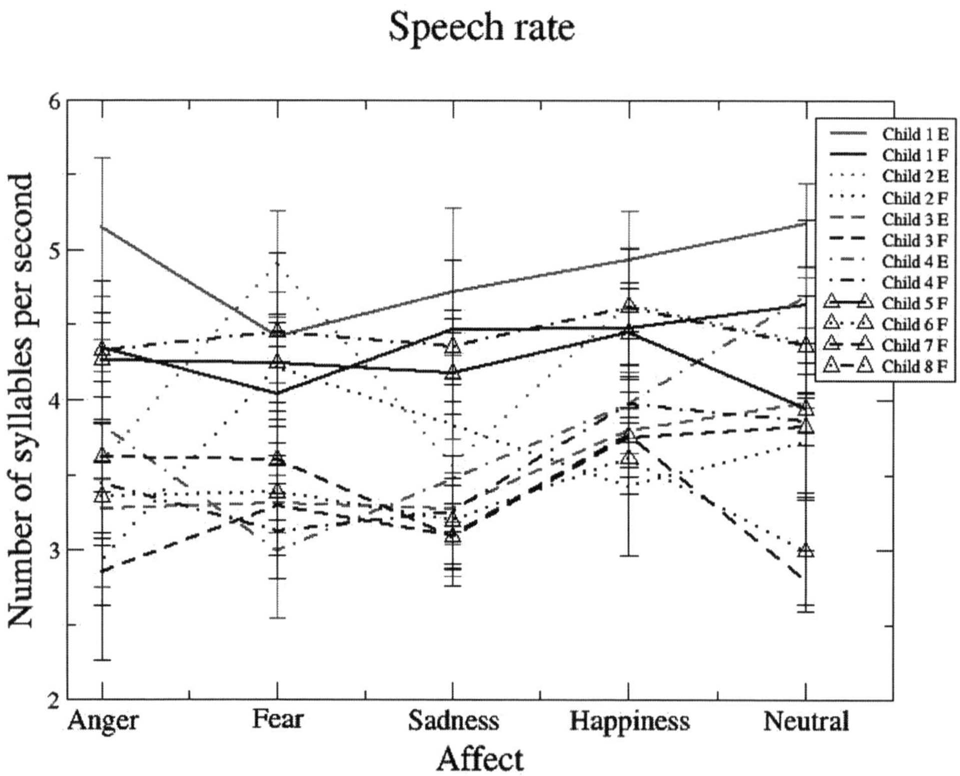

Figure 3–4. Results of speech rate for bilingual and French monolingual children. Gray represents English language, black—French language.

fers significantly from happiness and anger (similar lowest rate). In English, child 3 realizes neutral and happiness with the highest speech rate and it is significantly different from the others; in French, happiness has the highest rate and is differentiated from the other emotions, but neutral has the lowest rate, and is not significantly different from sadness and anger. Child 4 has the same realization pattern in both languages—happiness has the highest rate, but not significantly different from neutral and anger, and fear has the lowest rate, and not significantly different from sadness and anger. Monolingual child 5 has happiness with the highest rate, but not significantly different from fear and anger; sadness and neutral have the lowest rate. Child 6 has a similar realization. Child 7 differentiates only sadness from the other emotions with the lowest rate. Child 8 does not differentiate her emotions significantly with speech rate.

Discussion

Bilingual children use the analyzed acoustic parameters (pitch range, peak alignment, and speech rate) to differentiate some emotions in their two languages, as shown through a main effect of the factor language and/or through a significant interaction between the factors language and emotion. For all the children, at least one of the factors (factor language or interaction) is significant, and factor language is significant in 81.75%. Children 2, 3, and 4 separate happiness in their two languages in span, children 1 and 2 separate fear in span, and child 1 separates anger in span. Children 3 and 4 separate sadness and happiness in level. Child 1 separates happiness in peak alignment; child 4 separates sadness, happiness, and neutral in peak alignment in their two languages. Regarding pitch rate, child 1 separates anger in her two languages, child 2 separates happiness, and children 3 and 4 separate neutral. Thus, *happiness* is the only emotion that is differentiated by all the bilingual children, even though acoustic parameters of differentiation vary.

The majority of the children realize differences between emotions in each of the measurements taken in this study (monolingual child 6 does not differentiate her emotions by pitch range, and child 8 does by speech rate). The factor emotion is significant in 93.75% of the cases. Statistical post hoc tests show that there is a considerable amount of variability in these realizations across all the children. Nevertheless, it is possible to make some generalizations of the results. All the children realize fear with the highest level; it is also true for both the languages of bilingual children. Only child 3 makes an exception by having happiness with the highest level in French. Note that the significance and manner of fear differentiation from the other emotions vary across children. All the bilingual children realize neutral with the lowest level in French and English. French monolingual children 6, 7, and 8 realize anger with the lowest level; only child 5 has neutral with the lowest level, and it is not significantly different from her anger. In French, anger has the widest span in 7 children (the level of differentiation from the other emotions varies); monolingual child 7 has happiness with a slightly wider span than anger, but the difference is not significant. In English, children 1, 3, and 4 have happiness with the widest span, and it is significant for all the children.

Child 2 has fear with the highest span, which is significantly different.

In general, the results for peak alignment show less differentiation across emotions than for pitch range. Neutral is the only clearly separated emotion by monolingual French children, and by bilingual child 3. Children 1 and 2 differentiate happiness in English, and children 1, 2, and 4 differentiate fear in French (child 4 does both in English and French).

Speech rate results show that most children realize happiness with a high speech rate (child 2 has fear with the highest speech rate in French) and sadness with a low speech rate (children 1 and 2 have sadness in the group of emotions with a high speech rate in French). Fear is realized both with a high (child 2—in both languages; child 3—in French, four monolingual children) and low speech rate (child 1—in both languages, child 3 in English, child 4 in both languages). Bilingual child 4 realizes her emotions exactly with the same pattern in both languages. Monolingual children 5 and 6 have a similar realization pattern.

Thus, we observe three realization patterns of acoustic parameters for some affective states: similar pattern across all the children in both the languages (e.g., fear has the highest level across all the children); similar pattern across all the children only in one language (e.g., anger has the widest span across monolingual French children and across bilingual children in French); different realization pattern in the same language by bilingual and monolingual children [e.g., fear is realized both with a high (four French monolingual children, child 3 in French, child 2 in both languages) and low speech rate (child 1 in both languages, child 3 in English, child 4 in both languages)].

Conclusions

To the best of our knowledge, this study is a first attempt to look at the prosodic realizations of affective states by bilinguals. The developed methodology allowed us to collect a cross-linguistically comparable corpus of bilingual Scottish-French children and monolingual English and French children. Our preliminary results suggest that children use the chosen measures of pitch range, peak alignment, and speech rate to express emotions, and that bilingual children also use these measures to differentiate some emotions between their two languages. It appears that these measures may be effective in capturing cross-linguistic differences in affective speech.

In general, there is considerable variability across all the children, but it is also possible to see some common tendencies in child affective realizations. Scottish-French bilinguals show both differences and similarities compared to monolingual French children, depending on the acoustic parameters and affective states. There were observed three realization patterns of acoustic parameters for some affective states that were possible to generalize across children: similar pattern across all the children in both the languages; similar pattern across all the children only in one language; different realization patterns in the same language by bilingual and monolingual children. We cannot generalize further and make any firm conclusions about the reasons for the observed realization patterns until we have the results of monolingual Scottish-English children and other French and Scottish-French children from our corpus. However, once we obtain these data, we will be able to judge better our findings and to explore other important factors, such as the children's age and amount of language use and exposure for bilinguals.

Acknowledgments. We express our gratitude to all the children and their parents who participated in this study. We are also pleased to thank Dr. H. Ouerdane and Dr. O. Gordeeva for their assistance with automatization of data extraction and processing.

References

Abelin, A., & Allwood, J. Cross-linguistic interpretation of emotional prosody. In R. Cowie, E. Douglas-Cowie, & M. Schröder (Eds.), *Proceedings of the ISCA Workshop on Speech and Emotion*, September 5-7, 2000, Belfast, Ireland, 110-113. Retrieved January 28, 2008, from http://www.isca-speech.org/archive/speech_emotion/index.html

Aoyama, K., Flege, J. E., Guion, S. G., Akahane-Yamada, R., & Yamada, T. (2004). Perceived phonetic dissimilarity and L2 speech learning: The case of Japanese /r/ and English /l/ and /r/. *Journal of Phonetics*, *32*, 333-250.

Boula de Mareuil, P., Célérier, P., & Toen, J. Generation of emotions by a morphing technique in English, French and Spanish. *Proceedings of International Conference on Speech Prosody*, April 11-13, 2002, Aix-en-Provence, France, 187-190. Retrieved January 28, 2008, from http://www.isca-speech.org/archive/sp2002/index.html

Chen, A. J. (2005). *Universal and language-specific perception of paralinguistic intonational meaning*. Published doctoral dissertation, University of Utrecht publishing house, LOT dissertation series 102, Utrecht, Netherlands.

Clément, J. (1999). *Structure des représentations prosodiques. Développement normal et pathologique du traitement de la prosodie*. Unpublished doctoral dissertation, Université de Paris 5.

Field, T. M., & Walden, T. A. (1983). Production and discrimination of facial expressions by preschool children. *Child Development*, *53*, 1299-1311.

Ladd, D. R. (1996). *Intonational phonology*. Cambridge, UK: Cambridge University Press.

Mejvaldova, J. (2001). *Expressions prosodiques de certaines attitudes en tchèque et en français. Etude comparative*. Unpublished doctoral dissertation, Univerzita Karlova, Université de Paris 7.

Mennen, I. (2004). Bi-directional interference in the intonation of Dutch speakers of Greek. *Journal of Phonetics*, *32*, 543-563.

Patterson, D. (2000). A linguistic approach to pitch range modeling. Unpublished doctoral dissertation, University of Edinburgh, UK.

Rose, P. (1987). Considerations in the normalization of the fundamental frequency of linguistic tone. *Speech Communication*, *6*, 343-351.

Scherer, K. R., Banse, R., & Wallbott, H. G. (2001). Emotion inferences from vocal expression correlate across languages and cultures. *Journal of Cross-Cultural Psychology*, *32*(1), 76-92.

Van der Meulen, S., Janssen, P., & Den Os, E. (1997). Prosodic abilities in children with specific language impairment. *Journal of Communication Disorders*, *30*(3), 155-170.

CHAPTER 4

Conveyance of Emotion in Postlaryngectomy Communication

Philip C. Doyle

Abstract

This chapter has addressed the expression of emotion post-total laryngectomy. It is widely accepted that the conveyance of emotive states is manifest secondary to multiple actions of the human communicator, including physical postures, facial expressions, pitch, loudness, and cadence of speech, as well as many other factors. When disorder modifies or eliminates the ability for one to normally express emotions, regardless of the underlying causal factors, considerable disability is likely to occur. In the case of laryngectomy, the expression of emotion through common behaviors of laughing and crying are disrupted. However, despite the ability to understand the influence of laryngectomy on the physiology of these emotional acts, research in the area of conveying emotion postlaryngectomy appears to be wholly nonexistent in the literature.

Emotive vocal activities cannot be performed in normal fashion without a larynx; while isolated physiological behaviors in response to laughing and crying do appear in the individual who has been a laryngectomized individual, the cohesive normal response through the linkage of systems (respiratory system and upper airway along with a voicing source) is lost. When these isolated actions take place, vocalization is substituted for by the pulsatile respiratory response when laughing or crying, head movements associated with laughing, or the shedding of tears when crying.

Concerns related to the conveyance of emotion in those who have undergone laryngectomy for laryngeal cancer would appear to provide an important and fruitful area of empirical investigation, but such research is virtually nonexistent. Research of this type would not only appear to encourage interest from the perspective of interdisciplinary endeavors, but holds great promise in further understanding the impact of laryngectomy on the person within the social-communication context.

Conveyance of Emotion in Postlaryngectomy Communication

Introduction and Brief Review

Human communication and the related expression of emotion is a complex act that relies on numerous capabilities that are employed in the larger context of social behavior. The essence of any form of communication is based on a relatively simple objective, namely, to transfer and/or convey information to another person, transmission of which forms the expression of thoughts, feelings, and other internal and perceived external states of being.

In any communication interaction signs and signals, both verbal and nonverbal, are often highly integrated with one another. Take for example the use of simple hand gestures to facilitate emphasis when coupled with the spoken signal. Facial expressions, the tone of one's voice, head position, body posture, physical proximity, and many other factors must be considered as part of the communicative act (Ekman, 1997a; 1997b; Scherer & Ekman, 1983). Collectively, the expression of emotion is a psychobiological event for which multiple behaviors are necessary in order to facilitate effective and efficient communication between individuals (Darwin, 1965/1872; Ekman, 1999).

The Diversity of Factors that Influence Emotional Expression

The influence of such diverse factors as biology, physiology, cognition, neurology, and the like, on communication has been of interest to multiple disciplines including anthropology, ethnology, sociology, psychology, physiology, and numerous others for many years. While a number of emotions do exist and may be expressed by humans, they are not uniformly employed by all peoples of the world. But is it recognized that while some communication "universals" for the signaling of emotion may exist, others may be guided by specific needs or requirements (Ekman, 1993; 1999). That is, how we pursue the communicative act also must be considered in the context of one's age, gender, social milieu, cultural background and traditions, as well as many other influences (Ekman, 1972; 1993).

There is no doubt that those events which serve to either signal or embellish a communicative act must be considered in the larger description of how well one is able to communicate in the broadest sense. While some communicative behaviors may be shared across groups, other "features" may carry unique or special meaning in a given communication environment. A good case in point would be the collective experimental findings reported by several researchers who have noted that when confronted with photographs of specific facial expressions, judges from a variety of cultural backgrounds are able to provide an adequate and consistent verbal description of what they observe via the judgment method (Ekman, 1993). Yet other expressions are not judged as consistently. However, there appear to be two clear classes of emotion; they might be best defined as expressions of negative (e.g., sadness)[1] and positive (e.g., pride) emotions (Ekman, 1992). Not surprisingly, emotive responses have been shown to exist with patterns of activity in the autonomic nervous system (Ekman, Levenson, & Friesen, 1983) and may vary with age (Levenson, Cartensen, Friesen, & Ekman, 1991). The neurobiological aspects of emotion have become a very contemporary area of scientific research given significant technological advances specific to brain imaging (c.f. Davidson, 2001; Davidson & Irwin, 1999; Davidson, Maxwell, & Shuakman, 2004).

Interest in Emotion

Interest in the expression of emotion and potential physical correlates has been longstanding. In fact, more than 100 years ago Charles Darwin (1965/1872) pursued the concept of expression and emotion in his third book, *The Expression of Emotions in Man and Animals*. Not surprisingly, Darwin's efforts in this area provided an initial attempt to understand evolutionary linkages relative to the expression of emotional states.[2] This transfer of information is, however, multifold in both function and purpose.

Minimally, one must consider cognitive processes, physiologic components, and social constructs in the mediation of emotional states in a communication interaction (Ekman, 1999; Johnson-Laird & Oatley, 1992; Oatley & Johnson-Laird, 1987). Some forms of emotion such as crying are believed to share universal status relative to the group of expressions that represent one's emotional state. In contrast, other expressions of emotional status such facial postures may not be uniformly shared across some cultures and, hence, hold potential for misinterpretation when cultural factors are not considered. Additionally, variability may also be observed in what Ekman (1993)

[1]Ekman (1993) has also referred to negative emotional states as "unhappiness" emotions.

[2]Hopefully, reference to Darwin's work on expression and emotion and potential relationships of an evolutionary basis will not serve to create additional inane arguments relative to "intelligent design" for such behaviors. The reference only serves to acknowledge that interest in this broad academic area is characterized by a long history. I can only hope that such reference will not foster continuing debate for either church or state relative to emotional status.

has identified as the "display rules" for the representation of emotion by the individual. Display rules inform one relative to "cultural-specific prescriptions" of who, when, and how displays of emotion may be appropriate (Ekman, 1993, p. 384), hence facilitating correct interpretations of such emotions.

Within Western culture, we may acknowledge that many behaviors associated with the conveyance of emotion are commonly identified and interpreted (e.g., expressions of disgust, surprise, etc.). Ohman (1986) has suggested that the development of emotional representation must consider not only evolutionary contributors, but social learning constructs in order to fully understand emotional phenomena (Ekman, 1993; 1997a).

Because the expression of emotion typically involves integration with physical actions (e.g., frowning, raising vocal intensity), natural questions are raised concerning what occurs when the physical capacity to generate such changes is lost. Yet it also is important to understand that significant physical behaviors may coexist with emotional expression, even though these physical manifestations may not be volitional. Rather, in many instances, the literature would support the notion that physical correlates of emotion are involuntary. Whether they are voluntary or involuntary, however, multiple physical systems may need to be integrated in efforts to meet the demands of a particular expression. Doing so may be seen to facilitate the accurate representation of an emotion, which may be viewed as communicating more effectively (i.e., the likelihood that the "message" intended is received accurately). But it is important to realize that this communication often goes beyond simple verbal or auditory conveyance of information on one's emotional status.

Language and Emotion

Simpson (1967) has suggested that language is enhanced by the use of other signals and that these signals " . . . reflect the individual's physical, or more frequently, emotional state" (p. 39). Consequently, Simpson goes on to explicitly state that these signals do not " . . . name, discuss, abstract, or symbolize . . . ," but that they are " . . . emotional signals not discourse" (p. 39). For this reason, the linkage of communication (both verbal and nonverbal) and the need or desire to express emotion must be considered in the context of a "normal" communication system. That is, such assumptions are most likely based on the notion that these linkages of communication acts do not occur in those systems that are not normal. As stated by Ekman (1999, p. 2), " . . . the primary function of emotion is to mobilize the organism to deal quickly with important interpersonal encounters . . . "; thus, its functional significance to the state of being and the human condition is essential. It also may be readily argued that such a capacity serves a critical and perhaps mandatory function in the mediation of one's overall well-being. Ekman (1999, p. 3) goes on to extend his belief by stating that the expression of emotions "[is] crucial to the development and regulation of interpersonal relationships"; this point is critical to the present discussion.

Emotional Expression in Disordered Systems

States of abnormality or disorder to component systems essential for human communication cannot be understood fully if viewed unidimensionally; this suggestion is also true when considered relative to emotional expression. Concerns that center on features of communication that go beyond the verbal signal itself are critical. While definitive data on the capacity to express emotions have not been acquired or addressed extensively in the situation of disordered human communication systems, observational data do exist. This is particularly true for those populations that exhibit unique physical changes to facial structures.[3] When one considers these types of situations, it is not a stretch to justify that questions of this type are ripe for inquiry and have served to generate their own experimental set of methods (see Ekman, 1982). Concerns about what occurs when one's ability to adequately express emotional states is disrupted or lost because of an underlying impairment to a physiological or neurological subsystem appear to be quite natural. This question serves as the impetus for the present discussion. Therefore, the purpose of this chapter is to explore emotive expression in the context of a profound loss of a generating organ of voice as a result of total laryngectomy. To provide for reasonable discussion of this issue, several areas of topical interest are initially required.

First, basic information relative to total laryngectomy and the physical changes that occur as a result of this surgical treatment are presented. Second, a brief review of alternative methods of "verbal" communication that are employed postlaryngectomy will be presented. Third, although the concepts underlying questions about the conveyance of emotion have not been formally addressed in those who have been laryngectomized, there exists incidental and anecdotal information that is relevant to the present discussion and, therefore, deserves some attention. Lastly, coverage of potential opportunities to explore the area of communicating emotion in those treated for laryngeal cancer will be addressed. Collectively, it is hoped that the information provided will offer some extended insights into the level of communicative change that results from laryngectomy, changes that certainly extend beyond those influencing verbal communication proper.

Treatment for Laryngeal Cancer

Head and neck cancers as a general diagnostic class comprise less than 5% of all forms of malignant disease (American Cancer Society, 2004). Within this grouping, laryngeal cancers form approximately one quarter to one third of such diagnoses. Cancer of the larynx as a descriptive category is defined as those lesions that remain confined to the laryngeal structure proper. While this may include a lesion that extends superiorly into regions of the supraglottis, or interiorly into the subglottic region, for the purposes of the present discussion, we will focus on those lesions of the "glottic"

[3]One of the most obvious examples in the clinical literature would relate to those individuals who suffer the effects of damage or dysfunction to the facial nerve. In this condition, the muscles of facial animation are impaired for one half of the face. Differences between halves of the face are obvious and create multiple levels of disability for the person. However, many of these individuals report that they judge those whom they are communicating with to have significant problems in reading their facial expressions, thus disrupting communication efficiency. Another similar example may be gleaned from facial changes secondary to Parkinson's disease, where a characteristic "masklike" face is commonly observed.

larynx. Statistical data would suggest that of the entire group of laryngeal tumors, 75% occur on tissue of a vocal fold; hence, they are glottic in origin (Bailey, 1984). Although small, early lesions that are confined to a vocal fold may be treated with radiation therapy or very conservative surgical resections, lesions that extend outside of the vocal fold or invade cartilage often require more aggressive methods of treatment (Zeitels, 2005). For the purposes of the present treatise, it is the group of individuals who undergo the most aggressive surgical treatment option, namely total laryngectomy, who are of greatest interest.

Treatment Changes Associated with Total Laryngectomy

Total laryngectomy is a surgical procedure that necessitates complete surgical extirpation of the entire laryngeal framework. Thus, the normal anatomical and physiological relationship between the upper airway and the vocal tract (i.e., those structures of the pharynx and oral and nasal cavities) is completely disrupted. Because the larynx sits at the top of the trachea, surgical removal requires that the trachea is brought anteriorly to form a permanent tracheostoma in the anterior midline neck. Thus, following total laryngectomy there is no longer an anatomic or physiologic relationship between the oral cavity and respiratory system. This pre- and postsurgical relationship is depicted in Figure 4-1(a) and Figure 4-1(b).

As can be seen, following total laryngectomy, respiration no longer permits or requires that air passes through the mouth, nose, or vocal tract; respiration is now achieved via neck-breathing. As such, those who are laryngectomized will remain neck breathers for the remainder of their lives. It is this change that has clear and dramatic influences not only related to voice generation and subsequent speech production, but on the expression of basic emotions such as laughing and crying. There is a substantial and longstanding literature addressing the topic of postlaryngectomy voice and speech production (Diedrich & Youngstrom, 1966; Doyle, 1994; Doyle & Keith, 2005; Gardner, 1971; Graham, 1997; Salmon & Goldstein; 1978; Snidecor, 1978), but little information on emotional expression postlaryngectomy is available.

Therefore, in the context of the present discussion, I will address the potential impact that laryngectomy has on these two acts of emotional expression—laughing and crying. Prior to that discussion, however, it is necessary to briefly outline basic information concerning the methods and processes involved in the three primary methods of postlaryngectomy voice and speech production, namely, esophageal, tracheoesophageal, and electrolaryngeal modes. Knowledge related to each of these postlaryngectomy speech rehabilitation modes forms the foundation for additional understanding of the limitations experienced specific to emotional expression.

Methods of Postlaryngectomy Verbal Communication

Three methods or modes of postlaryngectomy verbal communication currently exist as rehabilitation options for those who lose their larynxes due to cancer. These methods are (a) esophageal speech, (b) tracheoesophageal (TE) speech, and

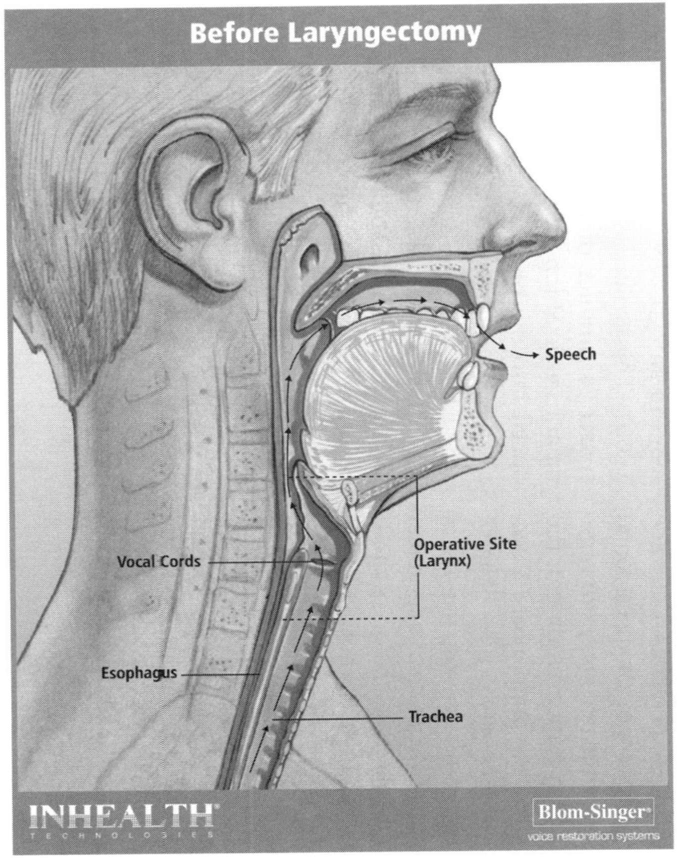

Figure 4–1(a). Graphic representation of normal anatomy and relationships between the airway and structures of the vocal tract. Reprinted with permission, InHealth Technologies, Carpenteria, CA.

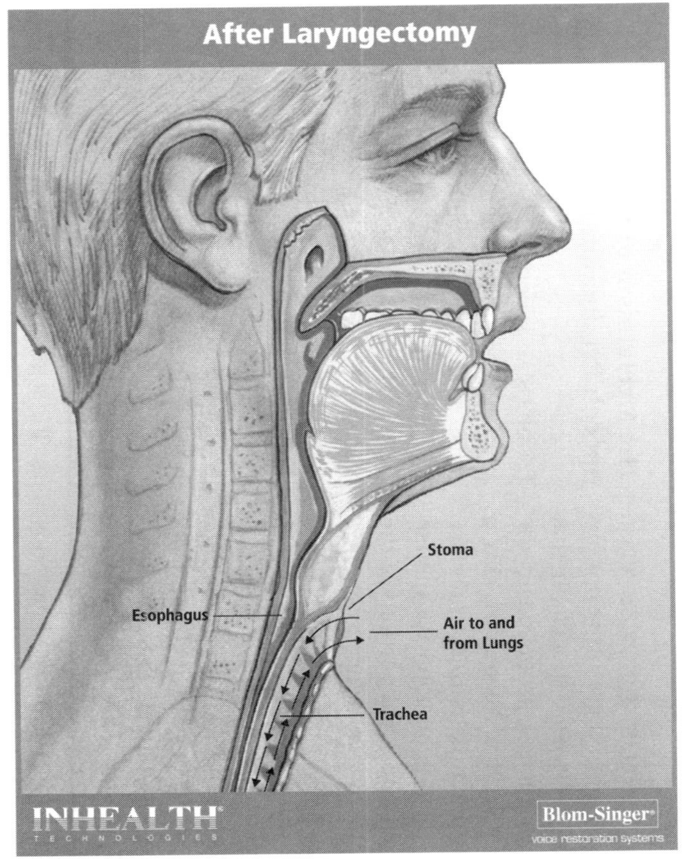

Figure 4–1(b). Graphic representation of postlaryngectomy anatomy. Note the separation between the primary airway and structures of the vocal tract, pharynx, and esophagus. Reprinted with permission, InHealth Technologies, Carpenteria, CA.

(c) electrolaryngeal or artificial laryngeal speech. As a group, these three options are termed *alaryngeal* speech in that this refers to speech produced in the absence of a larynx. All require that a new sound source is utilized to replace the loss of voice generation via the larynx. Because no residual portions of the larynx exist following laryngectomy, normal voice production is no longer possible postsurgically.

The first two methods, esophageal and TE speech, are categorized as *intrinsic* modes, while the last method, electrolaryngeal speech, is an *extrinsic* method (Weinberg, 1982). The distinction between these two classifications is based on the fact that intrinsic methods of alaryngeal speech rely on biological structures for the generation of the new alaryngeal voice. In the case of these two alaryngeal options, tissues of the transitional anatomical regions between the lower pharynx and upper esophagus serve as a vicarious mechanism of voice production. This biologic, alaryngeal sound source has been termed the *pharyngoesophageal* (PE) segment. Although the process of creating vibration of PE segment tissues differs between esophageal and TE speech, both rely on alaryngeal sound generation from this anatomical site. While a detailed discussion of these two voicing mechanisms is not appropriate within the context of this chapter, a brief description of the two modes will permit a greater understanding relative to concerns about conveyance of emotion in those who are laryngectomized. The distinction between these two methods will be addressed in the following two sections.

The Mechanism of Esophageal Speech Production

Esophageal speech is achieved when ambient air within the oral cavity is compressed and then moved in an inferior direction, thereby crossing the PE segment in the upper digestive pathway.[4] At rest, the PE segment is a tonically closed sphincteric structure. Air moving across the PE segment in response to an increase in pressure within the oral cavity due to voluntary compression then moves into the esophagus, which serves as a reservoir for this air charge. Once air is introduced into the esophagus, it can then be volitionally moved back across the PE segment through muscular contractions of thoracic and abdominal structures, and subsequently, esophageal voicing is initiated (Diedrich, 1968; Doyle, 1994). These muscular contractions serve to compress the reservoir, thus forcing it to move across the PE segment in an egressive fashion (Diedrich, 1968). This voiced alaryngeal sound source, a product of vibrating PE segment tissues (Shipp, 1970), is then introduced into the pharynx and remaining cavities of the vocal tract where it is articulated into the sounds of speech regardless of the speaker's language. Although a range of abilities in the successful acquisition and functional use of esophageal speech does exist, even the best speaker is required to regularly replenish the esophageal reservoir with air in an effort to maintain voicing for speech, which often disrupts the overall flow of speech (Doyle, 1994). The esophageal sound source has been well documented in the clinical literature rel-

[4]As a general rule, the PE segment retains tonicity postlaryngectomy, which necessitates that air must violate this anatomic sphincter in order to "charge" or insufflate the esophagus with air.

ative to characteristics in the frequency, intensity, and temporal domains (Doyle, 1994; Robbins, Fisher, Blom, & Singer, 1984; Weinberg, 1982; and others) as well as relative to a variety of aspects underlying speech intelligibility (Doyle, Danhauer, & Reed, 1988).

At this juncture, it is critical to acknowledge that esophageal speech production may be characterized by unusual relationships between the act of respiration and speech production when compared to normal processes. That is, normal laryngeal voice and speech production occurs as an egressive act—speech is generated during expiratory flow.[5] However, Isshiki and Snidecor (1965) demonstrated that esophageal speakers may utilize up to eight categories of respiratory-speech relationships. These phasic relationships are summarized in Table 4-1 and explicitly reveal that the normal pattern of speech production (i.e., inspiration preceding expiratory outflow for speech) is modified during esophageal speech and that expected relationships are often not observed. The reasons for these changes are multifactorial; however, the sum of Isshiki and Snidecor's (1965) data demonstrates that the normal pattern of respiratory control and phasic relations for the generation of verbal communication may be disrupted in myriad ways. Not only can esophageal voice be produced while air is being expelled from the lungs and tracheostoma, but voicing can occur on inspiration as well. In fact, what might be termed a paradoxical pattern of speech and breathing with eight

Table 4–1. Summary of phasic relationships between direction of airflow (inspiratory or expiratory) and voice generation in esophageal speakers

Type	Direction of Oronasal Airflow	Respiration	Voice Generation
1	In	EXP	No
2	In	EXP	Yes
3	In	INSP	No
4	In	INSP	Yes
5	Out	EXP	No
6	Out	EXP	Yes
7	Out	INSP	No
8	Out	INSP	Yes

Inspiratory = INS; Expiratory = EXP

Note. Adapted from "Air Intake and Usage in Esophageal Speech," by N. Isshiki and J. C. Snidecor, 1965, *Acta Oto-Laryngologica*, *59*, pp. 559–574.

[5]It is recognized that some languages do employ ingressive methods of sound production as a normal language-based requirement.

phase relationships, some asynchronous, has been documented (Figure 4-2). This concern has direct implications relative to how emotions such as laughing and crying may be displayed in those who undergo total laryngectomy and rely on esophageal speech as an alaryngeal method of communication. Consequently, once the other methods of alaryngeal speech are described, these implications will be further explored.

The Mechanism of Tracheoesophageal (TE) Speech Production

TE voice restoration has proven to be a viable postlaryngectomy rehabilitation option since its introduction in 1980 (Singer & Blom, 1980). TE speech can be classified as a surgical-prosthetic method of voice restoration in that it involves both a surgical procedure and use of a prosthetic device for voice and speech production. As noted earlier, total laryngectomy results in disconnection between structures of the primary airway, specifically the trachea, and those of the upper airway or vocal tract. Following laryngectomy, an anatomical relationship exists between the trachea and the esophagus, with the trachea located immediately anterior to the esophagus [see Figure 4-1(b)].

TE voice restoration involves the surgical creation of a *controlled midline tracheoesophageal puncture* across the common tissue wall between the trachea and esophagus in the upper region of the tracheostoma.[6] This puncture permits an anatomical communication between the primary airway and the esophagus (and its inherent capacity as an air reservoir). The TE puncture itself is then stented with a small, one-way valved voice prosthesis. The TE puncture voice prosthesis not only serves as a stent for the surgical puncture, but as a means of permitting tracheal air to be diverted into the esophageal reservoir when the tracheostoma is sealed during expiration. Thus, the TE puncture voice restoration method capitalizes on a surgical-prosthetic means of transferring pulmonary air into the esophagus. As pulmonary air is continuously transferred into the esophagus upon expiration, that air then moves across the PE segment where the (tracheo) esophageal voice source moves into the upper airway for articulation. Based on this description, it now becomes clear that TE speech is pulmonary powered esophageal speech; both esophageal and TE speech utilize the PE segment as a vicarious voicing source, but the approach and method to "charging" the esophageal reservoir differs.

Based on data contained in the experimental literature, the access to a pulmonary air supply clearly distinguishes esophageal from TE methods (Doyle, 1994; Doyle & Keith, 2005; Doyle et al., 1988; Robbins et al., 1984 and others). Despite the fact that both methods are intrinsic in nature (i.e., they both use a biological alaryngeal voice source), it is essential to note that the advantages observed in the TE voice signal are directly related to volumetric differences in the air supply used to power the PE segment.

[6] Viewing the circular tracheostoma from the front, and using a clock as an analogy, the TE puncture would be created in the area of 12 o'clock.

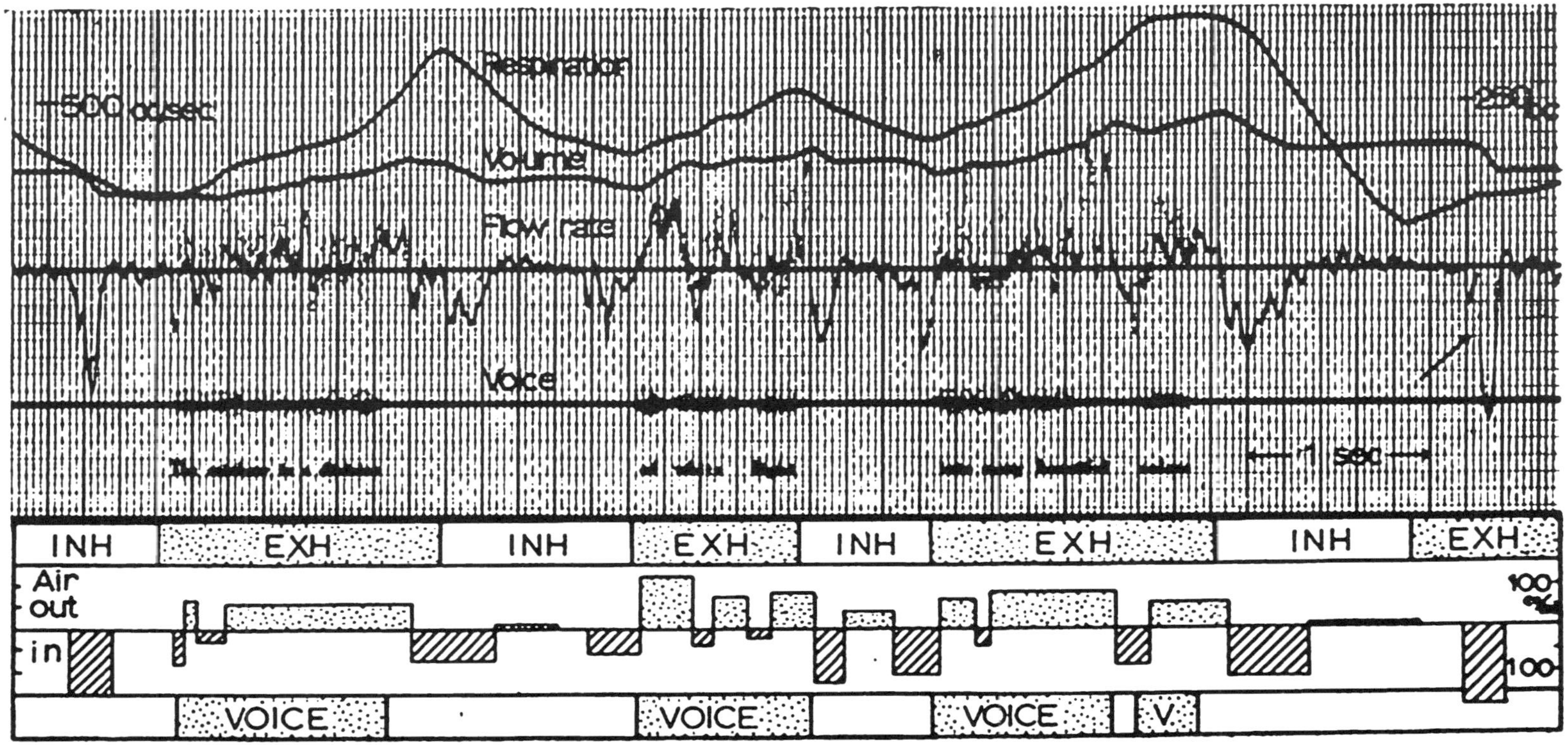

Figure 4–2. From top to bottom the traces represent (1) Respiratory. Inhalation is represented by the downward slope, exhalation by the upward curve. (2) Volume of air intake and exsufflation (each heavy graduation, consisting of five fine graduations, corresponds to 25 cc). Inward airflow is represented by the downward slope, outward flow by the upward slope. (3) Airflow rate traces above the baseline represent outward flow, below the line inward flow. Each heavy graduation corresponds to 50 cc per sec. (4) Voice. These recordings are schematically shown below by block diagrams. In the second row of the diagram, flow rate is represented by the height of the block, volume by the area. The arrow indicates an asynchronous air intake. *Note.* From *Speech Rehabilitation of the Laryngectomized* (2nd ed.), by J. C. Snidecor, 1978, Springfield, IL: Charles C. Thomas. Reprinted with permission.

Whereas the esophageal speaker frequently must replenish the esophageal reservoir, the TE speaker has a relatively endless supply of air to charge the reservoir Diedrich, 1968; Doyle, 1994[7] Advantages to TE speech relative to its intrinsic esophageal counterpart are replete in the clinical literature concerning alaryngeal speech (Izdebski, Reed, Ross, & Hilsinger, 1994; Robbins et al., 1984.

The Mechanism of Electrolaryngeal Speech Production

Up to this point, the discussion of alaryngeal methods of postlaryngectomy voice and speech production has focused on intrinsic modes. However, another option for postlaryngectomy communication does exist—use of an artificial larynx, or what is commonly referred to as an electrolarynx (EL). As noted, the EL is classified as an extrinsic mode of alaryngeal speech. The reason for this is that the voice source is now external to the speaker. In the case of EL speech, an external mechanical device is used to generate a sound source. This sound source is then transferred directly into the vocal tract using two potential approaches. The first of these is termed the transcervical (via the neck) approach, the second, an intraoral (via the oral cavity) approach. In order to distinguish these two approaches and the potential relevance to our discussion concerning the conveyance of emotion, a brief description of the mechanism for both is required.

When one uses a transcervical method of EL speech, the external source is placed on tissues of the neck, where the signal is then transferred across those tissues into the vocal tract where articulation will take place. In the case of the intraoral EL, the external sound source is transferred from a small diameter tube directly into the oral cavity via the mouth. The introduction of this EL sound source directly into the oral cavity is then articulated into the sounds of speech. Relative to both approaches to artificial laryngeal speech, the neck-type EL is more commonly used (Hillman, Walsh, Wolf, Fisher, & Hong, 1998). While both methods have considerable postlaryngectomy rehabilitative merit, there do exist a number of concerns about the quality of the signal produced (e.g., mechanical and robotic in nature), the use of an external device that is noticeable and potentially disruptive to others in the communication interaction, as well as potential reductions in overall speech intelligibility (Barney, 1958; Bennett & Weinberg, 1973; Doyle & Eadie, 2005; Meltzner et al., 2005; and others).

Comparing EL speech production with its intrinsic counterpart methods, one can obviously appreciate that the issue of coordinating respiratory functions with speech generation and output is potentially unique. While multiple phasic relationships have been documented for esophageal speech, TE speech mimics normal patterns of respiratory control in the context of speech production. However, the distinct and clear possibility that EL speech creates additional changes in

[7]Diedrich (1968) has suggested that that the volumetric capacity of the esophagus ranges between 40 and 80 cc; in contrast, the healthy adult pulmonary system has reasonable access to anywhere from 3000 to 5000 cc. At a minimum, the ability for the TE speaker to maintain continuous insufflation of the esophageal reservoir during an expiratory phase offers clear and distinct advantages that cross frequency, intensity, and durations domains.

how, or perhaps better stated where, speech occurs in the respiratory cycle does arise. In fact, clinical experience has shown that users of an EL, regardless of whether it be a neck-type or intraoral device, often suspend respiration altogether at points of speech output. This strategy is at times used to discourage the speaker from having respiratory noise compete with the EL signal. This same problem of "stoma noise" has been reported to be a real and significant impediment to successful acquisition of esophageal speech in that stoma noise or stoma blast secondary to excessive expiratory force may mask the less intense esophageal speech signal (Doyle, 1994).

In summary, three methods of postlaryngectomy speech rehabilitation exist, each with inherent advantages and disadvantages. Because of the disconnection between the primary airway and the structures comprising the vocal tract, secondary limitations specific to the respiratory system do emerge. The consequences of this disruption clearly have an effect on respiratory patterns, which may in turn create limitations in the conveyance of emotion following total laryngectomy. The essence of this disruption is seen primarily in alterations in the synchrony with which respiration and sound production may be achieved. However, the larger issue relative to the expression of emotional states in the present context is that the respiratory system is no longer linked to sound generating structures. When coupled with alterations in respiratory phase, the combined influence of these factors on emotional expression are substantial. Further information concerning associated problems that arise is presented in the subsequent section.

Problems Conveying Emotion: Postlaryngectomy Limitations and Restrictions

Evolving from our knowledge of the normal and postlaryngectomy speech production system, and regardless of alaryngeal mode, let's now consider two common acts of emotional expression as they might exist on a continuum, laughing and crying. Although both can be done volitionally and sometimes without true, internalized, and spontaneous emotional involvement (e.g., consider the polished actor), they more regularly exist as involuntary acts of emotional expression in response to a particular event or stimulus.

Laughing in Those Who Are Laryngectomized

The more pleasant of these two emotions, laughing, requires considerable integration of several physical structures.[8] The respiratory system in coordination with the abdomen and thoracic wall contribute greatly to the act of laughing. This involves active participation of a number of muscles in order to control movements associated with laughing. In the normal system, respiratory airflow is modulated through the upper airway and larynx, prior to moving into the vocal tract. In contrast, however, in those

[8]From a physiologic perspective, laughing and crying may share many common characteristics relative to airway and respiratory control mechanisms.

who are laryngectomized, while muscular movements associated with the act of laughing do occur, the product of this movement terminates through an open and unrestricted tracheostoma. For this reason, one might view the act of laughing in the individual who is laryngectomized as a paroxysmal respiratory event without vocalization of any form. More simply stated, laughing for those who are laryngectomized is tantamount to going through the respiratory motions without the benefit of acoustic speech output observed in the normal system. A common clinical complaint regarding this deficit is reported to be the lack of simple satisfaction of completing the act of laughing as it would have occurred normally.

Clearly, laughing may be characterized by variance relative to the intensity of the response and we have all observed the continuum from a subdued, light chuckle to the almost infectious belly-laugh. The duration of the response may be brief or extended, dependent upon the circumstances and how receptive and/or appropriate the behavior is for a given environment.

For the laryngectomized person, laughing is in essence manifest as solely a responsive change in breathing dynamics —short, quick inspiratory and expiratory movements secondary to adjustments in the abdominal and thoracic walls. Similarly, the disconnection from the ability to generate sound in response to respiratory actions is what creates the greatest level of loss for these individuals based on direct report from those who are laryngectomized. Consider laughing without the ability to make any type of vocalized noise and one can see that the conveyance of what might be viewed as a simple but primary human emotion is disrupted substantially. What this suggests to us in the case of laughing is that the ultimate satisfaction from this behavior is found in the direct linkage to and ultimate representation in some type of vocalization.[9] Shanks (1994) has recommended that attempts at compensating for the loss of normal laughter via use of a "body shake and thigh slapping," in addition to potential facilitation of this loss of emotional expression though "stoma exhalation concomitant with esophageal phonation" (p. 215) are of value. However, my own clinical interactions with those who are laryngectomized suggest that such levels of compensation are not satisfactory. This observation lends further credence to the suggestion that the loss of this ability to convey a common behavioral activity that is directly related to an affective state is reduced considerably if not entirely eliminated in the clinical population. Those who are laryngectomized frequently report that the loss of "normal" laughter is not insignificant relative to the nature and effectiveness of social interactions.

Crying in Those Who Are Laryngectomized

Despite sharing a number of features from a physiologic perspective, crying is indeed different from laughing. Similar to laughing, crying necessitates a substan-

[9]One need only consider his or her group of friends and acquaintances to accept the notion that the manner of how one laughs is indeed as unique as the human voice itself and carries considerable satisfaction to the individual.

tial contribution from respiratory muscles, both inspiratory and expiratory. This includes contributions from structures comprising the thoracic wall and the abdomen. As with laughing, durations of this emotional act may vary temporally relative to sequential events. However, crying is typically comprised of emotional vocalization, again varying in its acoustic properties, that in the normal system is synchronous with the respiratory cycle. Following laryngectomy, while respiratory actions may occur and tears may be shed in response to events that trigger crying, the collation of these behaviors with vocalization is lost. In my own clinical observations, many have informed me that while they may weep, they cannot sob. By definition, sobbing involves vocalization in some form during the expression of such an emotional state. Although tears may be shed in this circumstance, they cannot be integrated with vocalization via alaryngeal methods. Thus, the disconnection between vocalization capabilities and the respiratory system creates substantial limitations relative to conveying emotion through the act of crying.

One can see that the essential disruption between respiration and vocalization creates substantial difficulties specific to crying. As noted previously in relation laughing, the act of crying postlaryngectomy is incomplete. Again, the confirmation of this lack of satisfaction with the act of crying in those who are laryngectomized is common. The gravity of this problem, however, is much more significant than one might assume at face value. That is, recall that those who are laryngectomized have been diagnosed with a potentially life-threatening disease, they will more often that not be treated aggressively and quickly (frequently within days), which limits opportunities to verbally communicate prior to treatment, and perhaps most critically, they will lose normal communication entirely as a consequence of treatment. Although acquisition of one or more modes of alaryngeal speech is likely, voice and speech rehabilitation requires some time in many instances.[10] One need only consider the loss of one's ability to express oneself vocally through the use of language to understand the impact of laryngectomy during both the early and later periods of treatment, recovery, and rehabilitation. Yet the inability to *satisfactorily* realize emotional expression through the act of crying during this period provides a communicative purgatory that is almost certainly disabling. As such, losses in the ability to cry in a normal capacity following total laryngectomy must be regarded as a substantial and devastating personal loss to one's well-being.

Summary

This chapter has addressed the issue of the expression of emotion in individuals who have undergone total laryngectomy. It is widely accepted that the conveyance of emotion and emotional states is manifest secondary to multiple actions of the human communicator. This would include physical postures, facial expressions, pitch, loudness, and

[10]While EL and TE speech may be acquired relatively rapidly when compared to esophageal speech, one may not be fully communicative for at least some period of time early postoperatively, which restricts the ability to verbally communicate.

cadence of speech, as well as many other factors.

Regardless of the combination of events that occur in efforts to achieve and convey emotional states to others in the communicative context, it is widely agreed that physical, physiologic, neurologic, and social inputs are critical. When disorder modifies or eliminates the ability for one to normally express emotions, regardless of the underlying causal factors, considerable disability is likely. Minimally, the satisfaction with being able to move through the patterns that existed prior to the onset of a given disorder must be considered. For those who undergo laryngectomy for laryngeal cancer, the anatomic and physiologic changes are extensive. In addition to the loss of normal verbal communication, other behaviors of critical importance to one's well-being may be affected. In the case of laryngectomy, the expression of emotion through the common behaviors of laughing and crying are certainly disrupted. However, despite the ability to understand the influence of laryngectomy on the physiology of these emotional acts, research in the area of conveying emotion postlaryngectomy appears to be wholly nonexistent in the literature.

In the present context, two specific expressions of an emotional state, namely, laughing and crying, have been presented for consideration. While questions related to other emotions and their expression may be raised, the focus on laughing and crying is linked directly to one's respiratory system—a system that is permanently disrupted following laryngectomy. Based on anecdotal clinical observations and report, these two emotional activities cannot be performed in normal fashion without a larynx. While isolated physiological behaviors in response to laughing and crying do appear, the cohesive normal response through the linkage of systems (respiratory system and upper airway along with a voicing source) is lost. It does appear that while isolated actions can take place, for example, the pulsatile respiratory response in association with laughing or crying, head movements associated with laughing, or the shedding of tears when crying, the loss of system integration due to laryngectomy creates a significant loss for those who are laryngectomized.

When coupled with the inability to produce associated levels of voice (and laryngeal sound) generation in unison with laughing or crying, considerable personal and social disability results. Concerns related to the conveyance of emotion in those who have undergone laryngectomy for laryngeal cancer would appear to provide an important and fruitful area of empirical investigation. Research of this type would not only appear to have interest from the perspective of interdisciplinary endeavors, but holds great promise for further understanding the impact of laryngectomy on the person within the social-communication context. Neglecting to consider such expression (i.e., laughing and crying) as part of human communication is wholly incomplete and falls short of any effort to understand the essential objective of communication within our social world.

References

American Cancer Society. (2004). *Facts and figures*. New York: Author.

Bailey, B.J. (1984). *Surgery of the larynx*. Philadelphia: W.B. Saunders.

Barney, H. L. (1958). A discussion of some technical aspects of speech aids for postlaryngectomized patients. *Annals of Otology, Rhinology, and Laryngology*, *67*, 558-570.

Bennett, S., & Weinberg, B. (1973). Acceptability ratings of normal, esophageal, and artificial larynx speech. *Journal of Speech and Hearing Research*, *16*, 608-615.

Darwin, C. (1965). *The expression of the emotions in man and animals*. Chicago: University of Chicago Press. (Originally published 1872)

Davidson, R. J. (2001). Toward a biology of personality and emotion. *Annals of the New York Academy of Sciences*, *935*, 191-207.

Davidson, R. J., & Irwin, W. (1999). The functional neuroanatomy of emotion and affective style. *Trends in Cognitive Science*, *3*, 11-21.

Davidson, R. J., Maxwell, J. S., & Shackman, A. J. (2004). The privileged status of emotion in the brain. *Proceedings of the National Academy of Sciences of the United States of America*, *101*(33), 11915-11916.

Diedrich, W. M. (1968). The mechanism of esophageal speech. *Annals of the New York Academy of Sciences*, *155*, 303-317.

Diedrich, W., & Youngstrom, K. (1966). *Alaryngeal speech*. Springfield, IL: Charles C. Thomas.

Doyle, P. C. (1994). *Foundations of voice and speech rehabilitation following total laryngectomy.* San Diego, CA: Singular.

Doyle, P. C., Danhauer, J. L., & Reed, C. G. (1988). Listeners' perception of consonants produced by esophageal and tracheoesophageal talkers. *Journal of Speech and Hearing Disorders*, *53*, 400-407.

Doyle, P. C., & Eadie, T. L. (2005). The perceptual nature of alaryngeal speech. In P. C. Doyle & R. L. Keith (Eds.), *Contemporary considerations in the treatment and rehabilitation of head and neck cancer: Voice, speech, and swallowing* (pp. 113-140). Austin, TX: Pro-Ed.

Doyle, P. C., & Keith, R. L. (Eds.). (2005). *Contemporary considerations in the treatment and rehabilitation of head and neck cancer: Voice, speech, and swallowing.* Austin, TX: Pro-Ed.

Eadie, T. L. (2001). The ICIDH-2: Theoretical and clinical implications for speech-language pathology. *American Journal of Speech-Language Pathology*, *25*, 181-200.

Ekman, P. (1972). Universals and cultural differences in facial expressions of emotion. In J. Cole (Ed.), *Nebraska Symposium on Motivation* (pp. 207-283). Lincoln, NE: University of Nebraska Press.

Ekman, P. (1982). Methods for measuring facial action. In K. R. Scherer & P. Ekman (Eds.), *Handbook of methods in nonverbal behavioral research* (pp. 45-90). Cambridge, UK: Cambridge University Press.

Ekman, P. (1992). Facial expression of emotion: New findings, new questions. *Psychological Science*, *3*, 34-38.

Ekman, P. (1993). Facial expression of emotion. *American Psychologist*, *48*, 384-392.

Ekman, P. (1997). Expression or communication about emotion. In N. Segal, G. E. Weisfeld, & C. C. Weisfeld (Eds.), *Genetic, theological and evolutionary perspectives on human development: Essays in honor of Dr. Daniel G. Freedman* (pp. 34-38). Washington, DC: American Psychological Association.

Ekman, P. (1997). Should we call it expression or communication? *Innovations in Social Science Research*, *10*, 333-344.

Ekman, P. (1999). Basic emotions. In T. Dalgleish & M. Power (Eds.), *Handbook of cognition and emotion* (Chapter 16). Sussex, UK: John Wiley and Sons.

Ekman, P. (2003). Introduction. *Annals of the New York Academy of Sciences*, *1000*, 1-6.

Ekman, P., Levenson, R. W., & Friesen, W. V. (1983). Autonomic nervous system activity distinguishes between emotions. *Science*, *221*, 1208-1210.

Gardner, W. G. (1971). *Laryngectomee speech and rehabilitation.* Springfield, IL: Charles C. Thomas.

Graham, M. S. (1997). *The clinician's guide to alaryngeal speech therapy.* Boston: Butterworth-Heinemann.

Hillman, R. E., Walsh, M. J., Wolf, G. T., Fisher, S. G., & Hong, W. K. (1998). Functional outcomes following treatment for advanced laryngeal cancer. Part I—Voice preservation in advanced laryngeal cancer. Part II—Laryngectomy rehabilitation: The state of the art in the VA system. *Annals of Otology, Rhinology, and Laryngology, 172*(Suppl.), 1-27.

Isshiki, N., & Snidecor, J. C. (1965). Air intake and usage in esophageal speech. *Acta Oto-Laryngologica, 59*, 559-574.

Izdebski, K., Reed, C. G., Ross, J. C., & Hilsinger, R. L. (1994). Problems with tracheoesophageal fistula voice restoration in totally laryngectomized patients. A review of 95 cases. *Archives of Otolaryngology Head and Neck Surgery, 120*, 840-845.

Johnson-Laird, P. N., & Oatley, K. (1992). Basic emotions: A cognitive science approach to function, folk theory and empirical study. *Cognition and Emotion, 6*, 201-223.

Laukkanen, A-M., Vilkman, E., Alku, P., & Oksanen, H. (1996). Physical variations related to stress and emotional state: A preliminary study. *Journal of Phonetics, 24*, 313-335.

Levenson, R. W., Cartensen, L. L., Friesen, W. V., & Ekman, P. (1991). Emotion, physiology, and expression in old age. *Psychology and Aging, 6*, 28-35.

Meltzner, G., Hillman, R. E., Heaton, J. T., Houston, K. M., Kobler, J., & Qi, Y. (2005). Electrolaryngeal speech: The state of the art and future directions for development. In P. C. Doyle & R. L. Keith (Eds.), *Contemporary considerations in the treatment and rehabilitation of head and neck cancer: Voice, speech, and swallowing* (pp. 571-590). Austin, TX: Pro-Ed.

Oatley, K., & Johnson-Laird, P. N. (1987). Towards a cognitive theory of the emotions. *Cognition and Emotion, 1*, 29-50.

Ohman, A. (1986). Face the beast and fear the face: Animal and social fears as prototypes for evolutionary analyses of emotion. *Psychophysiology, 23*, 123-145.

Robbins, J., Fisher, H. B., Blom, E. D., & Singer, M. I. (1984). A comparative acoustic study of normal, esophageal, and tracheoesophageal speech. *Journal of Speech and Hearing Disorders, 49*, 202-210.

Salmon, S. J., & Goldstein, H. (1978). *The artificial larynx handbook.* New York: Grune & Stratton.

Shanks, J. C. (1994). Developing esophageal communication. In R. L. Keith & F. L. Darley (Eds.), *Laryngectomee rehabilitation* (3rd ed., pp. 205-217). Austin, TX: Pro-Ed.

Scherer, K. R., & Ekman, P. (1983). *Handbook of methods in nonverbal behavioral research.* Cambridge, UK: Cambridge University Press.

Shipp, T. (1970). EMG of pharyngoesophageal musculature during alaryngeal voice production. *Journal of Speech and Hearing Research, 13*, 184-192.

Simpson, G. G. (1967). *The meaning of evolution.* New Haven, CT: Yale University Press.

Singer, M. I., & Blom, E. D. (1980). An endoscopic technique for restoration of voice after laryngectomy. *Annals of Otology, Rhinology, and Laryngology, 89*, 529-533.

Snidecor, J. C. (1978). *Speech rehabilitation of the laryngectomized* (2nd ed.). Springfield, IL: Charles C. Thomas.

Snidecor, J. C., & Curry, E. T. (1960). How effectively can the laryngectomee expect to speak? *Laryngoscope, 70*, 62-67.

Weinberg, B. (1982). Speech after laryngectomy: An overview and review of acoustic and temporal characteristics of esophageal speech. In A. Sekey (Ed.), *Electroacoustic analysis and enhancement of alaryngeal speech* (pp. 5-48). Springfield, IL: Charles C. Thomas.

Weinberg, B., & Bosma, J. F. (1970). Similarities between glossopharyngeal breathing and injection methods of air intake for esophageal speech. *Journal of Speech and Hearing Disorders, 35*, 25-32.

Zeitels, S. M. (2005). Recent advances in the surgical treatment of laryngeal cancer. In P. C. Doyle & R. L. Keith (Eds.), *Contemporary considerations in the treatment and rehabilitation of head and neck cancer: Voice, speech, and swallowing* (pp. 171–194). Austin, TX: Pro-Ed.

CHAPTER 5

Impact of Cleft Lip and Palate (CLP) and Velopharyngeal Insufficiency (VPI) on Emotive Aspects of Voice and Speech

Maria A. Hortis-Dzierzbicka and Krzysztof Izdebski

Abstract

As a consequence of structural deficits introduced by cleft lip and/or palate (CLP) and velopharyngeal insufficiency (VPI), patients afflicted by these anomalies experience functional disturbances from birth, including feeding, breathing, hearing, facial expressions, and speech/voice production. These deficits may be long-lasting, despite advances in reconstructive and plastic surgery, including phoniatric and speech pathology rehabilitation, making many of these patients subject to multifactorial psychosocial stigmata for life. Here, we discuss the consequences of CLP and VPI on emotive production of voice and speech, a subject rarely given attention in world literature. Although our discussion is based on the Polish linguistic population, certain universals can be extrapolated. Based on our material, we present an opinion that anatomical and physiologic constraints present in CLP/VFI patients contribute greatly to the misdirected production of voice and speech, and when accompanied by unexpected and deviant facial gestures they further negatively affect the production of emotional intent by these patients. In addition to the intrinsically determined disturbances of the vocal tract mechanism, usage of compensatory maneuvers occurring during speech by these patients in an attempt to produce "the best possible speech" complicates vocalization and further distorts emotive aspects. As a consequence, not only is the emotive intent not produced as desired, but the output affected by these unintended distortions is subject to misinterpretation by the listeners, resulting in noncongruent responses, and thus causing additional conflict and embarrassment for the patient and the recipient, all impacting the fragile communication chain and affecting life expectations of CLP patients.

Introduction

In this chapter we focus on how CLP/VPI complex affects production of voice and speech, and how these intrinsic sensory motor deficits affect emotive vocal production and hence recognition of intended emotions.

Three major aspects are addressed here against the background of available literature. First, we discuss the fundamental points influencing neutral speech and voice production in these patients. Second, we discuss how distorted CLP communication affects the production of intended emotive expressions. Third, we discuss the psycho-social consequences for the speaker and the listener involved in emotive discourse. The material presented here is based on a specific ethnic and linguistic population (Poland), but the observations derived can be applied cross-culturally and can be used to form universal opinions.

Patients

The patient population discussed in this chapter is based on a unique cohort of nearly 200 new cases of male and female Polish children treated on a yearly basis in a centralized setting in Poland at the Warsaw Center for Craniofacial Disorders. The center team members comprise surgery, ENT/phoniatrics, orthodontics, speech therapy, and psychology. The basic surgical protocol (for unilateral cleft lip and palate) is introduced at 6 to 9 months of age using one-stage lip closure (modified Tennison-Randall) with primary ala nasi correction and hard (vomerplasty) and soft palate closure followed at about 2 years of age with alveolar bone grafting (iliac crest). Thanks to tight two-layer closure of all wounds by alveolus and minimally invasive anatomic restoration of clefted palatal musculature, excellent anatomical conditions are set for speech without disturbing craniofacial growth. The pharyngoplasty rate in our setting does not exceed 2–3% of cases (Hortis-Dzierzbicka, Kulewicz & Dudkiewicz, 2003; Hortis-Dzierzbicka, Dudkiewicz, Kulewicz, Piwowar & Surowiec, 2004). All patients operated on with the above-described one-stage method are followed for up to 20 years of age, or longer as dictated by individual cases by one of the authors of this report, who recently used the Eurocleft recommended criteria (Shaw, Semb, Nelson, Brattstrom, Moelsted, & Prahl-Anderson, 2001).

Background

Despite advances of surgery and postsurgical rehabilitation, many CLP patients continue to produce deviant facial and speech-phonatory gestures affecting both phonetic and phonologic components (Peterson-Falzone, Hardin-Jones, & Karnell, 2001; Watson, 2001). Therefore, despite even the most advanced and promising rehabilitation process, CLP communication may exhibit deficits in all components, that is, in speech, facial expressions, and phonation, the last occurring specifically as a compensatory consequence of disordered vocal tract affecting air pressure requirements.

Speech/Articulation

Speech articulation deficits occurring in CLP/VPI patients are the consequences of abnormal vocal tract in otherwise intellectually normal children who are "forced" by the naturally occurring forces to produce socially acceptable language-specific targets while using abnormal anatomy. These inherent anatomical deficits have profound consequences on the acquisition of expected expressive speech in general, and may cause the affected individual a loss of naturalness in speech and/or in vocalization, hence expressing vocally not only declarative speech but also speech- and voice-bound emotions, beyond automatic crying or laughter.

The articulatory errors encountered in the early stages of language development may become habitual with time despite ongoing treatment, and may form idiosyncratic speaking patterns, thus carrying serious social communicative consequences over the life span. Current scientific evidence suggests that early sound production is of paramount consequence to the overall communicative development of the child; hence, delays in the acquisition of "normal" sounds should be avoided at all costs, with surgical-rehabilitative regimen beginning no later than 13 months of age (Hardin-Jones & Jones, 2005)

Consequently, CLP and VPI speech quality reflects the origin and the extent of the anatomical deficits. Therefore, irrespective of the language group, CLP speech is typically characterized by open nasalization, nasal emissions, nasalization of bilabials, glottic overpressure, lack of oral voiced and voiceless consonants (the so-called vocalic or zero speech), coarticulation deficits, and unvoicing and devoicing of voiced segments. The specifics of these anatomical conditions and functional consequences are briefly outlined below.

For example, the deficits associated with nasopharynx abnormalities typically cause retroflexion of sounds and nasal production of dental sounds. VPI leads to hypernasality, while nasal cavity obstructions cause noise, friction, and hyponasality. Labiodental deficits introduce lateralization, palatalization, and dentalization of many consonants. In addition, aspiration, velarization, lateralizations, and laryngealization can be present. In all, speech production of the CLP/VPI child can be profoundly affected, including resonance, timing, loudness, vocal quality, and can cause secondary distortions of expected facial gestures, making in severe cases overall intelligibility extremely difficult and having profound effects on both the speaker and the listener.

It is also important to recall, specifically for the purposes of this chapter, that CLP speech is often accompanied by compensatory facial musculature mimicry affecting the nostrils, midface, and forehead. Similar compensatory mechanisms are found in patients with dystonia of the larynx and in so-called oral stutterers, who show recruitment on an involuntary basis of facial musculature in an attempt to release glottic overpressure (Izdebski, 1983), magnifying the bizarre and negatively perceived affect of their voice and speech. Presence of such acoustic deficits and facial grimacing affects not only the production of normative speech, but also may have profound influence on emotive communication as the distorted vocal and facial expressions may lead to confusing if not misconstrued perceptions of what kind of emotive expression was actually intended by the speaker.

The focus of this chapter is supposed to be on phonatory aspects of CLP patient communication; hence, we will now try to build a case that the sensory-motor and anatomical deficits inherent to the CLP condition impose significant effects on production of voice in general and thus further compound production of intended emotive vocal expressions.

Phonatory Disturbances in CLP Complex

The prevailing understanding of voice disturbances and voice quality in general in the CLP population is that phonatory quality in these patients is subject to compensatory glottic overpressure, as a consequence of compensating for intraoral pressure loss, because of the ill-functioning velopharyngeal sphincter (McWilliams & Paradise, 1973; Leder & Lerman, 1985). Therefore, the resultant excessive glottic compression and P_3 are blamed as responsible for creating organic mucosal vocal cord changes and formation of vocal cord nodes, as well as for the creation of other mucosal aberrations, as organic mucosal changes are found in up to 24% of the CP population (Marks, Barker, & Tardy, 1971). In a more direct work focusing on dysphonia in CPL population, 41% of these cases were found to exhibit audible dysphonia with 21% showing vocal cord mucosal changes (D'Antonio, Rice, & Fink, 1998).

Although the contributory factor for dysphonia in CLP patients can include other parameters, the general consensus is that Pio problems causing compensation of the vocal tract are the major culprit. The effects of upper vocal tract configuration on glottic wave shape have been studied in computer simulation (P. Alku, Horácek, M. Airas, & Laukkanen, 2005; Alku, Story, & Airas, 2006; Imatomi, 2005) and in various classes of professional voice users (Sjolander & Sundberg, 2004), and this relation is corroborated for cleft palate population in a recent work showing profound acoustic consequences on voice parameters because of nasal obstruction, adenoids, or CP conditions in contrast to a control population

(Niedzielska, 2005). The role of the narrowing of the pharynx in production of the so-called "throaty" voice quality (having negative emotional and injurious habitual connotations) has also been described recently (Laukkanen, Bjorkner, & Sundberg, 2005).

Thus, the so-called pressed or overpressured voice (Izdebski, 1983; 2008) as well as laborious and effortful phonation can be considered a sensitive indicator of upper vocal tract configuration problems including palatopharyngeal obstruction. Excessive phonatory effort and increased laryngeal resistance have also been discussed as a consequence of inadequate VP closure (Bernthal & Beukelman, 1977; Zajac, 1995), and since these pressure changes can lead to compensatory behavior of articulators within the entire vocal tract (including extra recruitment of facial musculature), they seem to add to the bizarreness and the unattractiveness or apparent unpleasantness of the CLP voice.

In contrast, the effects of breathiness caused by glottic hypoadduction seem to aid hypernasality, as it was shown that breathiness tends to moderate rather than to mask perceived hypernasality. And although breathiness raises mild hypernasality, it is also thought to reduce severe hypernasality. Breathiness is a more accepted form of vocalization than overpressure (Izdebski, 1983; 2008), with the latter leading to a perception of unpleasant strangled or angry voice, while breathiness can be understood as connoting a sense of confidence, intimacy, and even comfort; this is evident by the tendency of the voice-over industry to use a variety of breathy voice in various radio or TV commercials, whose goal is to instill customer confidence in a product.

Material

The material on which the rest of this discussion is based comprises observations of a cohort of nearly 1000 Polish children with CLP (AHD). The observations are based on longitudinal (up to 20 years' follow-up) interactions with these children beginning with the preoperative period and continuing to postoperative and rehabilitative years, including their entry into adolescent or early adult social life.

The attention is now focused on how these individuals strategize to express vocal emotions within the constraints imposed by the anatomical reality they face. Although our observations are limited to this specific socio-cultural environment, the findings appear to be carried across cultural and linguistic borders, as many other language group speakers, such as Flemish, Finnish, Swedish, and Marathi, just to mention a few, afflicted with CLP syndrome and described in the literature show similar consequences on verbal communication to Polish children (Hortis-Dzierzbicka & Stecko, 2001; Karling, Larson, Leanderson, & Henningsson, 1993; Pulkkinen, Ranta, Haapanen, Heliovaara, & Laitinen, 2002; Nandurkar, 2004; van Lierde, De Bodt, Baetens, Schrauwen, & Van Cauwenberge, 2003). The apparent universality of these observations can be further supported by the fact that the Polish population is representative of wide ethnic backgrounds, and often incorporates Slavic, Germanic, Jewish, Romany, and other Eastern European ethic mixes and cultural habits/traditions, and is also intermingled with other groups (Armenians, Hungarians, Latinos, and lately the Far Eastern, Arabic, and African cultures).

All subjects forming the clinical data corpus for this discussion were essentially monolingual but ethnically diversified speakers of the Polish language, who live and grew up in Poland and who are exposed to and expected to follow Polish emotive customs.

The Polish language belongs to a group of Western Slavic languages of the Indo-European language group, with modern Polish incorporating lexical items from classical languages (Latin, Greek, Sanskrit, Old Church Slavonic, etc.), and from modern languages such as French, Italian, German, English, Russian, Czech, Yiddish, and Turkish. Because the morpheme structure conditions, phonology, sound inventory, as well as prosody of these loan words may differ from Polish constraints, these foreign words are subjected to "Polonization" by assigning Polish pronunciation and prosodic features, and these foreign words may be written in such a way as to conform to the Polish orthographic rules (e.g., English *Shakespeare* becomes *Szekspir*, German *Scheibe* becomes *szajba*, etc.). This is despite certain universals Polish prosody shares with other distant language groups (Grabe & Karpinski, 2003). Moreover, because the Polish educational system requires learning foreign languages in school, and these requirements are not excused in the CLP population, CLP children are subjected to further communicative compromises.[1]

Furthermore, the Polish language comprises a rich inventory of voiced and voiceless phonemes, represented by eight vowels including two nasal vowels, and 36 consonantal phonemes (Hortis-Dzierzbicka & Stecko, 2001). Unique to the phonetic system of Polish language are long clusters of voiceless fricatives (e.g., *chszaszcz brzmi w trzcine w Szczebrzeszynie*), nasal and nasalized vowels, and so-called geminated consonant clusters (*rana* vs *ranna*) producing phonological and semantic distinctions. These general features can also be used opportunistically to produce emotive effects.

Being a Latin grammar-based language but with free word order; seven cases and multiple declensions, voices, and times; masculine, feminine, neuter genders; singular, plurals, and duals; a need for grammatical congruence; and a cultural habit of creating emotive diminutives on an ad hoc basis by inserting infixes, prefixes, and suffixes that elongate stems and shift prosody, the Polish language is complex to say the least. The usage of diminutive suffixes often utilizes palatalization and prosodic shifts, making the production of these phonatory-articulatory expressions challenging yet pleasant for any "normative" speaker, but extremely difficult for many of the CLP patients.

Of special interest to our topic are the so-called palatalization and velarization occurring widely in Polish (but also found in other languages), as they have emotive values. Also, the specific coarticulatory effects between labials and velars can be used to express emotions, and their presence in Polish phonology support the so-called "Duke of York" effects (essentially deemed to be impossible;

[1]Polish is currently spoken by about 38 million people in Poland and by about 8 million outside, making it the 25th most widely used language in the world. According to the U.S. 2001 census 667,414 Americans age 5 years and over reported Polish as the language spoken at home, which is about 1.4% of people who speak languages other than English, or 0.25% of the U.S. population.

McCarthy, 2002). To learn more about this phenomenon, the reader is referred to Rubach (2003).

Hypernasality

As in any language group, VPI and palatal dysfunctions introduced by cleft palate are causative of hypernasality. Notwithstanding the unquestionable progress in primary cleft surgery, persistent hypernasality continues to occur on the average in about 20% of cleft palate patients even after palatal reconstruction (Peterson-Falzone, Hardin-Jones, & Karnell, 2001).

Hypernasal quality is very easily detectable even by inexperienced listeners and may be read by a naïve population as a sign of mental retardation it may also subject the CLP children to teasing, bullying, and mocking by peers and schoolmates or even by adults. Because CLP hypernasality has also been implicated in raising subglottic air pressure and been shown to increase glottic resistance, the presence of hypernasality can make vocalization more overpressed and/or make phonation sound "hard," with both of these voice qualities carrying negative vocal image and negative emotive connotations.

In addition, some CLP speakers may try to mask or to reduce hypernasality by recruiting additional facial movements, often very intense and involving all muscles used for facial expression. This situation is demonstrated in Figure 5–1, which represents a repaired face of a 5-year-old girl with CP and VPI. It is seen that at rest (a) her face is in a neutral state and the expression on her face can be interpreted as being relatively restful and neutral, if not pleasant and esthetic in appearance; however, during the act of speaking (b), severe facial grimacing is noted. These facial grimaces are not purposeful but are used in a compensatory manner, specifically to increase the nasal airway resistance as evidenced by the narrowing of her nostrils. This form of compensation is consistent with the universal findings (Warren, Dalston, Morr, Hairfield, & Smith, 1989). One, however, cannot exclude the possibility that such compensatory facial grimacing may be

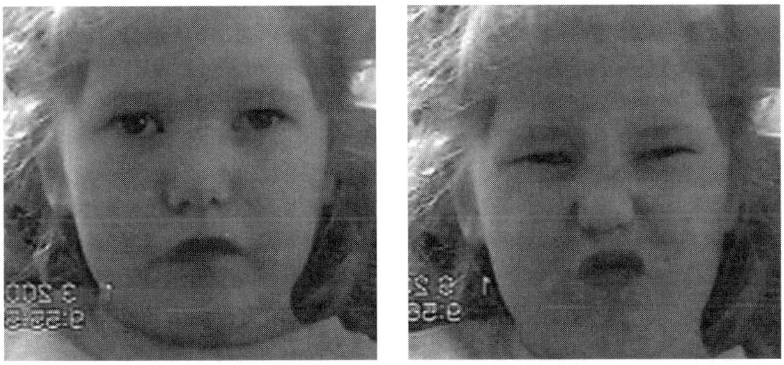

A. B.

Figure 5–1. Example of extremely vivid compensatory facial movement during speech in a 5-year-old girl with persistent VPI after primary repair of isolated cleft palate. **A.** Face at rest. **B.** Face during act of speaking.

interpreted by the uninitiated conversant as evidence of negative or skeptical emotions, in this case displeasure, or signaling negative emotive expressions, emotions that were not meant to be present.

The other extreme form of compensation occurring during speech of CP children with VPI is the so-called *zero* or *vocalic speech*, meaning that the afflicted child produces no other speech sounds besides vowels and nasal consonants with pressed hyperactive voice quality, making intelligibility very poor, and producing a strong negative reaction in the listener. These extreme conditions are not rare even in the speech of 4- to 6-year-old children with gross VPI.

Psychosocial Setting

The psychosocial cost of distorted communication is obvious: rejection by peers, often total. Although this volume focuses on phonatory aspects of emotions, isolating speech defects from phonation in CLP population is difficult, as this condition creates a unique scenario affecting all emotive expressions.

Assuming that the threshold of 3 years of age is paramount for the development of linguistic competence (Bryant & Colman, 1995; Flower & Izdebski, 1980; Lobacz, 1996), the anatomically determined lack of possibilities for acquiring normal phonetic and phonological inventory in the most dynamic period of the first 3 years of life is also considered to have a profoundly negative influence on the child's emotional development.

According to some research (Endriga & Kapp-Simon, 1999), behavior disorders in childhood and adolescence are commonly characterized as internalizing problems (e.g., shyness, somatization, and depression) and/or externalizing problems (e.g., disobedience, fighting, and impulsivity). Immediately from birth and from the early beginning of the preverbal stage of speech development, infants and toddlers use their voices and facial gestures as the means of emotional expression as they enter into social contact with their environment. (More on these early stages is found in Chapter 8 of this volume. Editor.)

Most papers dealing with psychosocial functioning of patients with orofacial clefts focus on facial disfigurement as the main cause of maladjustment and peer rejection (Canady, 1995; Markuson, Akerlind, & Paulin, 2001; McGregor, 1990; Reed, Robathan, Hockenhull, Rostill, Perrett, & Rees, 1999; Schneiderman & Harding, 1984; Tobiasen & Hiebert, 1993). In a recent study conducted by one of the authors on a large group (n = 124) of postadolescents and adults with CLP, the assessment of psychosocial functioning was found to be statistically significant not in relation to the severity of physical impairment, but rather to the social environment (Hortis-Dzierzbicka & Tarnowski, 2003).

Using assessment protocols, it became evident that even the smallest facial deformity (e.g., nasal tip deviation) may be a big psychological problem for a sensitive child, specifically in an unfriendly social or educational setting. Interestingly enough, with the progress of age towards maturation and with regard to dating and marriage, even a severe facial disfigurement was not found to be an obstacle in securing a partner. Instead, a significant correlation between severity of speech and voice disturbances and poor interpersonal relations as well as school and occupational underachievement was demonstrated. Furthermore, this study also demonstrated that all patients with poor speech intelligibility and articulation errors experienced teasing from peers, and they also provoked feelings of being different and ostracism (Hortis-Dzierzbicka & Tarnowski, 2003).

When considering the nature of emotional disorders in a given CLP case we must relate to each patient's own personality traits. However, in some CLP patients faces can lack expression and voice can be weak and flat or timid in a less active and responsive child (see Figure 5-2), portraying a neutral face with a downcast look. In other cases, the vivid facial mimics and the high-pitched or louder voice can reflect the high level of anxiety in response to the feeling of being rejected as a child, an adolescent, or an adult. Interestingly, high pitch contour has been classified as a submissive and insecure vocal trait (Grabe & Karpinski, 2003).

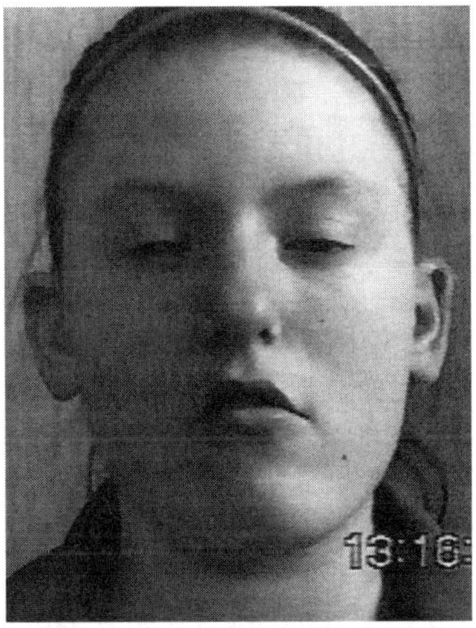

Figure 5–2. Flat animic face and downcast look in a 13-year-old girl with isolated cleft palate.

Attributed entirely to the lack of ability to generate proper Pio and reflected in the increase of Ps, the effects on loudness and pitch of voice can be interpreted as signs of excessive shyness and low self-esteem, although it may not be the case for every CLP child. Consequently, vocal nodules that are reported to occur in CLP may contribute to phonatory instability and cause aperiodicity or diplophonia (Izdebski, 2008), and these voice qualities may also be incorrectly interpreted as expression of aggressive vocal behavior or a socially maladjusted or rebellious child. This paradox may be justified further by the literature reporting cause-effect relationships between the occurrence of vocal nodules, vocal behavior, and so-called "A-type" personality traits in a non-CLP population of any age (Aronson, 1985; Boone & McFarlane, 1988), yet we could not locate any references on the possible relationship between the type of voice changes and personality in CLP patients.

The quality of hoarseness, breathiness, huskiness, or stridency in the CLP patient's voice can be to some extent also conditioned by a personality type, as one might expect a shy child to produce voice differently than a loud or aggressive child. Delays in lexical and phonological development secondary to persistent VPI and CLP related articulation disorders can also be associated in CP children with extremely low- or high-pitch voice production, depending in turn on a given child's personality and need to be understood and to communicate. Thus, voice quality can also serve as an indicator of peer, educational, and/or social status of the CLP patient as well as an indicator of physical attractiveness and of speech intelligibility index.

The Value of Phonation in CLP Population

The value of phonation in current society cannot be underestimated, and voice value is no longer restricted to singers, actors, preachers, or other professional voice users, but is of indisputable value to many people. It is now clear that voice and vocal emotions play an enormous role in social relations and may often be a factor in determining the extent of success, job placement, and societal status and even in the choice of a sexual partner or a mate. (For more on this subject see Chapters 13 and 15 in this volume.)

It is now evident that CLP voice quality can frequently be a cause of social exclusion (at all age stages) and can be a decisive factor in professional achievement or employment. When present, even discreetly, voice/speech problems can prevent the CLP patient from accessing the job market. Some of our patients report that even minor or discreet hypernasality and vocal stridency perceived by the listener on the phone can cause inquiry to the management by clients about the apparent deviancy of the speaker, or can simply result in a hang-up or aborted call or a request to speak to somebody else. (For more on the role of voice quality while on the phone see Chapter 8 of this volume.)

The voice and speech distortions present in CLP patients are often causative of reading difficulties, and are of importance in school settings for all CLP patients because of how teachers and peers react to their oral presentations (Richman, Eliason, & Lindgren, 1988). When a child with CLP is forced to talk or to read aloud in front of classmates, which is a particularly cruel task but which unfortunately happens rather frequently, this poses an enormous emotional burden on the child. In such a situation, a child with CLP may react by either increasing vocal efforts in an attempt to increase the chance of being understood, or by not being able to utter a single word. These efforts may manifest themselves in various types of vocal misuse, including excessive vocal hard attack, wrong voice pitch, excessive loudness, or combinations of all of these factors. If this defense behavior is frequently repeated it can create phonotrauma and form vocal fold edema, chronic laryngitis, vocal fatigue, muscular tension dysphonia, or vocal cord nodules. Those changes in turn will affect the voice quality, and the vicious circle continues.

Conclusions

The knowledge of how the voice in the CLP population hinders expression of emotions is not clear, judging from currently available literature. The data reviewed here show that vocalization in children with CLP may be tainted by intrinsic restrictions, hence providing false information about the emotive states of the speaker. We attempted here to show how important the knowledge of phonation is in consideration of how to improve treatment to provide the best anatomical condition for execution of nearly normal voice and speech. Based on our experience, we believe that early and properly executed palatal surgery may not only enable speech and language development under desirable anatomical and functional conditions, but can also prevent grave psychosocial maladjustment with all its consequences on the future well-being of the CLP population and aid in regulation of vocally emotive events, making the rehabilitative process more successful.

References

Alku, P., Horácek, J., Airas, M., & Laukkanen, A.-M. (2005).Assessment of glottal inverse filtering by using aeroelastic modeling of phonation and FE modeling of vocal tract. In C. Manfredi (Ed.), *Models and analysis of vocal emissions for biomedical applications, 4th International Workshop* (pp. 73–76), Firenze, Italy: Firenze University Press.

Alku, P., Story, B., & Airas, M. (2006). Estimation of the voice source from speech pressure signals: Evaluation of an inverse filtering technique using physical modeling of voice production. *Folia Phoniatrica et Logopaedia*, *58*(2), 102–113.

Aronson, A. E. (1985). *Clinical voice disorders* (2nd ed.). New York: Thieme-Stratton Inc., Brian C. Decker Division.

Bernthal, J. E., & Beukelman, D. R. (1977). The effect of changes in velopharyngeal orifice area on vocal intensity. *Cleft Palate Journal, 14*, 63–77.

Boone, D. R., & McFarlane, S. C. (1988). *The voice and voice therapy* (4th ed.). Englewood Cliffs, NJ: Prentice-Hall.

Bryant, P. A., & Colman, A. M. (1995). *Developmental psychology*. London: Longman Group.

Canady, J. W. (1995). Emotional effects of plastic surgery on the adolescent with a cleft. *Cleft Palate-Craniofacial Journal, 32*, 120–124.

D'Antonio, L., Muntz, H. R., Province, M. A., & Marsh, J. L. (1988). Laryngeal voice findings in patients with velopharyngeal dysfunction. *Laryngoscope, 98*, 432–438.

D'Antonio, L. L., Rice, R. D., Jr., & Fink, S. C. (1998). Evaluation of pharyngeal and laryngeal structure and function in patients with oculo-auriculo-vertebral spectrum. *Cleft Palate-Craniofacial Journal, 35*, 333–341.

Endriga, M. A., & Kapp-Simon, K. A. (1999). Psychological issues in craniofacial care: State of the art. *Cleft Palate-Craniofacial Journal, 36*, 3–11.

Flower, R. M., & Izdebski, K. (1979). *Common speech disorders in otolaryngologic practice*. American Academy of Otolaryngology, Rochester, Minn.

Grabe, E., & Karpinski, M. (2003, August 3–9). Universal and language specific aspects of intonation in English and Polish. In *Proceedings of the 15th International Congress of Phonetic Sciences* (Vol. 1, pp. 1061–1064)

Hardin-Jones, M. A., & Jones, D. L. (2005). Speech production of preschoolers with cleft palate. *Cleft Palate-Craniofacial Journal, 42*(1), 7–13.

Hortis-Dzierzbicka, M., Dudkiewicz, Z., Kulewicz, M., Surowiec, Z., & Piwowar, W. (2004, March). *Single stage lip and palate repair in UCLP—A within center study of three surgical modalities for hard palate repair*. Paper presented at the 61st Annual Meeting of the American Cleft Palate-Craniofacial Association, Chicago.

Hortis-Dzierzbicka, M., Kulewicz, M., & Dudkiewicz, Z. (2003, November). *Long term outcomes of one-stage surgical treatment of UCLP*. Paper presented at the VII European Craniofacial Congress, Bologna, Italy.

Hortis-Dzierzbicka, M., & Stecko, E. (2001). Cleft and Polish language—Neurophysiological and anatomical considerations. In Jan Lilja (Ed.), *Transactions of the 9th International Congress on Cleft Palate and Related Anomalies* (pp. 427–428). Gothenburg: Erlanders Novum.

Hortis-Dzierzbicka, M., & Tarnowski, A. (2003, November). *Investigations into later histories of children born with orofacial clefts*. Abstracts from the 7th European Craniofacial Congress, Bologna, Italy

Hortis-Dzierzbicka, M., Dudkiewica, Z., Kulewicz, M., Surowiec, Z., & Piwowar. W.

(2004, March). *Single stage lip and palate repair in UCLP—A within center study of three surgical modalities for hard palate repair.* Paper presented at the 61st Annual Meeting of the American Cleft Palate-Craniofacial Association, Chicago.

Imatomi, S. (2005). Effects of breathy voice source on ratings of hypernasality. *Cleft Palate-Craniofacial Journal, 42*, 641-648.

Izdebski, K. (1983). Overpressure and breathiness in spastic dysphonia. An acoustic (LTAS) and perceptual study. *Acta Otolaryngologica Scandinavia, 97,* 122-129.

Izdebski, K. (2008). Clinical voice assessment: The role and value of the phonatory function studies. In A. Lalwani (ed.), *Current diagnosis and treatment. Otolaryngology Head and Neck Surgery,.* (416-429). New York: McGraw Hill, Lange.

Karling, J., Larson, O., Leanderson, R., & Henningsson, G. (1993). Speech in unilateral and bilateral cleft palate patients from Stockholm. *Cleft Palate-Craniofacial Journal, 30*(1), 73-77.

Laukkanen, A. M., Björkner, E., & Sundberg, J. (2005). Throaty voice quality: Subglottal pressure, voice source, and formant characteristics. *Journal of Voice, 20*, 25-37.

Leder, S. B. & Lerman, J. W. (1985) Some acoustic evidence for vocal abuse in adult speakers with repaired cleft palate. *Laryngoscope, 95*, 837-840.

Łobacz, P. (1996). Polska fonologia dzieci ca. *Palate-Craniofacial Journal, 36,* 441-446. Warsaw, Poland: Ed. Energeia.

McWilliams B. J. & Paradise, L. P. (1973). Educational, Occupational, and mariatal status of cleft palate adults. *Cleft Palate Journal, 10*, 223-229.

Marks, C. R., Barker, K., & Tardy, M. E., Jr. (1971). Prevalence of perceived acoustic deviations related to laryngeal function among subjects with palatal anomalies. *Cleft Palate Journal, 8*, 201-211.

Markuson, A., Akerlind, I., & Paulin, G. (2001). Quality of life in adults with repaired complete cleft lip and palate. *Cleft Palate-Craniofacial Journal, 38*, 379-385.

McGregor, F. C. (1990). Facial disfigurement: Problems and management of social interaction and implications for mental health. *Aesthetic Plastic Surgery, 14*, 249-257.

McWilliams, B. J., Bluestone, C. D., & Musgrave, R. H. (1969). Diagnostic implications of vocal cord nodules in children with cleft palate. *Laryngoscope, 79*, 2072-2080.

McWilliams, B. J., Lavorato, A. S., & Bluestone, C. D. (1973). Vocal cord abnormalities in children with velopharyngeal valving problems. *Laryngoscope, 11*, 1745-1753.

Nandurkar, A. (2002). Nasalance measures in Marathi consonant-vowel-consonant syllables with pressure consonants produced by children with and without cleft lip and palate. *Cleft Palate-Craniofacial Journal, 39*(1), 59-65.

Niedzielska, G. (2005). Acoustic estimation of voice when incorrect resonance function of the nose takes place. *International Journal of Pediatric Otorhinolaryngology, 69*(8), 1065-1069.

Peterson-Falzone, S., Hardin-Jones, M., & Karnell, M. (2001). *Cleft palate speech* (3rd ed.). St. Louis, MO: Mosby.

Pulkkinen, J., Ranta, R., Haapanen, M. L., Heliovaara, A., & Laitinen, J. (2002). Associations between lateral cephalometric dimensions and misarticulations of Finnish dental consonants in cleft lip/palate children. *Folia Phoniatrica et Logopaedia, 54*(5), 240-246.

Reed, J., Robathan, M., Hockenhull, A., Rostill, H., Perrett, D., & Lees, A. (1999). Children's attitudes toward interacting with peers with different craniofacial anomalies. *Cleft Palate-Craniofacial Journal, 36*, 441-446.

Richman, L. C., Eliason, M. J., & Lindgren, S. (1988). Reading disability in children with clefts. *Cleft Palate Journal, 25*, 21-25.

Rubach, J. (2003, November). *Linguistic Inquiry, 34*(4), 601-629(29).

Schneiderman, C. R., & Harding, J. B. (1984). Social ratings of children with cleft lip by school peers. *Cleft Palate Journal, 21*, 219-223.

Shaw, W., Semb, G., Nelson, P., Brattstrom, V., Molsted, K., & Prahl-Andersen, B. (2001). *The Eurocleft Project 1996-2000. Standards of care for cleft lip & palate in Europe.* Amsterdam: IOS Press.

Sjölander, P., & Sundberg, J. (2004). Spectrum effects of subglottal pressure variation in professional baritone singers. *Journal of the Acoustical Society of America, 115*(3), 1270-1273.

Stathopoulos, E. T. (1986). Relationship between intraoral air pressure and vocal intensity in children and adults. *Journal of Speech and Hearing Disorders, 29*, 71-74.

Tobiasen, J. M., & Hiebert, J. M. (1993). Combined effects of severity of cleft impairment and facial attractiveness on social perception: An experimental study. *Cleft Palate-Craniofacial Journal, 30*, 82-86.

Van Lierde, K. M., De Bodt, M., Baetens, I., Schrauwen, V., & Van Cauwenberge, P. (2003). Outcome of treatment regarding articulation, resonance and voice in Flemish adults with unilateral and bilateral cleft palate. *Folia Phoniatrica et Logopaedia, 55*(2), 80-90.

Warren, D. W., Dalston, R. M., Morr, K. E., Hairfield, W. M., & Smith, L. R. (1989). The speech regulating system: Temporal and aerodynamic responses to velopharyngeal inadequacy. *Journal of Speech and Hearing Research, 32*, 566-575.

Watson, A. C., Sell, D. A., & Grunwell, P. (2001). Management of cleft lip and palate. London: Whurr.

Zajac, D. J. (1995). Laryngeal airway resistance in children with cleft palate and adequate velopharyngeal function. *Cleft Palate-Craniofacial Journal, 32*, 138-144.

CHAPTER 6

The Estill Voice Model: Physiology of Emotion

Kimberly M. Steinhauer and Jo Estill

Abstract

The Estill Voice Model evolved over the past 25 years. The model comprises two levels: (1) *Compulsory Figures for Voice Control*© and (2) *Figure Combinations for Six Voice Qualities*,© through which the tools for concise production of a myriad of voice qualities are provided to anyone who can make a sound. Many of the qualities are derived from basic, primal, and universal emotional prompts that are practiced throughout the model. Estill Voice Model may be defined as *emotion on pitch* and offers specific options for all vocalists of all genres to communicate their vocal emotions both safely and effectively.

Introduction

Voice motor control involves a complex relationship among anatomy, physiology, environment, and task that becomes more complicated when taken to the expert level—acting or singing. The number of voice qualities produced from the dynamic interactions among these systems is limitless, and inspires heated debate when voice professionals attempt to explain voice quality or singing. For example, *singing* can be anything from a

Russian lament, an Anglican choir boy chant, an American country music ballad, to an African song of worship and praise. In this instance, the definition of singing would vary on the basis of stylistic and emotional impact on the voice quality. If not careful, the esthetic bias of the *definer* can greatly sway the forthcoming *definition* and, thus, the results of *scientific* research on voice quality.

Voice pedagogues have explained singing as a sustained vocalization powered by airflow via the respiratory system, converted to a sound source via oscillation of the two vocal folds, and filtered via resonant properties of the vocal tract. This simplistic representation works until the degrees of freedom are factored in for each subsystem of voice. In other words, the sound generated by the vocal folds is dependent upon their length, tension, and mass in isolation or a combination thereof. Usually, lengthening the vocal folds will increase the tension and decrease the mass that, in turn, will facilitate a higher rate of oscillation—or higher pitch. However, if a singer deliberately holds the mass *degree of freedom* at a constant thickness to produce a powerful pop ballad, Broadway belt, or Shakespearean monologue, then lengthening the vocal folds alone may not be enough to increase the pitch. Another mechanism, such as increased activity in the vocalis muscle, might be engaged to sing higher.

The Estill Voice Model was the first comprehensive system to address this daunting issue of degrees of freedom in voice motor control by isolating the *craft* of voice production from the *artistry* and *performance magic*. In the Compulsory Figures for Voice Control (Estill, 1982; 1992; 1997a; 1997b; Klimek, Obert, & Steinhauer, 2005a; 2005b), 13 anatomical structures were identified as integral to the production of voice quality; i.e., manipulating the degrees of freedom for each structure independently resulted in categorical changes in voice quality. Estill patterned the exercises for the Compulsory Figures after the training regimen of ice skaters, in which they moved their blades in various positions to create initial basic shapes that led to artistic masterpieces. With the Compulsory Figures for Voice Control, the first level in the model, speakers and singers create specific sounds by moving each structure into one of two or three positions (degrees of freedom) for artistic vocal expression (Figure 6–1). In the next level, the Figures are combined to produce six basic voice qualities that Estill used as a framework for her research. This research for the Estill Voice Model began with multiple studies of one subject producing many repetitions of all vocalizations, as found in psychoacoustic paradigms (Estill, 1983; 1984; Estill, Kobayashi, Honda, & Kakita, 1990; Honda & Estill, 1986); however, ensuing seminal publications documented these voice quality variations across many subjects and tasks (Colton & Estill, 1981; Yanagisawa, Citardi, & Estill, 1996; Yanagisawa, Estill, Kmucha, & Leder, 1989; Yanagisawa, Kmucha, & Estill, 1990a; 1990b; Yanagisawa, Mambrino, Estill, & Talkin, 1991).

Structures manipulated in the Estill Voice Model include true vocal folds, false vocal folds, aryepiglottic sphincter, velum, vertebral posture, laryngeal height, cricoid cartilage, thyroid cartilage, tongue, lips, and jaw. Presently, we are aware that purely isolated movement of laryngeal structures is improbable; however, distinct and categorical perceptual changes are achieved when producing each option for each Figure as independently as possible

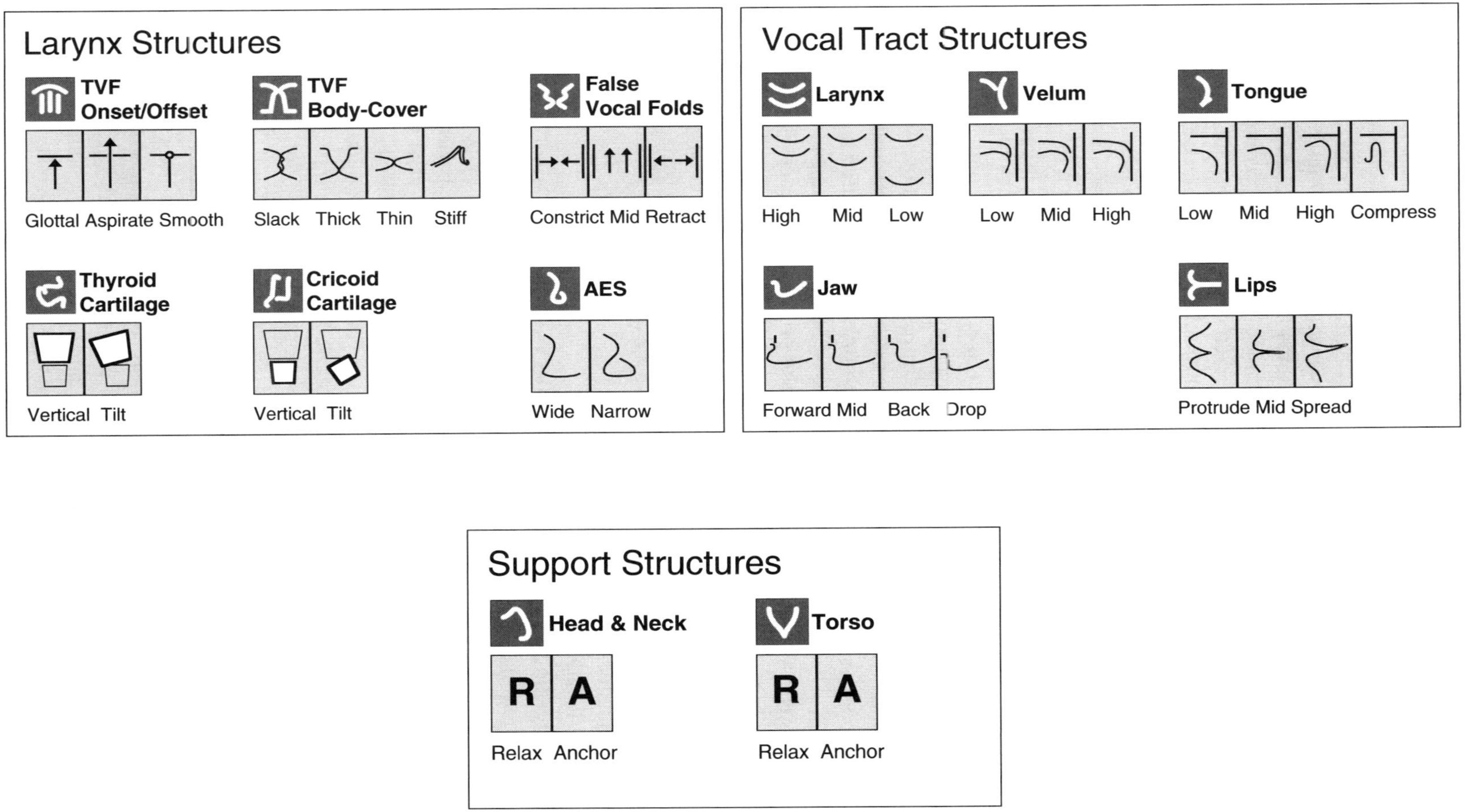

Figure 6–1. Overview of voice structures and options for the Compulsory Figures for Voice Control.

(Colton & Estill, 1981). In the Estill Voice Model, the production and teaching of each Figure is verified not only by auditory perceptual sound of the quality, but also by bodily kinesthetic perception of effort, visuo-perceptual acoustic feedback, and videoendoscopy. The following summary of the Estill Voice Model begins with the Compulsory Figures for Voice Control, Level One, and moves to Figure Combinations for Six Voice Qualities, Level Two. Interestingly, almost all of the Compulsory Figures for Voice Control are elicited via emotional prompts such as laugh, whine, or sob; therefore, the essential emotional physiology associated with each voice quality is also included.

The Estill Voice Model: Compulsory Figures for Voice Control

People are heard to vocalize in many different voice qualities that vary according to geographic location, language, culture, education, speaking environment, audience, and emotional state. An investigation of each of the voice qualities posed such a formidable task that Colton and Estill (1981) proposed studying a limited number of voice qualities associated with different genres of music. This early research led to the genesis of the Estill Voice Model and the specific exercises designed to isolate voice quality variations according to anatomy and physiology called Compulsory Figures for Voice Control (CFVC). Although she sang "The Sound of Music," Estill was more interested in "The Sound of Muscles."

Originally, the CFVC were presented hierarchically according to their contributions to Power, Source, and Filter properties of voice motor control, as consistent with the theory by Fant (1960). However, recent theories of dynamical systems (Kelso, 1995; Wallace, 1996) embrace voice motor control as more interactive and heterarchical than initially implied by the Source-Filter Theory. Therefore, the CFVC currently are organized by anatomical position of the 13 structures and their relationship to the larynx, vocal tract, or support (see Figure 6-1 and Figure 6-2). The description of each figure includes the options for each exercise and the accompanying emotional percept for the Estill Voice Model. Estill presents the options for each Figure categorically to maximally exploit the corresponding differences in voice quality; of course, the changes attributed to the production of each Figure can be produced on a categorical or continuous spectrum. Finally, Estill intends that each option for each CFVC be produced across the range for every pitch and every vowel.

True Vocal Folds: Onset/Offset

The true vocal folds (TVF) can be controlled by the delicate balance of intrinsic laryngeal muscles at the onset and offset of any tone (Moore, 1938; Steinhauer, Grayhack, Smiley-Oyen, Shaiman, & McNeil, 2004). The three TVF onset/offset options include: *glottal, aspirate*, and *smooth*. Each option is explained according to tone onset; however, the exact configurations can be applied to stopping the sound at the end of vocalization, as well. In the glottal onset, the TVF are adducted tightly before releasing the air for phonation, resulting in a pop as in the surprised exclamation, "Uh-Oh!" In the aspirate onset, the TVF are not

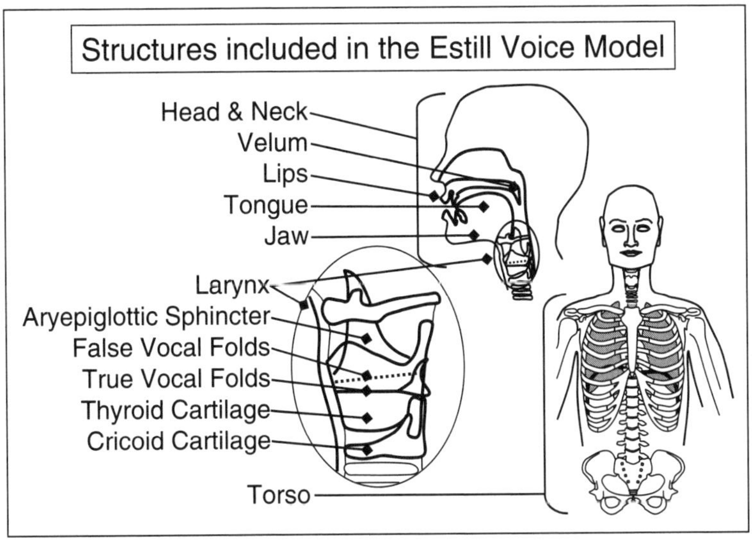

Figure 6–2. Anatomical structures controlled in the Estill Voice Model.

tightly adducted and allow an audible air stream to precede the phonation in two manners: abrupt and gradual. The TVF may suddenly close following the airflow producing an *aspirate abrupt* onset sounding like the jolly exclamation from Santa Claus' "Ho, Ho, Ho!" Or the TVF may carefully adduct after the airflow producing an *aspirate gradual* onset sounding like the sexy ingénue á la Marilyn Monroe in "Happy Birthday, Mr. President." In the smooth onset, the airflow and TVF adduction are coordinated simultaneously to produce easy voicing. The smooth onset is heard in Western classical singing to initiate a pure, clearly suspended vowel as in the first phrase of Schubert's "Ave Maria."

False Vocal Folds

Highly controversial is Estill's inclusion of the false vocal folds (FVF) in the model. Early on, Estill observed independent control of the true and false vocal folds during various vocal functions (Yanagisawa et al., 1990a). Further study confirmed the isolated manipulation of these structures in even more subjects (Yanagisawa et al., 1996). The exact mechanism for retraction of the FVF is unclear, although Kotby and Haugen (1970) observed long ago that extrinsic muscles, such as the sternothyroid, may be responsible. The three options for FVF control include: *constrict, mid*, and *retract*. When the FVF constrict, they adduct and produce a harsh, guttural sound elicited through effortful bearing down. In a mid position, the FVF are comfortably abducted and the resulting tone is relatively clear. To retract the FVF, a speaker must pretend to silently laugh or cry with high emotion (but never constriction) while producing the tone to obtain maximal abduction. *FVF retraction* promotes healthy, safe vocalization by freeing the TVF to oscillate in any configuration, and thus diminishing detrimental constrictive compression in the laryngeal vestibule that may occur when accessing tenuous voice qualities or even higher pitches.

True Vocal Folds: Body-Cover

In the body-cover model of vocal fold vibration (Hirano, 1974), Hirano assigned a functional grouping to the complex morphology of the TVF layers that Estill integrated into this Figure. In addition, the complex relationship among TVF length, tension, and mass involved in producing pitch, quality, and intensity (Hirano, Vennard, & Ohala, 1970) was also incorporated into this second CFVC exploiting TVF. The four options for TVF: body-cover include: *thick, thin, stiff,* and *slack*. Although these descriptors obviously mix TVF mass (thick, thin) with tension properties (stiff, slack), the terms imply separate percepts that remain meaningful across disciplines and for that reason have remained as a part of the Estill Voice Model (Estill & Moore, 1975; Honda & Estill, 1986).

In *thick TVF: body-cover*, the body mass is full and the cover is pliant. This configuration leads to a vibratory cycle with a long closed. Thick TVF productions sound like a loud modal speech quality or a chest voice singing quality. The emotive percept is authoritative, sincere, and heard in the voice of news broadcasters.

A *thin TVF: body-cover* quality is produced by decreasing vocal fold body mass and still maintaining a pliant flexible cover. The closed phase for the thin vibratory cycle is shorter than that for the thick production, thus eliciting a soft but clear voice quality as in upper class, snobby British speech or in a non-breathy, pure singing "head voice."

A *stiff TVF: body-cover* occurs by elongating and tightening both the body and cover, thus leading to the shortest closed phase. The production of the stiff TVF may be facilitated by a higher posterior plane of the TVF due to the apex of the arytenoid cartilages rocking backward (Hollien, 1983). The resulting soft, breathy voice quality is categorized as both weak and sexy and heard as a breathy falsetto singing voice. Also, a shift in TVF plane causing an abrupt change in mass from thick to thin results in a yodel. Clearly, TVF: body-cover is related closely to the register notion in voice production; however, Estill posits that, unlike registers, these previous three conditions of TVF: body-cover are *not* dependent upon the fundamental frequency (F_0) of vocal fold vibration and can be produced throughout the entire pitch range with varying degrees of difficulty and risk.

Slack was added recently as an option to TVF: body-cover. In this condition, vocal fold body and cover are loose resulting in pulselike vibrations indicative of vocal fry. A disengaged, relaxed phonation is emoted in slack productions. Existing research has shown that vocal fry is produced only at a low F_0; however, more research may bear otherwise.

Thyroid Cartilage

The thyroid cartilage, as part of the larger laryngeal framework, is known to tilt forward with high pitches, yet it can be tilted forward at any F_0 or be held constant within a vertical plane (Honda & Estill, 1986). Possible mechanisms for thyroid positioning include a delicate balance between extrinsic and intrinsic laryngeal muscles that either stabilize or free the cartilage to tilt for a desired size of the crico-thyroid space (Kotby & Haugen, 1970). The two options for thyroid cartilage include *vertical* and *tilt*. The vertical thyroid position elicits a thicker voice quality void of sweetness, yet a "real" speech quality necessary for pop and folk singing. Since the vocal folds are connected anteriorly to the thyroid notch, maintaining a vertical position of the thyroid cartilage at higher pitches is a challenge. The tilted thyroid position generates a clarity and sweetness in the tone due to the lengthening of the vocal folds that can be triggered by whimpering. The thyroid tilt also creates the pure tone common to classical bel canto singing.

Cricoid Cartilage

Another alternative for manipulating the crico-thyroid space is via the cricoid cartilage Figure. TVF configurations will be affected by cricoid position because the arytenoids sit atop the cricoid lamina. The two options for cricoid cartilage include *vertical* and *tilt*. The basic condition of vertical cricoid cartilage occurs naturally in quiet breathing and almost all other voice qualities. In cricoid cartilage tilt, the anterior portion of the cricoid tilts forward, thus raising the posterior lamina, moving the arytenoids forward, and shortening and thickening the TVF. The result of this motion is a loud, but unconstricted, shout for joy that can be elicited with a "*Yay!*" The cricoid tilt enables the belter to maintain the powerful thick TVF: body-cover throughout the entire pitch range. The underlying mechanics of cricoid tilting is not anatomically obvious (Kotby & Haugen, 1970), yet this posture is observed often in videoendoscopy of the belt voice quality (Yanagisawa et al., 1989).

Larynx

The entire vocal tract can be lengthened or shortened using the Larynx CFVF. The three options for larynx are based upon position in the vocal tract, and include: *mid, low,* and *high*. Mid larynx occurs during quiet breathing and the production of a neutral modal speech. High larynx is produced by contraction of the same supra-laryngeal muscles that raise the larynx for swallowing. The sound created by the short vocal tract of the high larynx is bright and naive like that of the munchkins singing in *The Wizard of Oz*. A low larynx is achieved via contraction of the infrahyoid muscles. This lowering lengthens the vocal tract and in turn darkens the sound substantially as in sobbed speech or opera singing.

Velum

The velum (soft palate) functions like a door that opens or closes the entranceway from the oropharynx (mouth) to the nasopharynx (nose). This doorway is called the velopharyngeal port and its position greatly affects voice quality (Yanagisawa, Mambrino, Estill, & Talkin, 1991). Three options for velum control include: *low, mid,* and *high*. In low velum, the palatopharyngeus, palatoglossus, and possibly the tensor veli palatini combine to lower the velum and open the velopharyngeal port totally so that the resulting sound is a nasal consonant such as *m, n,* or *ng*. When the coordination between these structures balances for the mid velum option, the velopharyngeal port is half open and the corresponding percept is a nasalized vowel found in French or Spanish or the sound of deaf speech. Mid velum singing is acceptable as a color in Broadway, country, or some folk singing. The high velum option is accomplished via contraction of the levator veli palatini and superior pharyngeal constrictor. This action closes the velopharyngeal port and leads to a totally oral, open sound used in almost all speech or song.

Tongue

The manipulation of the tongue in the CFVC concerns mainly the dorsum and can change the shape of the vocal tract, thus leading to changes in voice quality (Honda, Hirai, Estill, & Takahura, 1995). The four options for tongue include: *high, mid, low,* and compressed. In the high tongue option, the dorsum of the tongue remains lifted high against the hard palate as in the vowel /i/. The percept is bright for the production of all vowels and consonants. In the mid tongue option, the dorsum is in a central position in the oral cavity. The percept is a neutral, Standard American English phonetic quality. In the low tongue option, the dorsum is pressed low and flat leading to a dark quality because the pushing down on the tongue dorsum may lead to lowering the larynx. Low tongue is the only tongue posture that compromises the integrity of the vowel. In the compressed tongue option, the dorsum is pushed forward and the tongue tip curled back. This option expands the pharynx in the anteroposterior position, thus providing a darker tone without lowering the larynx. Compressed tongue is especially useful to opera singers who desire a dark tone but need to maintain the *squillo* or ring in the voice produced with a higher larynx position.

Aryepiglottic Sphincter

Manipulating the size of the epilaryngeal space above the true vocal folds via the aryepiglottic sphincter can greatly affect the brightness and power in voice quality. The two options for aryepiglottic sphincter include *wide* and *narrow*. Vocalizations with a wide aryepiglottic sphincter sound warm and rounded. In the narrow aryepiglottic sphincter condition, the epilaryngeal space gets smaller leading to a loud, bright (some say annoying) twang percept that sounds like a witch cackling or a duck quacking. The voice is amplified with piercing intensity because of an increase in energy between 2.8 and 4.3 kHz that corresponds with the resonant frequency of the external auditory meatus; as a result, fundamental frequencies below 1.0 kHz receive a boost of 15–20 dB in sound transmitted to the middle ear without an increase in vocal effort by the speaker (Yanagisawa et al., 1989). The arrow aryepiglottic sphincter CFVC has been exploited by expert speakers and opera singers to boost vocal resonance or *squillo* and is referred to as the speaker's ring or singer's formant (Yanagisawa et al., 1989; Yanagisawa et al., 1996).

Jaw

Moving the lower jaw (mandible) in various positions can affect the color of the voice, extraneous facial and neck tension, and sometimes the intelligibility of the speech. Options for the jaw CFVC include: *forward, mid, back,* and *drop.* With forward jaw, the chin is jutted forward moving the lower teeth in front of the upper teeth, producing an unrefined percept like that heard in old New York gangster films. The mid jaw condition is produced by slightly releasing the jaw in a relaxed position that optimizes jaw alignment. This mid jaw posture, in which the temporomandibular joint (TMJ) moves freely without extraneous tension, is the desired option for most speakers and singers. In the back jaw option, the lower teeth are pulled far back behind the upper teeth in a pronounced overbite. The resulting vocal percept is a full, dark color that is sometimes exploited by Western classical singers. The actor using back jaw sounds and appears a bit dimwitted. In the drop jaw condition, the jaw is lowered as far as possible producing a dark and sometimes "hooty" sound.

Lips

Lip position affects the length of the vocal tract and therefore affects the resonant tone of the speaker. The three options for lips can vary continuously, yet are presented in the Estill Voice Model categorically and include: *protrude, mid,* and *spread.* A speaker using the protrude lip CFVC extends the lips far forward of the face, thus lengthening the tube of the vocal tract, lowering corresponding vowel formants, and darkening the voice quality that is identified as "high-brow." In the mid lip position, the lips are neutral or relaxed for a normal speech or singing quality. The spread lip option is produced by smiling broadly, which in turn shortens the vocal tract and brightens the tone that sounds and looks sunny or happy.

Head and Neck

A tenet of the Estill Voice Model states that as the skeletal structures of the head and neck are anchored or braced, the smaller muscles that control the vocal mechanism work optimally to fine-tune adjustments within this stable external framework (Estill, 1990). Outcomes of head and neck control are postural alignment and intensity modification. The primary muscles recruited for head and neck anchoring are in the nasopharynx (velum), the nape of the neck, and the sides of the neck (sternocleidomastoid). The two options for head and neck anchoring include relax and anchor. In the relax head and neck state, the cervical vertebrae are somewhat curved and compressed leading to suboptimal posture and an "unsupported," flat voice quality. By contrast, the anchor head and neck option engages the sternocleidomastoid and velum, thereby aligning the cervical vertebrae for a "supported" voice quality that increases in intensity and energy.

Torso

As in head and neck control, the muscles recruited for torso control act as a postural anchor so that the respiratory muscles work efficiently. Estill identified the latissimus dorsi, the pectoralis major, and the quadratus lumborum as possible torso anchoring muscles. The two conditions for torso anchoring include *relax* and *anchor*. The relax condition is assumed by sitting or standing in a comfortably upright posture without slumping. The resulting sound is characterized as "nice" but not exciting. In the torso anchor position, the shoulders drop slightly and the sternum lifts while the rib cage widens and elevates for maximal production. The experience noted by speakers during the torso anchor is a feeling of breath support and energized, intense vocalizations, also noted in head and neck anchor.

Additional Elements of Compulsory Figures for Voice Control

Effort

One overarching element of CFVC concerns the subjective effort employed in the control of each of the above anatomical structures. In the Estill Voice Model, effort level is identified in each of the structures and not limited to pulmonary force (Colton & Estill, 1981; Estill, 1982). In addition, effort extends from minimum to most comfortable to maximum and is not necessarily associated with sound intensity but with the amount of work sensed at each structure. Thus, a loud tone, as in belting, can require a great effort in various parts of the total instrument, yet remain at a most comfortable vocal effort (MCVE) at the larynx. Often, the resulting production of belting is judged by the performer to be "effortless" or "easy."

Using the concept of magnitude estimation and magnitude production developed by S. S. Stevens (1940), vocalists assign numbers to each task and sense effort in several forms. Effort can be steady, as in anchoring; variable, as in accessing different frequencies in the singing of a musical scale; or periodic, as in the firm articulation of consonants in repeated syllables. These types of effort may occur simultaneously and should be monitored to varying degrees by the performer. The rules for monitoring effort in CFVC include: (a) locate the work; (b) assign it a number (1 to 10, or 1 to infinity); (c) maintain the number while singing, speaking, or producing specific relaxation maneuvers in other parts of the body. Effort monitoring is used constantly, especially at the larynx, so that trauma or risk to the vocal folds is minimized during production of every Figure.

Breath

One glaring and provocative omission in the Compulsory Figures for Voice Control is breathing exercises. Estill maintains that the breath will "free vary" depending upon the configuration of the larynx and resonators for a particular quality (Estill, 1982). Support for this hypothesis is found in early research on prephonatory tuning of the larynx (Gould & Okamura, 1974) that showed motor unit activity in the larynx preceded that of the respiratory muscles even before a sound was made. Current Dynamical theories (Kelso, 1995; Wallace, 1996) that promote organic reorganization of systems according to motor targets also provide a framework that embraces this tenet. Although a specific Figure for breath does not exist, monitoring and observing respiratory consequences of each CFVC is encouraged throughout the model.

The Estill Voice Model: Figure Combinations for Six Voice Qualities

Although the possibilities for voice quality variation provided by the Compulsory Figures for Voice Control are limitless, Estill chose six distinct and arbitrary Figure combinations to study: speech, falsetto, sob, twang, opera, and belting. The scientific framework used to select and operationalize these qualities began with investigations by Colton and Estill (1981) into the physiologic, acoustic, and perceptual characteristics of voice quality. The Estill Voice Model began with four qualities (speech, sob, twang, and opera) and by 1986 (Honda & Estill, 1986) two more qualities (falsetto and belt) were added. Estill emphasized continuously that the voice qualities are color variations that are *not* frequency dependent and can be produced throughout the entire pitch range (Estill, Fujimura, Sawada, & Beechler, 1994). This explanation delineates the voice qualitics from the common definition of a voice register that is frequency dependent. Figure 6-3 shows Figure "recipes" for the six voice qualities. Each quality in the model has been operationalized on six levels: physiology, acoustics, perception, risks, limitations, and applications. For the purposes of this chapter, the voice qualities will be described according to all levels, with the exception of physiology, which is already represented in Figure 6-3.

Speech Quality

Speech quality, identified as modal speech by voice scientists, is heard in everyday conversation, particularly from TV newscasters and radio announcers. Singers describe it as "chest voice" and use speech quality in folk songs, jazz, pop, early music, musical theater, and even opera recitative.

STRUCTURE OPTIONS — ESTILL VOICE MODEL — WORKSHEET — LEVEL TWO: Six Voice Qualities

	TVF1			FVF			TVF2				THY		CRI		AES		LARYNX			TONGUE				VELUM			JAW				LIPS			H&N		TOR	
OPTIONS	glottal	aspirate	smooth	constrict	mid	retract	slack	thick	thin	stiff	vertical	tilt	vertical	tilt	wide	narrow	low	mid	high	low	mid	high	compress	low	mid	high	forward	mid	back	drop	protrude	mid	spread	relax (R)	anchor (A)	relax (R)	anchor (A)
Speech	X				X			X			X		X		X			X			X					X		X				X		X		X	
Falsetto		X			X					X	X		X		X			X			X					X		X				X		X		X	
Sob			X			X			X			X			X		X					X				X		X				X			X		X
Twang-N			X			X			X			X	X			X			X			X			X			X				X		X		X	
Twang			X			X			X			X	X			X			X			X				X		X				X		X		X	
Opera			X			X		X↔	X			X	X			X	X						X			X		X				X			X		X
Belting	X					X		X			X			X		X			X			X				X		X				X			X		X

EFFORT DIAL MIN MAX

KEY TO ABBREVIATIONS
TVF1 = True Vocal Fold: Onset/Offset FVF = False Vocal Folds TVF2 = True Vocal Fold: Body-Cover THY = Thyroid Cartilage CRI = Cricoid Cartilage AES = Aryepiglottic Sphincter H&N = Head & Neck TOR = Torso

Figure 6–3. Figure combinations for six voice qualities in the Estill Voice Model.

Acoustics

The power spectra reveal a negative slope in the amplitude of the partials.

Perception

The sound has a comfortable presence and is easily heard in the lower pitch range.

Risks

Since the true vocal folds need to oscillate with a thick mass, the risk of constriction rises when speech quality is produced at higher pitches.

Limitations

Speech quality is most effective and powerful in the lower part of the pitch range. The tone is thinner and unpleasing in the upper range.

Applications

Speech quality enables highly intelligible diction; therefore, this color is effective for music in which a speechlike sound is desired for expression of the lyrics, e.g., pop music, patter songs, opera recitative.

Falsetto Quality

Falsetto quality is the soft, breathy voice heard in the higher ranges of male a cappella groups, boy choirs, and by Julia Child and Marilyn Monroe. The common definition of falsetto implies that this quality is only produced at high pitches, but not in the Estill Voice Model.

Acoustics

Falsetto productions reveal very little intensity above 1 kHz and much interharmonic noise.

Perception

Falsetto is flutelike and conveys a purity or naiveté in tone. Falsetto has no vibrato and resembles a blown tone.

Risks

There is very little risk to falsetto due to the minimal closed phase of vocal fold oscillation.

Limitations

Falsetto is more powerful in the higher pitches, but it generally lacks intensity of sound and emotion.

Applications

Men can sing falsetto for treble voice parts, and this quality is useful for stylistic expression in early music, Celtic, and pop singing.

Sob Quality

Sob quality is the sound associated with dynamically suppressed but intensely soft sobbing. The low larynx contributes to the very dark sound and can be heard in Russian choral pieces, medieval chanting, and very soft lullabies.

Acoustics

Sob quality spectra reveal low amplitude in the higher partials and minimal interharmonic noise.

Perception

The sob quality appears distant, dark, repressed, muffled, and extremely soft to the listener.

Risks

The thin true vocal folds barely adduct in sob quality, leading to very little risk in production.

Limitations

Sob quality is never loud.

Applications

Sob quality is ideal for soft singing, especially "marking" during a musical rehearsal and Lied singing. The pianissimo extremes of the messa di voce are facilitated quite effectively with this quality.

Twang Quality

Twang quality is commonly used for speaking in noisy environments or large rooms. The sound is reedy and piercing and described as unpleasant and annoying to those listeners who use a quieter mode for communication. In the Estill Voice Model, twang is operationalized as either nasal or oral in order to emphasize that this piercing color often referred to as nasal can in fact be produced in both manners; therefore, the model provides a recipe for nasal twang and for oral twang. The following explanation covers both types of productions.

Acoustics

The hallmark characteristic of both nasal and oral twang is a spectral increase in intensity between 2.5 and 3.5 kHz due to the narrowing of the aryepiglottic sphincter. This frequency region is known as the *singer's formant* and is exploited by power speakers and singers.

Perception

Listeners describe this quality as penetrating, brassy, bright, twangy, and nasal; however, the physiologic production can be nasal or oral depending upon velar position during the narrowing of the aryepiglottic sphincter for the twang quality.

Risks

The risks of twang quality are minimal *if* retraction of the false vocal folds is maintained during the production. Narrowing of the epilaryngeal space may trigger increased oscillation of the true vocal folds due to a dynamical interaction between source and filter properties of voice production (Titze & Story, 1996); therefore, effort at the true vocal fold is always monitored for safety.

Limitations

Twang is difficult to produce at lower pitches and is always *loud*.

Applications

Pure twang can be used for character voices and is used in various amounts in country and folk singing. Also, twang has been used successfully as a treatment for hypophonic voice due to vocal fold paralysis or paresis (Lombard, 2001; Steinhauer, Lombard, & Eichhorn, 2005).

Opera Quality

Although descriptions of opera singing vary widely, the Estill Voice Model defines *opera quality* as the full, rich, powerful classical quality with ring or *squillo*. The Seven-Part Figure for Opera Quality (Estill,

1997; Estill & Colton, 2001; Klimek et al., 2005b) clearly produces the sound Estill describes as opera in this model. The early perceptual research in opera quality (Colton & Estill, 1981) revealed that it was misidentified as other qualities including speech, sob, and twang. Estill posited that the incorrect naming of this quality was due to the fact that opera is a mixture of many qualities and is dynamic in nature depending upon the theatrical context.

Acoustics

Spectral peaks around 1 kHz and 3 kHz are present in opera productions. Vibrato, as modulating frequency and amplitude, is always evident.

Perception

Listeners perceive opera quality as a dark and brilliant "trained" sound that is always accompanied by vibrato.

Risks

Since the opera quality is such a highly intense sound with a thicker mass and longer closed phase than the other qualities, the risks of vocal fold trauma increase if effort monitoring at the true vocal folds is minimized.

Limitations

Opera is not suitable for all genres of music, and vibrato can become extreme if not evaluated often.

Applications

Opera quality can "cut through" a large orchestral accompaniment due to the addition of *squillo* via aryepiglottic narrowing. This quality is demanded in operas by Verdi or Wagner or with heavily orchestrated scores. It is heard sometimes in Shakespearean speech.

Belt Quality

Belt is the loud quality made famous by Ethel Merman and heard on playgrounds, in ethnic speech, school cafeterias, market places, noisy environments, or outdoor political events. The quality is alarmingly loud if produced in a small space.

Acoustics

Overall, belting reveals higher amplitudes throughout the spectrum as a whole.

Perception

Belt quality is loud, bright, and brassy—although less so than pure twang.

Risks

Due to the long closed phase and very thick oscillating mass of the true vocal folds, the risk of trauma is high if optimum conditions are not maintained.

Limitations

Belting is always loud. A change in intensity results in a switch to another quality.

Applications

The excitement of belting is heard often in American musical theater, rock, pop, and gospel music.

Conclusion

The Estill Voice Model evolved over the past 25 years into a comprehensive system for evaluating, teaching, and producing voice qualities. The two levels of the model, Compulsory Figures for Voice Control and Figure Combinations for Six Voice Qualities, provide the tools for concise production of a myriad of voice qualities and are available to anyone who can make a sound. Many of the qualities are elicited from basic, primal, and universal emotional prompts that are practiced throughout the model. Estill began her journey explaining the anatomy and physiology behind the emotion; still presently, singing in the Estill Voice Model may be defined as *emotion on pitch*. The Estill Voice Model offers specific options for all vocalists of all genres to communicate their emotion both safely and effectively.

Acknowledgment. The authors are indebted to Mary McDonald Klimek for producing the figure illustrations.

References

Colton, R. H., & Estill, J. (1981). Elements of voice quality: Perceptual, acoustic and physiological aspects. In N. Lass (Ed.), *Speech and language: Advances in basic research and practice* (pp. 311-403). New York: Academic Press.

Estill, J. (1982). The control of voice quality. In V. Lawrence (Ed.), *Transcripts of the 11th Symposium: Care of the Professional Voice* (pp. 152-168). New York: The Voice Foundation.

Estill, J. (1983). The control of pitch and voice quality, Part I: An EMG study of supralaryngeal muscles. In V. Lawrence (Ed.), *Transcripts of the 11th Symposium: Care of the Professional Voice* (pp. 152-168). New York: The Voice Foundation.

Estill, J. (1984). The control of pitch and quality, Part II: An EMG study of infrahyoid muscles. In V. Lawrence (Ed.), *Transcripts of the 11th Symposium: Care of the Professional Voice* (pp. 152-168). New York: The Voice Foundation.

Estill, J. (1990). Lateral x-rays of the anchoring posture in six voice qualities. [Unpublished data].

Estill, J. (1992). *Basic figures and exercise manual.* New York: Imagetech.

Klimek, M., Obert, K. & Steinhauer, K. (2005). *The Estill Voice Training System Level One: Compulsory figures for voice control.* Pittsburgh, PA: Estill Voice Training Systems International.

Klimek, M., Obert, K. & Steinhauer, K. (2005). *The Estill Voice Training System Level Two: Figure combinations for six voice qualities*. Pittsburgh, PA: Estill Voice Training Systems International.

Estill, J., & Colton, R. (2001). *Seven physiological steps to an opera quality*. Paper presented at the 30th Annual Symposium: Care of the Professional Voice, Philadelphia.

Estill, J., Fujimura, O., Sawada, A., & Beechler, K. (1994). Temporal perturbation and voice qualities. In P. Davis & N. Fletcher (Ed.), *Vocal fold physiology: Controlling complexity and chaos* (pp. 237-252). San Diego, CA: Singular.

Estill, J., Kobayashi, N., Honda, K., & Kakita, Y. (1990). A study on respiratory and glottal controls in six western singing qualities: Airflow and intensity measurement in professional singing. In H. Fujisaki & S. Furui (Eds.), *Proceedings of the 1990 International Conference on Spoken Language Processing* (pp. 169-172). Kobe, Japan: Acoustical Society of Japan.

Estill, J., & Moore, G. P. (1975). Fast films of three voice modes: A preliminary look at one frequency at two degrees of vocal effort. [Unpublished data].

Fant, G. (1960). *Acoustic theory of speech production*. The Hague, Netherlands: Mouton.

Gould, W. J., & Okamura, H. (1974). Interrelationships between voice and laryngeal mucosal reflexes. In B. Wyke (Ed.), *Ventilatory and phonatory control systems* (pp. 347-359). Oxford, UK: Oxford University Press.

Hirano, M. (1974). Morphological structure of the vocal cord as a vibrator and its variations. *Folia Phoniatrica, 26*, 89-94.

Hirano, M., Vennard, W., & Ohala, J. (1970). Regulation of register, pitch and intensity of voice: An electromyographic investigation of intrinsic laryngeal muscles. *Folia Phoniatrica, 22*, 1-20.

Hollien, H. (1983). In search of vocal frequency control. In D. Bless & J. Abbs (Eds.), *Vocal fold physiology: Contemporary research and clinical issues* (pp. 361-367). San Diego, CA: College Hill Press.

Honda, K., & Estill, J. (1986). Pitch control in six voice qualities: An EMG study. In M. Sawashima (Ed.), *Proceedings of the XXth Congress of the International Association of Logopedics and Phoniatrics* (p. 307). Tokyo.

Honda, K., Hirai, H., Estill, J., & Takahura, Y. (1995). Contribution of vocal tract shape to voice quality: MRI data and articulatory modeling. In O. Fujimura & M. Hirano (Eds.), *Vocal fold physiology: Voice quality control* (pp. 23-38). San Diego, CA: Singular.

Kelso, J. A. S. (1995). *Dynamic patterns: The self organization of brain and behavior*. Cambridge, MA: MIT Press.

Klimek, M. M., Obert, K. B., & Steinhauer, K. (2005). *The Estill Voice Training System, Level One: Compulsory Figures for Voice Control.* Pittsburgh, PA: Think Voice International.

Klimek, M. M., Obert, K. B., & Steinhauer, K. (2005). *The Estill Voice Training System, Level Two: Figure Combinations for Six Voice Qualities.* Pittsburgh, PA: Think Voice International.

Kotby, M. N., & Haugen, L. K. (1970). Attempts at evaluation of the function of various laryngeal muscles in the light of muscle and nerve stimulation experiments in man. *Acta Otolaryngologica, 70*, 419-427.

Kotby, M. N., & Haugen, L. K. (1970). The mechanics of laryngeal function. *Acta Otolaryngologica, 70*, 203-211.

Lombard, L. L. (2001,). *Pilot study of new voice therapy techniques for the hypofunctional voice*. Paper presented at the 30th Annual Symposium: Care of the Professional Voice, Philadelphia.

Moore, P. (1938). Motion picture studies of the vocal folds and vocal attacks. *Journal of Speech and Hearing Disorders, 3*, 235-238.

Steinhauer, K., Grayhack, J., Smiley-Oyen, A., Shaiman, S., & McNeil, M. (2004). The relationship among voice onset, voice quality, and fundamental frequency: A dynamical perspective. *Journal of Voice, 18*(4), 432-442.

Steinhauer, K., Lombard, L. L., & Eichhorn (2005). *Voice motor learning in the aging adult: Increasing power in hypofunctional voice.* Paper presented at the Ohio Voice Association, Columbus, OH.

Stevens, S. S. (1940). Problems and methods of psychophysics. *Psychological Bulletin, 54*, 177-196.

Titze, I. R., & Story, B. H. (1996). Acoustic interactions of the voice source with the lower vocal tract. *Journal of the Acoustical Society of America, 101*(4), 2234-2243.

Wallace, S. A. (1996). Dynamic pattern perspective of rhythmic movement: An introduction. In H. N. Zelaznik (Ed.), *Advances in motor learning and control* (pp. 155-194). Champaign, IL: Human Kinetics.

Yanagisawa, E., Citardi, M., & Estill, J. (1996). Videoendoscopic analysis of laryngeal function during laughter. *Annals of Otology, Rhinology, and Laryngology, 105*(7), 545-549.

Yanagisawa, E., Estill, J., Kmucha, S. T., & Leder, S. B. (1989). The contribution of aryepiglottic constriction to "ringing" voice quality—A videolaryngoscopic study. *Journal of Voice, 3*, 342-350.

Yanagisawa, E., Kmucha, S. T., & Estill, J. (1990). Endolaryngeal changes during high intensity phonation: Video laryngoscopic observations. *Journal of Voice*, *3*, 342-350.

Yanagisawa, E., Kmucha, S. T., & Estill, J. (1990). The role of the soft palate in laryngeal function and in selected voice qualities. *Annals of Otology, Rhinology, and Laryngology*, *99*, 18-28.

Yanagisawa, E., Mambrino, L., Estill, J., & Talkin, D. (1991). Supraglottic contributions to pitch raising. *Annals of Otology, Rhinology, and Laryngology*, *100*, 19-30.

Yanagisawa, E., Mambrino, L., Estill, J., & Talkin, D. (1991). The voluntary control of the soft palate. [Unpublished research video].

CHAPTER 7

Neurology and Clinical Considerations of Affective Prosody

Marilee Monnot, Diana Orbelo, Julie Testa, and Elliott Ross

Overview

Prosody is a paralinguistic aspect of language that is embedded into articulate speech through acoustical features of pitch, loudness, and rhythm. It imparts information beyond that transmitted by word choice and grammar (Bolinger, 1980; Crystal, 1975; Kent & Read, 1992; Monrad-Krohn, 1963; Ross, 2000). Prosodic systems include *linguistic* prosody that helps to clarify semantics and syntax, *dialectical* prosody that underlies regional pronunciation variations, and *idiosyncratic* prosody that reveals personal identity (Monrad-Krohn, 1948; Ross, 2000). *Affective* prosody, the focus of this chapter, gives the listener information about the speaker's emotional and attitudinal state, and allows the speaker to convey the same. Many studies show that if the linguistic message is at odds with its affective prosodic content, the affective prosodic message invariably takes precedence in adults (Ackerman, 1983; Bolinger, 1972). Thus, the ability to modulate affective prosody is an essential element of face-to-face communication. Research suggests that modulation of affective prosody is a dominant and lateralized function of the right hemisphere (Bowers, Bauer, & Heilman, 1993; Bowers, Coslet, Bauer, Speedie, & Heilman, 1987; Buchanan et al., 2000; Gorelick & Ross, 1987; Heilman, 1984; Heilman, Scholes, & Watson, 1975; Ross, Thompson, & Yenkosky, 1997). When this ability is disrupted by focal brain lesions, psychosocial difficulties may ensue (Ross, 1982; Ross & Mesulam, 1979).

Linguistic prosody shares some of the same perceptual features of affective prosody but is used for semantic purposes and to clarify potentially ambiguous syntax (Monrad-Krohn, 1963). For example, if the word *subject* is used as a noun, it receives stress on the first syllable (*sub*ject), whereas if *subject* is used as a verb it receives stress on the second syllable (sub*ject*). Linguistic prosody is also used for syntactic clarification where prosodic emphasis and pausing substitute for punctuation; e.g., "The woman and her daughter in *pink* . . . approached the stage," or "The woman . . . and her *daughter* in pink . . . approached the stage." Linguistic prosody appears to be incompletely lateralized to the left hemisphere (Behrens, 1985; Pell, 1998; Ross, 1988; Ryalls, 1988). Other paralinguistic aspects of communication also include thematic inference and the use of connotation (unusual word meanings) and nonliteral phrases (idioms) and certain kinesic activities such as facial expressions and gestures (body language), all of which appear to be modulated by the right hemisphere (Critchley, 1939; Cicone, Wapner, Foldi, Zurif, & Gardner, 1979; Monrad-Krohn, 1948). However, pantomime, which conveys specific semantic information, is disrupted by left hemisphere lesions that cause aphasic deficits (Gainotti & Lemmo, 1976; Seron, van der Kaa, Remitz, & Van der Linden, 1979).

Functional-Anatomic Correlations of Affective Prosody in Right Brain Damage

Initial studies in patients with focal right brain damage (RBD) due to ischemic stroke using CT scan localizations suggested that the organization of the affective prosodic aspects of language in the right hemisphere was similar to the organization of the propositional (semantic-linguistic) aspects of language in the left hemisphere (Ross, 1981). Patients were assessed qualitatively for their ability to spontaneously impart affective prosody into their speech and for their ability to repeat sentences with appropriate affective prosody and comprehend affect in the voice and facial gestures of the examiner. Specific combinations of affective prosodic deficits occurred following focal lesions in the right hemisphere that were analogous to the functional-anatomic clustering of aphasic deficits observed after focal left brain damage (Benson, 1979). These particular syndromes were called *aprosodias* and appropriate modifiers were used to classify the aprosodias into different syndromes, similar to the aphasias, such as motor, sensory, global, and transcortical types. In a follow-up study, using blinded evaluations, patients with focal right brain lesions again displayed various deficits in affective language that corresponded with the aprosodic classifications and localizations published previously (Gorelick & Ross, 1987). Figure 7-1 shows cortical distribution of ischemic strokes in right brain damaged patients, sorted by affective prosodic performance. In addition, the prevalence of aprosodia following right brain damage was equal to the prevalence of aphasia following left brain damage, emphasizing that the aprosodias are common rather than rare syndromes. A more recent study using quantitative measures of affective prosody and MRI scanning for lesion localization has confirmed these patterns in patients with focal ischemic injury during the acute/sub-acute post-stroke phase of injury (Ross, Orbelo, Burgard, & Hansel, 1998). If patients are studied in the chronic phase of recovery,

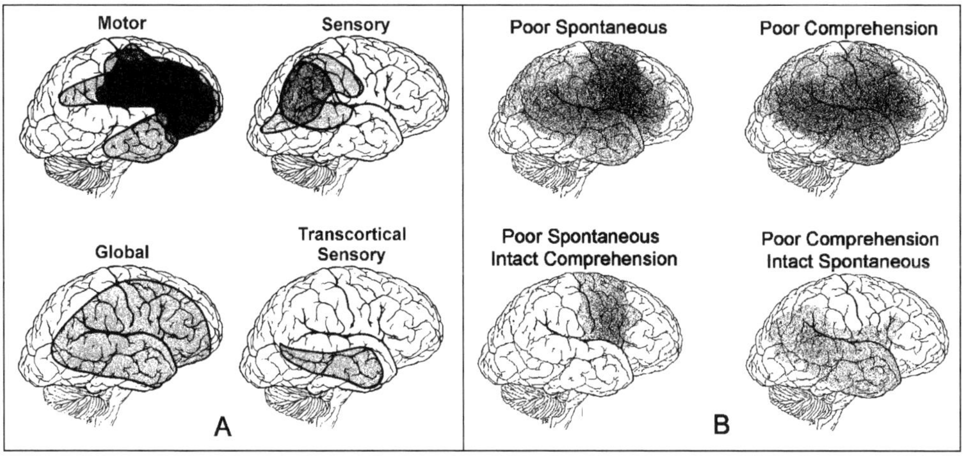

Figure 7–1. Cortical distribution of ischemic strokes in right brain damaged patients, sorted by affective prosodic performance. Composite **A** shows cortical distribution of lesions causing various types of aprosodias based on qualitative bedside examinations and CT scan localizations [adapted from "The Aprosodias: Functional-Anatomical Organization of the Affective Components of Language in the Right Hemisphere," by E. D. Ross, 1981, *Archives of Neurology*, *38*, pp. 561–569, and "The Aprosodias: Further Functional-Anatomic Evidence for the Organization of Affective Language in the Right Hemisphere," by P. B. Gorelick and E. D. Ross, 1987, *Journal of Neurology, Neurosurgery, and Psychiatry*, *50*, pp. 553–560); composite **B** shows cortical distribution of lesions associated with deficits in spontaneous production and comprehension of affect prosody based on results from the Aprosodia Battery and MRI scan localizations (adapted from "Lateralization of Affective Prosody in Brain and the Callosal Integration of Hemispheric Language Functions," by E. D. Ross, R. D. Thompson, and J. Yenkosky, 1997, *Brain and Language*, *56*, pp. 27–54, and "Functional-Anatomic Correlates of Aprosodic Deficits in Patients with Right Brain Damage," by E. D. Ross, D. M. Orbelo, M. Burgard, and S. Hansel, 1998, *Neurology*, *50*(Suppl. 4), A363.]

greater than 6 months post-stroke, these localization patterns do not hold (Baum & Pell, 1997; Pell & Baum, 1997) because of brain reorganization (Ross, 2003) similar to what has been observed in patients with aphasias (Goodglass, 1993).

Lateralization of Affective Prosody

The terms *dominant* and *lateralized* brain function have different neurological implications. A brain function is considered dominant if a unilateral lesion produces a behavioral deficit that subtends both sides of space (Denny-Brown, 1954; Denny-Brown & Horenstein, 1952). For a function to be considered lateralized, it must also be shown that the behavioral deficit does not occur following lesions of the opposite hemisphere. This concept is illustrated in the seminal publications by Paul Broca. Soon after his initial discovery that damage to the foot of the left third frontal convolution caused loss of articulate speech (Broca, 1861), Broca reported that similar lesions in the right hemisphere did not result in loss of articulate speech (Broca, 1865), thus establishing that articulation was both a dominant and highly lateralized function. However, the degree of lateralization of affective prosody has been questioned because some researchers have reported that aphasic patients with left hemisphere lesions may also have affective prosodic deficits (Cancelliere & Kertesz, 1990; De Bleser & Poeck, 1985; Pell, 1998).

Based on the well-known clinical observation that aphasic deficits may complicate formal testing of cognitive abilities, the Aprosodia Battery was developed (Ross et al., 1997). Its purpose was to determine if affective prosodic deficits in patients with left brain damage (LBD) would improve under conditions of progressively reduced verbal-articulatory demands. The original battery was composed of four subtests assessing spontaneous *production, repetition, comprehension,* and *discrimination* of affective prosody. Spontaneous production is assessed by recording the speech of subjects who are asked to discuss emotional events in their life. The ability of subjects to spontaneously impart affective prosody can be measured either quantitatively, using acoustical measures to determine how well the subjects vary their fundamental frequency over time (intonation), or qualitatively by judges (Ross et al., 1997; Monnot, Lovallo, Nixon, & Ross, 2002). *Repetition* is assessed by having subjects repeat what they hear in recorded standardized exemplars of utterances with six different emotions (happy, sad, angry, surprised, disinterested/bored, and neutral) using three set of carriers of affective intonation. The first set, Word, uses a completely articulated sentence, *I am going to the other movies*, which the subjects attempt to mimic using random variations of the six emotions and, in addition, two stress patterns, one with emphasis on *am* and the other with emphasis on *other,* for a total of 12 exemplars. In the next two subtests, the verbal-articulatory content is sequentially reduced using utterances with similar emotional and stress patterns. The Monosyllabic subtest uses 12 utterances with *ba ba ba ba ba* as the carrier of affect prosody and the Asyllabic subtest uses 12 utterances with *aaaaahhhhh* as the carrier of affective prosody. The subject's vocalizations are recorded for later acoustical analysis or can be judged qualitatively. The *comprehension* of affective prosody is assessed by having subjects listen to the aforementioned recordings in which each exemplar is presented twice for a total of 24 sentences per set. After each exemplar subjects decide which one of the six emotions they heard. The fourth subtest, Discrimination, presents 24 *pairs* of exemplars from the Word subtest that have undergone low-pass acoustical filtering to remove articulatory information. Subjects must indicate if the two sentences in each pair project the *same* or *different* emotions. Standardization studies of the Aprosodia Battery in adults are presented in Table7-1. In addition, 15 young adults 20–30 years of age underwent test-retesting separated by 3 months. Statistical analysis indicated no significant differences in scores between the two testing sessions, indicating that the Aprosodia Battery is reliable.

In a study of patients with single focal ischemic infarctions, LBD patients showed significant improvement in their ability to both comprehend and repeat affective prosody as the verbal-articulatory demands were reduced, whereas right brain damaged patients showed no improve-

Table 7–1. Aprosodia Battery Comprehension Subtest Scores

Decade of life	Word	Monosyllabic	Asyllabic	Discrimination
20 to 29 yrs.	22.57 (1.20)	22.10 (1.29)	22.63 (2.56)	22.34 (2.34)
30 to 39 yrs.	22.22 (1.39)	22.23 (1.42)	22.15 (1.34)	22.31 (1.55)
40 to 49 yrs.	21.60 (2.32)	21.67 (1.50)	20.07 (2.89)	20.87 (1.51)
50 to 59 yrs.	21.50 (1.91)	21.63 (1.60)	20.50 (2.62)	20.86 (2.87)
60 to 69 yrs.	20.61 (3.08)	20.37 (2.38)	18.22 (4.21)	20.04 (2.85)
70 to 79 yrs.	20.72 (2.30)	18.90 (2.69)	16.04 (4.14)	20.16 (2.69)
80 to 89 yrs.	20.34 (1.04)	17.20 (3.27)	15.60 (4.95)	18.00 (4.85)

Aprosodia Battery comprehension mean (and standard deviation scores) by subtest and by decade of life; results show the steady decline in average ability to identify emotion in the voice.

ment in their performance (Figure 7-2) (Ross et al., 1997). In addition, the affective prosodic deficits in LBD patients were not associated with the presence or severity of aphasic deficits, and had no relationship to the cortical distribution of the lesions. However, lesions involving the deep white matter adjacent to the corpus callosum best predicted affective prosodic disturbances in patients with LBD. This suggests that the predominant mechanism underlying affective prosodic deficits following LBD is loss of callosal integration of the dominantly lateralized language functions represented in each hemisphere (LBD/Callosal profile) (Ross et al., 1997). The appropriate coordination of both linguistic and affective aspects of language infers a healthy callosal transfer of information enabling the hemispheres to produce articulate speech with appropriate affective prosody that is temporally coherent (Ross, Harney, deLacoste-Utamsing, & Purdy, 1981; Speedie, Coslett, & Heilman, 1984; Ross et al., 1997). The left hemisphere must apprise the right hemisphere of which words will be articulated and their rate in order for the proper application of stress and intonation to be delivered, and the right hemisphere must inform the left hemisphere of certain affective requirements in order to introduce emotional meaning into the propositional string. The predominant mechanism underlying affective prosodic deficits following RBD appears to be loss of affective communicative representations resulting in the inability to dominantly modulate affective prosody (RBD/Aprosodic profile) (Blonder, Bowers, & Heilman, 1991; Bowers et al., 1987; Bowers et al., 1993).

Clinical Aspects of Affective Prosody

Right hemisphere lesions that result in problems processing affective prosody may cause social and emotional difficulties (Ross, 1982; Ross & Mesulam, 1979). The social difficulties that result are based upon the patient's inability to impart affect into speech and/or to understand

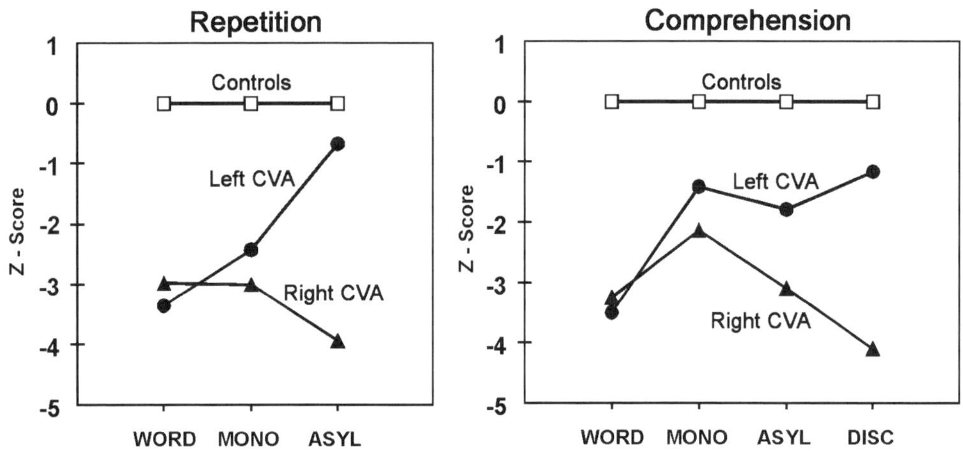

Figure 7–2. Patterns of results on the Repetition and Comprehension components of the Aprosodia Battery for stroke patients. Patterns of Repetition and Comprehension deficits in affective prosody observed in patients with left brain damage (LBD) and right brain damage (RBD) compared to age-matched controls as measured by the Aprosodia Battery; Z-scores represent transformation of raw scores based on control means and standard deviations; Repetition results are based on acoustical analysis of how well individuals manipulated their fundamental frequency to produce intonation contours; Comprehension results are based on number of exemplars correctly identified out of 24 stimuli per subset; based on repeated-measure ANOVAs, statistical results show highly robust main effects and interactions [adapted from "Lateralization of Affective Prosody in Brain and the Callosal Integration of Hemispheric Language Functions," by E. D. Ross, R. D. Thompson, and J. Yenkosky, 1997, *Brain and Language*, *56*, pp. 27–54, and "Functional-Anatomic Correlates of Aprosodic Deficits in Patients with Right Brain Damage," by E. D. Ross, D. M. Orbelo, M. Burgard, and S. Hansel, 1998, *Neurology*, *50*(suppl. 4), A363.]

affect in the speech of others. Thus, neurological irregularities may underlie behavioral differences, which have been attributed to socialization processes in certain clinical conditions. Individuals insensitive to social nuances and unskilled in social interactions may be less able *neurologically* to perceive and process attributes, such as affective prosody that imparts important pragmatic, social, and emotional information during discourse. Recently, several clinical conditions with prominent behavioral signs and symptoms have been shown to have significant deficits in modulating affective prosody. These include schizophrenia (Ross et al., 2001; and also Leitman et al., 2005; Mitchell & Crow, 2005), early exposure to alcohol (Monnot, 2002; Monnot, Lovallo, et al., 2002; Monnot, Nixon, Lovallo, & Ross, 2001), and Alzheimer's disease (AD) (Testa, Beatty, Gleason, Orbelo, & Ross, 2001).

Schizophrenia and Affective Prosody

Although schizophrenia has been ascribed traditionally to compromise of left hemisphere cognitive systems, various investigators have argued that it is a bihemispheric disease (Mitchell & Crow, 2005; Ross et al., 2001). One of the major arguments for a right hemispheric deficit in schizophrenia has been the consistent documentation of affective prosodic deficits, which could underlie their difficulties involving emotional judgment and poor socialization. Thus, an essential question to resolve, given the issues surrounding the lateralization of affective prosody in brain (see above), was whether the affective prosodic disturbances in schizophrenia are similar to profiles associated with LBD or RBD, or simply a unique variation. Data were collected from 45 chronic, medication-stabilized, schizophrenic patients and compared with results for 10 patients with focal LBD, 9 patients with focal RBD, and 19 controls (Ross et al., 2001). Schizophrenic and aphasic symptoms were evaluated using standard assessment tools. Based on patients with impaired performance on the Aphasia Battery (AB), schizophrenics were statistically identical to patients with RBD and robustly different from those with LBD. Thirty-eight schizophrenic patients (84.4%) were found to have some type of affective prosodic deficit with 64.4% demonstrating significant difficulties comprehending affective prosody. In comparison, only 15.5% of the schizophrenics had mild aphasic problems on the Western Aphasia Battery. These results underscore that schizophrenics have major deficits involving right hemisphere cognitive and behavioral systems. When schizophrenic symptoms and prosodic deficits were examined using a principal component analysis, comprehension and repetition loaded uniquely as a separate factor. Thus, affective prosodic deficits may also represent a cardinal symptom of schizophrenia because they are highly prevalent and not associated statistically with traditional clusters of schizophrenic symptoms (Ross et al., 2001).

Alcohol Abuse and Affective Prosody

Much has been written about psychological effects of alcohol abuse on adults, and the physiological, anatomical, and functional damage to offspring resulting from alcohol abuse by the mother during pregnancy (Jones, Smith, Ulleland, & Streissguth, 1973; Mattson & Rilcy, 1999). Traditional *left* hemisphere cognitive deficits and brain shrinkage in chronic heavy drinkers have been documented by neuropsychological assessments and imaging studies (Cala et al., 1983; Holloway, 1994; Nixon & Phillips, 1999; Oscar-Berman, 1985; Parsons, 1998). Parenthetically, *right* hemisphere visual spatial skills also have been shown to be affected by alcohol abuse (Parsons & Nixon, 1998). Another "nontraditional" skill found to be altered by alcohol abuse is interpersonal problem-solving (Nixon, Tivis & Parsons, 1992). However, emotion cognition in alcohol abusers has not been studied until very recently, including affective prosodic abilities, despite their importance in social interaction and communication (Kornreich et al., 1998; Kornreich et al., 2002; Kornreich, Blairy, Philippot, Dan, et al., 2001; Kornreich, Blairy, Philippot, Hess, et al., 2001; Oscar-Berman, Hancock, Mildworf, Hutner, & Weber, 1990; Philippot et al., 1999). Because affective prosodic processing is an essential component for psychosocial competency, it was thought that this cognitive skill might also be affected by alcohol abuse. Therefore, a study was conducted assessing the affective prosodic abilities in 82 subjects ranging in age from 25 to 58 years (Monnot et al., 2001; Monnot, Lovallo, et al., 2002). Twenty-nine males and 3 females meeting DSM-IV criteria for an alcohol use disorder with a median 39 days of sobriety (ALC), 11 males with a probable history of fetal alcohol *exposure* (FAexp), and 41 age-matched control subjects were tested using the Aprosodia Battery. ALC and FAexp groups were significantly less accurate at affective prosodic comprehension compared to controls. The ALC group scored −2 SD and the FAexp group scored −5 SD below the control group mean (Figure 7-3). Multiple regression analysis, using nine alcohol use variables to model affective prosodic comprehension, resulted in four significant regressors related to both (a) early bingeing behaviors and (b) chronicity of alcohol abuse [$F(5,37) = 27.3$, R^2Adjusted = .78, $p < .0000$]. These alcohol-exposed subjects appeared to be deficient in the ability to understand emotional valence in the speech of others, resulting in errors of judgment, which could explain their well-known difficulties involving social communication and interactions. Yet, despite their poor performance on affective prosodic comprehension, ALC and FAexp groups performed almost identi-

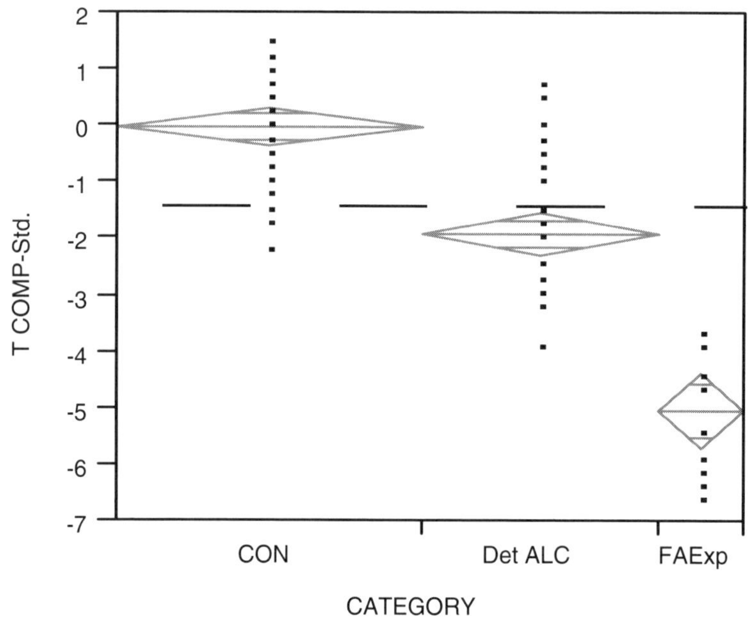

Figure 7–3. Aprosodia Battery standardized scores and means diamonds for three groups. T Comp-Std. = total correct responses on the Aprosodia Battery Comprehension subtests of Word, Monosyllabic, and Asyllabic (standardized using control subject scores); CON = control subjects; Det ALC = detoxified alcoholics; FAExp = alcoholic and non-alcoholic subjects with putative fetal alcohol exposure; greater width of means diamonds indicates greater statistical significance; ANOVA groups are statistically different when means diamonds do not overlap.

cally to the control group on vocabulary, abstract reasoning, and basic cognitive functions, as measured by the Shipley Institute of Living Scales. This information, along with publications showing that emotional facial expression recognition is also deficient in detoxified alcoholics, indicates that emotion cognition is damaged by early alcohol abuse (Kornreich et al., 1998; Kornreich et al., 2002; Kornreich, Blairy, Philippot, Dan, et al., 2001; Kornreich, Blairy, Philippot, Hess, et al., 2001).

In addition, alcoholics also appear to be deficient in vocal production of affect (Monnot, Orbelo, et al., 2001). Four experienced raters listened to the vocal production of the 82 subjects in the alcohol abuse study (described above) and identified what emotion was projected using a forced choice of the six emotions represented in the Aprosodia Battery. Their inter-rater reliability correlation was 0.82. Results showed detoxified alcoholics were significantly impaired in their ability to produce understandable and accurate emotion in their speech [F (2,54) = 7.0, p = .0036]. In addition, these pragmatic ratings of subjects' ability to inject emotion into the voice show a positive, significant relationship to acoustic analyses assessing fundamental frequency variability [F (2,54) = 24.58, R^2Adjusted = 0.52, p < .0001]. A regression analysis showed a significant association between the Comprehension and Production components of the Aprosodia Battery for all 82 subjects [F (1,54) = 9.27, p < .003]. Subjects' sex, education, ethnic origin, and other drugs of abuse were not predictive of results. However, age was negatively associated with accuracy of affective prosodic repetition [F (1,54) = 4.96, p < .03] (Monnot, 2002; Monnot, Orbelo, et al., 2001). These results indicate that detoxified alcoholics (and those with putative prenatal exposure) are impaired in their ability to produce understandable affective prosody in speech and to comprehend emotion in the voice of a communication partner and, thus, this may explain partially the poor social skills and altered personal and work relationships so often noted in alcoholics.

Alzheimer's Disease and Affective Prosody

Alzheimer's disease (AD) is a progressive neurodegenerative disease characterized by declines in memory and cognitive abilities, such as language and problem solving (McKhann, Folstein, Katzman, Price, & Stadlan, 1984). In addition to these cognitive deficits, some patients with AD experience disturbances in behavior, mood, and emotional regulation (Cummings, 1996; Piccininni, Baldereschi, Zaccara, & Inzitari, 2005; Shimabukuro & Matsuoka, 2005; Zubenko & McPherson, 2003). Patients with AD can have difficulty expressing and comprehending emotional information through facial expressions and affective prosody (Albert, 1991; Allender, 1989; Bucks, 2004; Cadieux, 1997; Cohen & Brosgole, 1988; Hargrave & Stone, 2002; Lavenu, 2005; Roberts, 1996), which worsen as dementia severity increases, and these deficits have been associated with mood and behavior disturbances (Allender, 1989; Roberts, 1996).

From a pathological standpoint, affective prosody deficits should reflect the underlying distribution and severity of neurofibrillary tangles. It is well known that in late-onset AD, pathological changes first appear in the medial and orbitofrontal limbic system, then the medial and orbitofrontal limbic-associated cortices and posterior neocortices, and finally the frontal neocortices (Braak, 1991, 1994; Foster, 1994; Haxby & Koss, 1988). Based on the localization of prosodic deficits (Ross, 1981; Rosset al., 1997), and the known AD pathological stages, it would be expected that affective prosody comprehension deficits would occur early in AD due to changes in posterior neocortical areas, followed by repetition deficits and then deficits in spontaneous production as disease severity progresses to involve the frontal neocortices, similar to the documented pattern of how aphasic deficits unfold in AD (Appell & Fisman, 1982; Cummings, Benson, Hill, & Read, 1985; Faber-Langendoen et al., 1988; Murdoch, Wilks, & Boyle, 1987).

We assessed the affective prosodic performance in mildly, moderately, and severely demented AD patients to determine the patterns of deficits and the association of these deficits with cognitive changes, neuropsychiatric problems, and onset of aphasic symptoms (Testa et al., 1998). Twenty-seven patients with AD and 20 normal controls, matched for age and education, completed a test battery consisting of a thorough neuropsychological evaluation, including the Aprosodia Battery (Ross et al., 1997). All AD patients met NINCDS-ADRDA criteria for probable AD (McKhann et al., 1984) and all controls scored > 26 on the Mini-Mental State Examination (MMSE). Our findings indicated that AD patients had significant deficits in processing affective prosody compared to normal, healthy elderly comparison subjects. *Comprehension* deficits were significantly greater than deficits in repetition or discrimination, occurred very early in the disease process before the appearance of aphasic or anomic disturbances, and were strongly associated with severity of dementia. Comprehension of affective prosody, a putative right posterior temporal function, was impaired in mildly demented patients and worsened as the disease entered the moderate and severe stages. Affective prosody *repetition*, a peri-Sylvian function, and *spontaneous production* of affective prosody, an anterior-superior Sylvian function, were relatively preserved in mildly demented patients. Although repetition deficits emerged as patients became more demented, spontaneous production of affective prosody in natural conversation was not affected in most patients, regardless of the level of dementia severity.

In addition to affective prosody deficits, AD patients exhibited significantly greater neuropsychiatric behaviors. Both patients and their caregivers endorsed that AD patients had more depressive symptoms than controls. Patients with prosodic deficits were more likely to have higher ratings of psychiatric problems, including apathy and irritability, than patients without prosodic deficits. These findings indicate that AD patients with abnormal affective-prosodic performance have higher incidence of behavioral problems than those with normal performance.

Much as been published on propositional language deficits which accompany AD. It is known that transcortical sensory and sensory aphasias occur long before the onset of nonfluent speech (Appell & Fisman, 1982; Cummings et al., 1985; Faber-Langendoen et al., 1988; Murdoch, et al., 1987). However, few comparisons of prosodic deficits to aphasic changes in AD have been published. In our study (Testa et al., 2001) the resultant pattern of prosodic deficits paralleled previously documented patterns of aphasic deficits in AD (Table 7-2) with a critical difference: prosodic comprehension deficits occurred much earlier and were more prevalent than aphasic comprehension deficits. Additionally, impaired affective prosody repetition and comprehension, but not aphasic deficits, were associated with increased frequency and severity of behavioral changes. In contrast, AD patients with normal affective-prosodic performance were significantly less demented, had normal linguistic abilities, and displayed fewer neuropsychiatric behaviors.

These findings suggest that even mildly demented patients with AD may be limited in their ability to interpret social-emotional messages and may be at greater risk for neuropsychiatric problems. Diminished ability to process emotional information may have numerous implications for AD patients and their families including greater caregiver, personal, and marital stress and increased behavioral disturbances. Because emotional communication is vital in establishing and maintaining interpersonal relationships, it is imperative that clinicians detect early deficits in emotional communication in AD patients to better help families and patients cope with these changes.

Advanced Age and Affective Prosody

While studying numerous populations with affective prosodic deficits in our VA Affective Communication Research Laboratory, we observed that *healthy* older individuals appeared to make more errors compared to *healthy* younger subjects on the Comprehension portion of the Aprosodia Battery, a finding also supported by qualitative observations in the literature (Brosgole, 1995; Cohen & Brosgole, 1988; Kiss & Ennis, 2001; Oscar-Berman, 1985; Tompkins & Flowers,

Table 7–2. Classification of Alzheimer's disease patients by aprosodia type: Relationship of aprosodic syndromes to cognition and behavior in AD

Tests of Cognition and Behavior	None (n = 6)	Transcortical Sensory (n = 14)	Sensory (n = 7)
MMSE*	23.3[a]	16.8[a,b]	14.7[b]
WAB-AQ	94.9	87.4	83.9
UCLA*	5.2[a]	17.6[a,b]	25.6[b]
Apathy	0.2[a]	2.8[a,b]	5.3[b]
Irritability	0.6[a]	2.0[a,b]	4.9[b]
GDS-Caregiver Report	14.8	14.8	20.4
GDS-Patient Report	6.5	5.6	10.9

Note. MMSE = Mini-Mental State Examination; WAB-AQ = Western Aphasia Battery—Aphasia Quotient; UCLA = UCLA Neuropsychiatric Inventory; GDS = Geriatric Depression Scale.

*$p < .05$.

[a,ab,b]indicate post-hoc relationships $\alpha < 0.05$.

1985). Therefore, we conducted a post hoc quantitative study of Aprosodia Battery scores across ages using individuals who had served as healthy controls for our previous studies (Orbelo, Testa, & Ross, 2003). Sixty-nine subjects (29 men and 40 women) completed the Aprosodia Battery and regression analyses were used to model age based on their performance. For spontaneous affective prosody and repetition no deficits were observed in relationship to age. Three of the four Comprehension tasks showed significant aging effects (p-values $< .001$). Specifically, Monosyllabic Comprehension resulted in a moderate effect size ($R^2 = 0.21$), Asyllabic Comprehension resulted in large effect size ($R^2 = 0.42$); and Discrimination had a moderate effect size ($R^2 = 0.16$). Thus with age, older individuals show a decrement in their ability to comprehend affective prosody under reduced verbal-articulatory demands that is consistent with a right-hemisphere aging process because the pattern is similar to what has been observed in patients with RBD (Ross et al., 1997). Of interest in regards to this observation is the recent documentation of selective loss of both white and gray matter with aging that predominantly involves the right hemisphere, especially the temporal neocortex (Resnick, Kraut, Zonderman, & Davatzikos, 2003).

In a follow-up study, we explored other possible reasons for elderly subjects' poorer performance on tasks with progressively reduced verbal articulatory content. Because hearing loss and general cognitive decline is prevalent in the elderly, we conducted a prospective study of 62 elderly subjects ages 65 to 80 years (Orbelo, Grim, Talbott, & Ross, 2005). The subjects' hearing was assessed by standard means and their neuropsychological status was assessed using the Stroop Test and the Repeatable Battery for the Assessment of Neuropsychological Status (RBANS). Using multiple stepwise regression analysis to model affective prosodic results, hearing loss had no predictive value on Aprosodia Battery comprehension scores. The Stroop and RBANS subtest scores were able to account for only 10% to 22% of the variability in the Aprosodia Battery comprehension scores, suggesting that this battery is assessing skills that are less dependent on memory and attention, and more dependent on the right hemisphere's ability to process affective prosody.

Summary

Affective prosody, a dominant and lateralized function of the right hemisphere, is an essential element in meaningful face-to-face discourse. Deficits in the ability to produce appropriate emotion/attitude in the voice, and/or to comprehend properly and quickly it in others, leave the individual vulnerable to communication mistakes. These social interaction deficits may result in emotional distress and interpersonal inadequacy. Clinicians must be aware of these problems so they can provide appropriate diagnosis and treatment for their patients and families.

Acknowledgements. The work presented in this chapter involving the Aprosodia Battery and its application for assessment of various clinical populations, including brain-damaged patients, schizophrenics, AD patients, alcohol exposed individuals, and aged controls, was supported in part by grants to Dr.

Ross from the Merit Review Board, Medical Research Service, Department of Veterans Affairs, Washington, DC; the EJLB Foundation, Montreal, Canada; the Oklahoma Center for the Advancement of Science and Technology, Oklahoma City, OK; and the Neuropsychiatric Research Institute, Fargo, ND.

References

Ackerman, B. (1983). Form and function in children's understanding of ironic utterances. *Journal of Experimental Child Psychology*, *35*, 487-508.

Albert, M. C. C., & Koff, E. (1991). Perception of affect in patients with dementia of the Alzheimer type. *Archives of Neurology*, *48*, 791-795.

Allender, J. K. A. (1989). Processing of emotional cues in patients with dementia of the Alzheimer's type. *International Journal of Neuroscience*, *46*, 147-155.

American Psychiatric Association. (2000). *Diagnostic and statistical manual of mental disorders* (4th ed.). Washington, DC: Author.

Appell, J. K. A., & Fisman, M. (1982). A study of language functioning in Alzheimer patients. *Brain and Language*, *17*, 73-91.

Baum, S. R., & Pell, M. D. (1997). Production of affective prosody and linguistic prosody by brain-damaged patients. *Aphasiology*, *11*, 177-198.

Behrens, S. J. (1985, November). The perception of stress and lateralization of prosody. *Brain and Language*, *26*(2), 332-348.

Benson, D. (1979). *Aphasia, alexia, and agraphia*. New York: Churchill Livingstone.

Blonder, L. X., Bowers, D., & Heilman, K. M. (1991). The role of the right hemisphere in emotional communication. *Brain*, *114*, 1115-1127.

Bolinger, D. (1972). *Intonation*. Hardmondsworth, UK: Penguin.

Bolinger, D. (1980). *Language: The loaded weapon*. London: Longman Group.

Bowers, D., Bauer, R. M., & Heilman, K. M. (1993). The nonverbal affect lexicon: Theoretical perspectives from neuropsychological studies of affect perception. *Neuropsychology*, *7*, 433-444.

Bowers, D., Coslet, H. B., Bauer, R. M., Speedie, L. J., & Heilman, K. M. (1987). Comprehension of emotional prosody following unilateral hemispheric lesions: Processing defect versus distraction defect. *Neuropsychologia*, *25*, 317-328.

Braak, H., Braak, E. (1991). Neuropathological staging of Alzheimer-related changes. *Acta Neuropathologica* *82*(4), 239-259.

Braak, H., Braak, E. (1994). Pathology of Alzheimer's disease. In D. Calne (Ed.), *Neurodegenerative diseases* (pp. 585-613). Philadelphia: Saunders.

Broca, P. (1861). Remarques sur le siege de la faculte du langage articule, suives d'une observation d'aphemie. *The cerebral cortex*. Springfield, MO: Thomas. (translated by Von Bonin, G., 1960)

Broca, P. (1865). Du siege de la faculte du langage articule. *Bulletin de la Société d'Anthropologie de Paris*, *6*, 337-393.

Brosgole, L. Weisman, J. (1995). Mood recognition across the ages. *International Journal of Neuroscience*, *82*(3-4), 169-189.

Buchanan, T. W., Lutz, K., Mirzazade, S., Specht, K., Shah, N. J., Zilles, K., et al. (2000). Recognition of emotional prosody and verbal components of spoken language: An *f*MRI study. *Cognitive Brain Research*, *9*, 227-238.

Bucks, R. S. (2004). Emotion processing in Alzheimer's disease. *Aging and Mental Health*, *8*(3), 222-232.

Cadieux, N., Greve, K. (1997). Emotion processing in Alzheimer's disease. *Journal of the International Neuropsychological Society*, *3*, 411-419.

Cala, L. A., Jones, B., Burns, P., Davis, R. E., Stenhouse, N., & Mastaglia, F. L. (1983). Results of computerized tomography, psychometric testing and dietary studies in social drinkers, with emphasis on reversibility after abstinence. *Medical Journal of Australia, 17,2*(6), 264-269.

Cancelliere, A. E. B., & Kertesz, A. (1990). Lesion localization in acquired deficits of emotional expression and comprehension. *Brain & Language, 13*, 133-147.

Cicone, M., Wapner, W., Foldi, N., Zurif, E., & Gardner, H. (1979). The relationship between gesture and language in aphasic communication. *Brain and Language, 8*, 324-349.

Cohen, E., & Brosgole, L. (1988). Visual and auditory affect recognition in senile and normal elderly persons. *International Journal of Neuroscience, 43*, 89-101.

Concelliere, A. B., & Kertesz, A. (1990). Lesion localization in acquired deficits of emotional expression and comprehension. *Brain and Cognition, 13*, 133-147.

Critchley, M. (1939). *The language of gesture.* London: Edward Arnold.

Crystal, D. (1975). *The English tone of voice.* New York: St. Martin's Press.

Cummings, J., Benson, F., Hill, M. A., & Read, S. (1985). Aphasia in dementia of the Alzheimer type. *Neurology, 35*, 394-397.

Cummings, J. L., Kaufer, D. (1996). Neuropsychiatric aspects of Alzheimer's disease: The cholinergic hypothesis revisited. *Neurology, 47*, 876-883.

DeBleser, R. & Poeck, K. (1985). Analysis of prosody in the spontaneous speech of patients with CV-recurring utterances, *Cortex, 21*, 405-416.

Denny-Brown, D., Banker, B. Q. (1954). Amorphosynthesis from left parietal lesion. *Archives of Neurology and Psychiatry, 71*, 302-313.

Denny-Brown, D., Meyer, J., & Horenstein, S. (1952). The significance of perceptual rivalry resulting from parietal lesion. *Brain, 75*, 433-471.

Faber-Langendoen, K., Morris, J. C., Knesevich, J. W., LaBarge, E., Miller, J. P., & Berg, L. (1988). Aphasia in senile dementia of the Alzheimer type. *Annals of Neurology, 23*, 365-370.

Foster, N. (1994). PET imaging. In R. Katzman & K. Bick (Eds.), *Alzheimer disease* (pp. 87-103). New York: Raven Press.

Gainotti, G., & Lemmo, M. (1976). Comprehension of symbolic gestures in aphasia. *Brain and Language, 3*, 451-460.

Goodglass, H. G. (1993). *Understanding aphasia.* New York: Grune & Stratton.

Gorelick, P. B., & Ross, E. D. (1987). The aprosodias: Further functional-anatomic evidence for the organization of affective language in the right hemisphere. *Journal of Neurology, Neurosurgery, and Psychiatry, 50*, 553-560.

Hargrave, R., Maddock, R.J., & Stone, V. (2002). Impaired recognition of facial expressions of emotion in Alzheimer's disease. *Journal of Neuropsychiatry and Clinical Neuroscience, 14*(1), 64-71.

Haxby, J., Grady, C.L., & Koss, E. (1988). Heterogeneous anterior-posterior metabolic patterns in dementia of the Alzheimer type. *Neurology, 38*, 1853-1863.

Heilman, K. (1984). Comprehension of affective and nonaffective prosody. *Neurology, 34*, 917-921.

Heilman, K. M., & Gilmore, R. L. (1998). Cortical influences in emotion. *Journal of Clinical Neurophysiology, 15*(5), 409-423.

Heilman, K. M., Scholes, R., & Watson, R. T. (1975). Auditory affective agnosia: Disturbed comprehension of affective speech. *Journal of Neurology, Neurosurgery, and Psychiatry, 38*, 69-72.

Holloway, F. (1994). *Low-dose alcohol effects on human behavior and performance: A review of post-1984 research.* Oklahoma City: Office of Aviation Medicine, F.A.A.

Jones, K. L., Smith, D. W., Ulleland, C. N., & Streissguth, A. P. (1973). Pattern of malformation in offspring of chronic alcoholic mothers. *Lancet, 1*(815), 1267-1271.

Kent, R. D., & Read, C. (1992). *The acoustic analysis of speech.* San Diego, CA: Singular Publishing Group.

Kiss, I., & Ennis, T. (2001). Age-related decline in perception of prosodic affect. *Applied Neuropsychology, 8*(4), 251-254.

Kornreich, C., Blairy, S., Philippot, P., Dan, B., Foisy, M., Hess, U., et al. (2001). Emotional facial expression recognition compared in two pathological conditions: Obsessive compulsive disorder and alcoholism. *Psychiatry Research, 102*, 235-248.

Kornreich, C., Blairy, S., Philippot, P., Hess, U., Noel, X., Streel, E., et al. (2001). Deficits in emotional facial expression recognition are still present after mid- to long-term abstinence in alcoholic patients. *Journal of Studies on Alcohol, 62*, 533-542.

Kornreich, C., Philippot, P., Foisy, M., Blairy, S., Raynaud, E., Dan, B., et al. (2002). Impaired emotional facial expression recognition is associated with interpersonal problems in alcoholism. *Alcohol and Alcoholism, 37*(4), 394-400.

Kornreich, C., Philippot, P., Verpoorten, C., Dan, B., Baert, I., Le Bon, O., et al. (1998). Alcoholism and emotional reactivity: More heterogeneous film-induced emotional response in newly detoxified alcoholics compared to controls—A preliminary study. *Addictive Behaviors, 23*(3), 413-418.

Lavenu, I., Pasquier F. (2005). Perception of emotion on faces in frontotemporal dementia and Alzheimer's disease: A longitudinal study. *Dementia and Geriatric Cognitive Disorders, 19*(1), 37-41.

Leitman, D. I., Foxe, J. J., Butler, P. D., Saperstein, A., Revheim, N., & Javitt, D. C. (2005). Sensory contributions to impaired prosodic processing in schizophrenia. *Biological Psychiatry, 58*(1), 56-61.

Mattson, S. N., & Riley, E. P. (1999, July). Implicit and explicit memory functioning in children with heavy prenatal alcohol exposure. *Journal of International Neuropsychological Society, 5*(5), 462-471.

McKhann, G., Drachman, D., Folstein. M., Katzman, R., Price, D., Stadlan, E. M. (1984). Clinical diagnosis of Alzheimer's disease: Report of the NINCDS-ADRDA work group under the auspices of Department of Health and Human Services Task Force on Alzheimer's Disease. *Neurology, 34*, 939-944.

Mitchell, R. L., & Crow, T. J. (2005). Right hemisphere language functions and schizophrenia: The forgotten hemisphere? *Brain, 128*(Pt. 5), 963-978.

Monnot, M., Lovallo, W., Nixon, S., & Ross, E. (2002). Neurological basis of deficits in affective prosody comprehension among alcoholics and fetal alcohol exposed adults. *Journal of Neuropsychiatry and Clinical Neurosciences, 14*(3), 321-328.

Monnot, M., Nixon, S., Lovallo, W., & Ross, E. (2001). Abnormal emotional perception in alcoholics: Deficits in comprehension of affective prosody. *Alcoholism: Clinical and Experimental Research, 25*(3), 362-369.

Monnot, M., Orbelo, D., & Ross, E. (2001, April). *Affective prosodic production in alcoholics*. Paper presented at the Social Cognitive Neuroscience Symposium, University of California, Los Angeles.

Monnot, M., Orbelo, D., Riccardo, L., Sikka, S., & Ross, E. (2002). Acoustic analyses support subjective judgments of vocal emotion. In P. Ekman, J. Campos, R. Davidson, & R. de Waal (Eds.), *Emotion inside and out: 130 years after Darwin's.* Expression of the Emotions in Man and Animals (pp. 288-292). New York: New York Academy of Sciences.

Monrad-Krohn, G. H. (1948). Dysprosody or altered "melody of language." *Brain, 70*, 405-415.

Monrad-Krohn, G. H. (1963). The third element of speech: Prosody and its disorders. In L. Halpern (Ed.), *Problems in dynamic neurology* (pp. 101-118). Jerusalem: Hebrew University Press.

Murdoch, B. C. H., Wilks, V., & Boyle, R. S. (1987). Language disorders in dementia of the Alzheimer type. *Brain and Language, 31*, 122-137.

Nixon, S. J., & Phillips, J. A. (1999). Neurocognitive deficits and recovery in chronic alcohol abuse. *CNS Spectrums, 4*(1), 95-108.

Nixon, S. J., Tivis, R., & Parsons, O. (1992). Interpersonal problem-solving in male and female alcoholics. *Alcoholism: Clinical and Experimental Research, 16*(4), 684-687.

Orbelo, D., Grim, M. A., Talbott, R. E., & Ross, E. D. (2005). Impaired comprehension of affective prosody in elderly subjects is not explained by age-related hearing loss or age-related cognitive decline. *Journal of Geriatric Neurology and Psychiatry, 18*, 25-32.

Orbelo, D. M., Testa, J. A., & Ross, E. D. (2003). Age-related impairments in comprehending affective prosody: Comparison to brain damaged subjects. *Journal of Geriatric Psychiatry and Neurology, 16*, 44-52.

Oscar-Berman, M. (1985). Neuropsychological consequences of alcohol abuse: Questions, hypotheses and models. In O. Parsons, N. Butters, & P. Nathan (Eds.), *Neuropsychology of alcoholism: Implications for diagnosis and treatment*. New York: Guilford.

Oscar-Berman, M., Hancock, M., Mildworf, B., Hutner, N., & Weber, D.A. (1990). Emotional perception and memory in alcoholism and aging. *Alcohol: Clinical and Experimental Research, 14*(3), 383-393.

Parsons, O. A. (1998). Neurocognitive deficits in alcoholics and social drinkers: A continuum? *Alcoholism: Clinical and Experimental Research, 22*(4), 954-961.

Parsons, O. A., & Nixon, S. J. (1998, March). Cognitive functioning in sober social drinkers: A review of the research since 1986. *Journal of Studies on Alcohol*, 180-190.

Pell, M. D. (1998, August). Recognition of prosody following unilateral brain lesion: Influence of functional and structural attributes of prosodic contours. *Neuropsychologia, 36*(8), 701-715.

Pell, M. D., & Baum, S. R. (1997). The ability to perceive and comprehend intonation in linguistic and affective contexts by brain-damaged patients. *Brain and Language, 57*, 80-99.

Philippot, P., Kornreich, C., Blairy, S., Baert, I., Den Dulk, A., Le Bon, O., et al. (1999). Alcoholics' deficits in the decoding of emotional facial expression. *Alcoholism: Clinical and Experimental Research, 23*(6), 1031-1038

Piccininni, M., DiCarlo, A., Baldereschi, M., Zaccara, G., Inzitari, D. (2005). Behavioral and psychological symptoms in Alzheimer's disease: Frequency and relationship with duration and severity of the disease. *Dementia and Geriatric Cognitive Disorders, 19*(5-6), 276-281.

Resnick, S., Kraut, M. A., Zonderman, A. B., & Davatzikos, C. (2003). Longitudinal magnetic resonance imaging studies of older adults: A shrinking brain. *Journal of Neuroscience, 23*(8), 3295-3301.

Roberts, V. (1996). Prosody impairment and associated affective and behavioral disturbances in Alzheimer's disease. *Neurology, 47*, 1482-1488.

Ross, E. D. (1981). The aprosodias: Functional-anatomical organization of the affective components of language in the right hemisphere. *Archives of Neurology, 38*, 561-569.

Ross, E. D. (1982). The divided self. *The Sciences, 22*, 8-12.

Ross, E. D. (2000). Affective prosody and the aprosodias. In M. M. Mesulam (Ed.), *Principles of behavioral and cognitive neurology* (pp. 316-331). New York: Oxford University Press.

Ross, E. D., Harney, J., deLacoste-Utamsing, M. C., & Purdy, P. (1981). How the brain integrates affective and propositional language into a unified behavioral function: Hypothesis based on clinico-anatomical evidence. *Archives of Neurology, 38*, 745-748.

Ross, E. D., & Mesulam, M. M. (1979). Dominant language functions of the right hemisphere? Prosody and emotional gesturing. *Archives of Neurology, 36*, 144-148.

Ross, E. D., Orbelo, D. M., Burgard, M., & Hansel, S. (1998). Functional-anatomic correlates of aprosodic deficits in patients with right brain damage. *Neurology, 50*(Suppl. 4), A363.

Ross, E. D., Orbelo, D., Cartwright, J., Hansel, S., Burgard, M., Testa, J., et al. (2001). Affective-prosodic deficits in schizophrenia: Profiles of patients with brain damage and comparison with relation to schizophrenic symptoms. *Journal of Neurology, Neurosurgery, and Psychiatry*, *70*, 597-604.

Ross, E. D., Thompson, R. D., & Yenkosky, J. (1997). Lateralization of affective prosody in brain and the callosal integration of hemispheric language functions. *Brain and Language*, *56*, 27-54.

Ryalls, J. (1988). Concerning right-hemisphere dominance for affective language. *Archives of Neurology*, *45*, 337-338.

Seron, X., van der Kaa, M. A., Remitz, A., & Van der Linden, M. (1979). Pantomime interpretation and aphasia. *Neuropsychologia*, *17*, 661-668.

Shimabukuro, J., Awata, S., Matsuoka, H. (2005). Behavioral and psychological symptoms of dementia characteristic of mild Alzheimer patients. *Psychiatry and Clinical Neuroscience*, *59*, 274-279.

Speedie, L. J., Coslett, B., et al. (1984). Repetition of affective prosody in mixed transcortical aphasia. *Archives of Neurology*, *41*, 268-270.

Spreen, O., & Strauss, E. (1998). *A compendium of neuropsychological tests: Administration, norms, and commentary.* Oxford, UK: Oxford University Press.

Testa, J., Beatty, W., Gleason, A. C., Orbelo, D. M., & Ross, E. D. (2001). Impaired affective prosody in AD: Relationship to aphasic deficits and emotional behaviors. *Neurology*, *57*(8), 1474-1481.

Tompkins, C., & Flowers, C. R. (1985). Perception of emotional intonation by brain-damaged adults: The influence of task processing levels. *Journal of Speech and Hearing Research*, *28*, 527-538.

Trauner, D. A., Ballantyne, A., Fridland, S., & Chase, C. (1996, March). Disorders of affective and linguistic prosody in children after early unilateral brain damage. *Annals of Neurology*, *39*(3), 361-367.

Warrier, C. M., Zatorre, R. J. (2004). Right temporal cortex is critical for utilization of melodic contextual cues in a pitch constancy task. *Brain*, *127*(7), 1616-1625.

Zubenko, G. S., Zubenko, W. N., McPherson, S. (2003). A collaborative study of the emergence and clinical features of the major depressive syndrome of Alzheimer's disease. *American Journal of Psychiatry*, *160*, 857-866.

CHAPTER 8

Pathologic Phonation Connotes and Evokes Wrong Emotive Reactions in Listeners

Krzysztof Izdebski

Abstract

Pathologic phonation is typically divided into organic, neurological, and functional subgroups, each of which can generate more or less specific vocal characteristics, although a wide overlap is expected. Nonetheless, the acoustic features of some of the specific dysphonic qualities can approximate acoustic features of emotional vocalization produced by "normals"; hence, they can mimic some specific emotive states, for example, joy, anger, sadness, fear, etc. The emotional "distance" towards which certain pathological voices tend to gravitate when perceived by naïve listeners is explored here on the basis of reported reactions of the dysphonic patients they experience daily in communicative situations.

Introduction

It is commonly agreed that certain voice qualities, prosodic features, and temporal vocal characteristics are associated on an almost universal basis with perception of specific emotions, like anger, joy, fear, happiness, and sadness (Shearer, Banse, & Wallbott, 2001). When vocalization is affected by pathological processes, the resultant dysphonic voice assumes deviant qualities, some of which may approximate the voice qualities associated with various emotive states. Hence, even during an emotionally neutral speaking condition a dysphonic patient may sound as if he or she is expressing a specific emotion, when indeed there is no such intent on the part of the afflicted speaker. The situation may be even more convoluted when the vocal condition does not match the gender of the speaker. Moreover, with certain pathological conditions, this incongruence is more pronounced when speaking on the phone, and may be amplified further in face-to-face conversation, the latter occurring when the accompanying facial expressions bring the total percept (voice-face-posture) closer to the assumed emotional quality, or when they are in conflict with the acoustic signal produced.

The scenario of voice-gender mismatch is typical when a female voice drops to a low F_0, whether due to polypoidal vocal cords, or a virilized voice, or a person who looks female but has a male voice quality (in a transgender patient; Flower & Izdebski, 1979; Izdebski, 2007).

The emotional mismatch scenario can be present in a variety of dysphonias, and can be amplified further in neurological cases such as in the various dystonias and dyskinesias, in various craniofacial anomalies, or in Parkinsonian syndrome patients, where facial expressions do not match the intended vocal signals. This mismatch, when present in nonpathologic populations, is known as the McGurk effect (McGurk & MacDonald, 1976).

In this chapter I will discuss how the pathologic voice may be misinterpreted by the naïve listener as being indicative of a "wrong" emotional or physical state that is not representative of the dysphonic patient. I will demonstrate that this scenario often brings serious embarrassment to the afflicted patient (the producer) and the listener alike, and in many cases carries profound psychosocial consequences for the afflicted patient (Krischke et al., 2005).

Vocal Movement Dysphonias

Typical vocal movement dysphonias include focal dystonia of the larynx represented by adductor (ADDSD) and abductor (ABDSD) spasmodic dysphonia, vocal tremor, or mixed ADDSD with VoT (Izdebski, 1981; 1992; 1997; Izdebski & Ward, 1997). In all these conditions, symptoms are organized phonetotopically, meaning that the voice can be normal or abnormal depending on predictable F_0/dB levels or as a function of phonemic context (Izdebski, 1996; 2007).

ADDSD

The distinguishing quality of ADDSD is vocal overpressure (Izdebski, 1992). Overpressure results from increased glottic compression and increased subglottic pressure (Alku, Svec, Vilkman, & Sram, 2000; Shipp, Izdebski, & Schutte, 1988).

Overpressured voice quality can give an impression of disturbed, angry, and hostile emotive character (Izdebski, 1981).

These patients, regardless of gender, may be referred to as producing a bizarre sound that evokes negative and fearful reactions in the uninitiated listener. When speaking on the phone, some of these patients are asked if they are unable to breathe, if they are crying, are in pain, are angry, are being strangled, or are emotional, and the conversation may end quite abruptly. These patients often fear talking on the phone as they have experienced listeners' unwillingness to continue discourse.

Interestingly, the members of the family of ADDSD patients are typically extremely tolerant and accepting of their vocal handicaps, though ADDSD patients themselves are often embarrassed and may withdraw from public speaking in the presence of the spouse in a nonfamilial setting, even when they know that there is no rejection from the family.

When overpressure is accompanied by facial grimacing (which in ADDSD cases is of compensatory nature), the typically evoked emotion is that of pain or discomfort. However, because of the nature of dystonia, the voice quality and facial expressions of these patients may actually match the intended emotional states when these are experienced by the speaker, making an uninitiated listener even more confused when participating in a communication process with these patients. It is worthwhile to notice that the bizarreness of the voicing process in ADDSD patients was instrumental in the diagnosis of ADDSD (and ABDSD) as a "hysterical dysphonia" (for review, see Izdebski, 1981). When vocal arrests are present, in addition to overpressure, the evoked emotion may be that of fear, stuttering, stress, and anxiety.

ABDSD

ABDSD is a counterpart of ADDSD, and patients afflicted with this disorder may produce normal sustained phonation, but become dysphonic in the context of speech containing voiceless-voiced segments (e.g., he saw half . . .) by de- or unvoicing the vocalic segment that follows the voiceless sound. This sounds as if the speaker is running out of air in a hissy, semi-aspirated way, or is gasping for air, and the associated voice quality evokes a perception of effort.

This feature also seems to evoke a perception of semi-silent crying, exhaustion, sobbing, desperation, depression, pain, and/or despair. If the face struggles as well, pain is typically perceived as severe and acute.

These acoustic vocal features impact speech intelligibility in both ADDSD and ABDSD in a significant way at times and frustrate both the speaker and the listener, because words that are uttered can take on different meanings (e.g., penny can become benny, hair can be perceived as air) in addition to voice quality distortions. Severe cases can render a patient truly a vocal cripple (Izdebski, 1981), having profound socioeconomic consequences.

Vocal Tremor (VoT)

VoT introduces 5–6 Hz oscillations to the voice signal independently of the frequency and intensity of the F_0. VoT is also global and, contrary to ADDSD, affects all laryngeal tasks, be it speech or nonspeech (Barkmeier & Case, 2000; Izdebski, 1992). The 5–6 Hz rate is similar to the rate of vibrato present in artistic voice ornamentation (Dejonkere,

Hirano & Sundberg, 1995). While vibrato connotes positive emotions and is valued artistically, the 5–6 Hz pathologic VoT found in vocal tremor patients is an unwelcome acoustic feature.

When this rate affects either amplitude/frequency or both, the voice may sound as a wobble or may be equated with microtremor, and microtremor in speech is associated with nervousness and deception (Shipp & Izdebski, 1981). Hence, the shaky-wobbly voice can evoke connotations of psychological stress, nervousness, insecurity, reduced self-esteem, aging, and even deception.

Parkinsonian Syndrome (PS)

The Parkinsonian voice tremor is really not distinguishable, on the basis of tremor rate alone, from other forms of VoT (Izdebski, 2004), but can be more variable than, for example, the essential voice tremor. As in all voice patients, phonation of VoT patients is often met on the phone with "Are you OK?" and connotes a perception of emotional distress including fear and crying, never laughter or joy, though the rate of laughter is also 5–6 Hz (Provine, 1978).

Tardive Dyskinesia (TD)

Voice associated with TD can combine features of overpressure, instability, prosodic variability, and hydrophonia (wet voice quality), and vocalization and speech (often quite dysarthric) can be accompanied by very severe facial contortions. This makes for a devastating combination, often evoking not only an emotion of pity, but also of pain, fear, and emotional instability. (More on this subject can be found in Chapter 17 of these volumes).

Other Vocal Pathologies

Cerebral Palsy (CP)

Patients with CP, in addition to dysarthria, produce thin, high-pitched, weak, and aperiodic voice accompanied by facial grimacing. Because the gait of the CP patient is also often affected, the vocal-speech-visual signals do not stick out as in the dystonia or TD cases, since the orofacial movements fit, so to speak, the overall diagnostic picture. Consequently, in live face-to-face situations, the CP voice, though clearly abnormal and capable of emoting pain, crying, or pity, is not judged as harshly as when heard on the phone, or as in those clinical entities that display a normative visual picture at rest but produce abnormalities during phonation and speech as, for example, TD patients. Therefore, CP patients do not tend to hide vocally.

Unilateral Vocal Cord Paralysis (UVCP)

UVCP of pure recurrent laryngeal nerve (RLN) etiology typically causes problems with glottic approximation and produces differential vibrating pattern between the vocal cord, translating vocally to an increase in breathiness, limitations of loudness, reduction of duration, and introduction of diplophonia or polyphonia; when combined with superior laryngeal nerve (SLN) injury, additional vocal thinness and pitch limitations in the upper range are formed (Izdebski, 2007; Izdebski & Murry, 1980; Izdebski & Ward, 1997).

Breathiness (specifically when mixed with vocal roughness) can be used purposefully to produce a seductive voice if the air loss is mild, or a so-called confidential voice when associated with soft volume (Colton & Casper, 1996), but breathiness can evoke a perception of sickness, despair, exhaustion, and secrecy when it is more severe or paradoxically the effect of confidence or calmness. This is evidenced in the commercial use of such voices to promote various products. The topic of voice and advertising is discussed in more details elsewhere (Izdebski, 2008).

When RLN is combined with SLN injury, the posterior glottis is not approximated (Izdebski, 2007), and this adds thinness to the voice and creates an impression of an aged speaker (Sulter, Schutte, & Miller, 1996). This condition has been referred to in clinical settings as the geriatric falsetto voice.

In severe cases, the voice quality of combined RLN and SLN paralysis patients can evoke the sensation of an obscene caller, causing people to hang up the phone after listening to only a short phrase, like "Hello." Why? Because this nerve injury combination causes the glottis to be open and the posterior commissure unapproximated, and invites ventricular vocal fold compensation (von Doersten, Izdebski, Ross, & Cruz, 1993), hence causing severe breathiness and vibratory instability and an inability to elevate F_0, making the voice a worse case of the "Godfather's voice."

Curiously, certain types of breathy voices that appear to be pathologic in nature are considered either attractive or pleasant by the advertising industry, and are used commercially to promote confidence, trust, knowledge, or simply sex. This is evidenced by these voice qualities being used in promoting such diverse products as hospitals, insurance, or seductive films. Though it may seem quite questionable wisdom, the advertising industry is not in agreement, as judged by the frequent usage of such voices in commercials.

Mucosal Organic Phonatory Lesions

Emotions associated with seductiveness and sexuality can be evoked by a female voice when organic swellings of the vocal cord mucosa are present. Such changes account for asymmetrical vibrations, underclosure of the posterior glottic commissure, friction, noise, and breathy air escape.

Interestingly, when a thin and breathy voice is produced by a female actress, it is usually done for the purposes of evoking naïveté, dumbness, adult infantile behavior, and triviality. This may be intentional and may be in fact quite derogatory in its purpose. Some of these sensations may be heard when listening to Marilyn Monroe singing "Mr. President."

False Vocal Fold (FVF) Phonation

When the FVF (vermicular folds) interfere with production of the voice by the true vocal cords, or when the FVF actually produce voice alone or in combination with the TVC vibration, the resultant voice is harsh and aperiodic, but can be loud and can show some prosodic flexibility. Patients producing this type of voice are often asked if they are sick, ill, have a cold, or what is wrong with them. The quality of this voice thus produces a negative sensation and sometimes appears to be equated with fear.

Although not necessarily correct, FVF voice can be labeled perceptually by nonspecialists as a throaty voice, or a Louis Armstrong voice, which has quite a different pattern and characteristics from the FVF phonation (Izdebski, 2007), and it is also different from the so-called pharyngealized or laryngo-pharyngealized voice quality (Laver,1980; Nolan, 1983). According to a recent study, throaty voice was contrasted with a habitual one in the same speakers acting as their own controls (Laukkanen, Bjornkner, & Sundberg, 2006). These throaty voices may be considered either as harmful or even undesirable and were defined as throaty based on altered format positions, lower LTAS levels in the F_0 range (considered to reflect hyperfunctional) phonation type, and raised F_0 in both male and female speakers.

This recent work from Scandinavia can be related to an earlier work in which tense, throaty, and nasal voice qualities were simulated by two male and two female actors (Addington, 1968). The results indicated that throatiness in male voices gave the impression of a realistic and mature person, but in the females the voice was associated with reduced intelligence, increased masculinity, laziness, lack of emotions, ugliness, and carelessness. Tense voices in male speakers gave an impression of an older and more quarrelsome person, while tense female voices evoked the impression of a younger, more emotional, and a less intelligent person. Breathy male voice was interpreted to reflect a young and artistic person, while breathy female voice was linked to a feminine and pretty appearance. On the other hand, gender differences for nasality were absent, as nasality evoked many negative impressions for both genders.

Vocal Cord Stiffness (VCS)

When one vocal cord is stiff and the other vibrates, the voice can be perceived as normal and fails only somewhat at loud levels. But when stiffness is combined with aperiodicity, ventricular contraction, and noise, a harsh quality is perceived and this seems to evoke emotions of rudeness, defiance, and suspicion of criminality. This may be approaching the so-called Godfather's voice, and can be found in patients with widespread organic findings, including carcinoma, and in those whose lesions affect the anterior commissure only (Dedo & Izdebski, 1982).

Alaryngeal Voice (AV)

Alaryngeal voice is produced by totally laryngectomized patients (Izdebski, Reed, Ross, & Hilsinger, 1994). Essentially two types of voice are produced, artificial or physiologic. Artificial voice is produced when the patient uses either an intraoral or surface electrolarynx. Physiologic voice is produced by injection or tracheoesophageal puncture technique.

Using an electrolarynx or Tokyo artificial device as a sound source seems to evoke strangeness and a distant, robotlike quality. This type of voice is often liked and accepted by children, but may be unpleasant for adults.

The physiologic esophageal injection voice can be perceived as unpleasant or even repulsive as it is often rudely called the "burp voice."

The buccal voice may evoke the sound of a cartoon voice, as if produced by a dwarf or a munchkin, and is typically difficult to understand on the phone. In pathological cases, this voice is not considered pleasant or attractive. However, when buccal voice, like the Mickey Mouse-type voice, is produced by a laryngeal speaker for the purposes of entertainment, the quality is considered pleasant and attractive.

Among the alaryngeal voices, the most positive emotions are evoked when a patient is fitted with a tracheoesophageal (TEP) voice prosthesis (Izdebski et al., 1994), indicating that in TEP voice, vocal pleasantness improves significantly, as are the social acceptance and intelligibility of the TEP voice on and off the phone.

Functional Voice Problems (FVP)

Functional voice can evoke an array of emotions, as the voice qualities associated with this condition are extremely wide (Kotby, Titze , Saleh, & Berry, 1993). Whisper aphonia seems to connote pain, displeasure, surprise, and astonishment. Generalized FVP with reduced volume, range, and rate can connote depressive emotions and pain. Ingressive dysphonia seems to evoke surprise and curiosity, while persistent puberophonia in a male evokes insecurity and weakness.

Conversely, polypoidal thickening of the vocal cord mucosa (Izdebski, 2007; Dedo & Izdebski, 1982) (in a female patient evokes a tough, demanding, and decisive image, perhaps because it approximates the male voice. Aperiodicity introduced by vocal cord masses can be equated with roughness and seductive emotions.

Summary

In summary, pathologic voice production can evoke emotions that have not been intended by the speaker because of the intrinsic content of the acoustic features of such a voice. Though some of these pathological voices may be unpleasant, others may be both pleasant and attractive. The information presented here is based on my long-term clinical experience with dysphonic patients, and was intended to be more or less a generalized "teaser" to evoke in a reader a desire for more in-depth research.

References

Addington, D. W. (1968).The relationship of selected vocal characteristics to personality perception. *Speech Monographs, XXXV*, 492-503.

Alku, P., Svec, J. G., Vilkman, E., & Sram, F. (2000). Analysis of voice production in breathy normal and pressed phonation by comparing inverse filtering and videokymography. In B. Yuan, T. Huang, & X. Tang (Eds.), *Proceedings from the 6th International Conference on Spoken Language Processing* (ICSLP 2000, Vol. 3). Beijing, China: Military Friendship Publishers.

Aminoff, M., Izdebski, K., & Dedo, H. H. (1978). Clinical aspects of spasmodic dysphonia. *Journal of Neurology, Neurosurgery, and Psychiatry, 41*, 361-365.

Barkmeier, J. M., & Case, J. L. (2000). Differential diagnosis of adductor-type spasmodic dysphonia, vocal tremor, and muscle tension dysphonia. Speech therapy and rehabilitation. *Current Opinion in Otolaryngology & Head & Neck Surgery*, *8*(3), 174-179.

Colton, R. H., & Casper, J. K. (1996). *Understanding voice problems: A physiological perspective for diagnosis and treatment* (2nd ed.). Baltimore: Williams & Wilkins.

Dedo, H. H., & Izdebski, K. (1982). Hoarseness. In G. Gates (Ed.), *Current therapy in otolaryngology, head and neck surgery* (pp. 339-344). St. Louis, MO: B.C. Decker-Mosby.

Dejonkere, P. H., Hirano, M., & Sundberg, J. (1995). *Vibrato.* San Diego, CA: Singular.

Flower, R. M., & Izdebski, K. (1979). *Common speech disorders in otolaryngologic practice.* Rochester, MN: American Academy of Otolaryngology.

Izdebski, K. (1981). Spastic dysphonia. In J. Darby (Ed.), *Speech evaluation in medicine and psychiatry: Vol. II, Medicine* (pp. 105-127). New York: Gruene and Stratton.

Izdebski, K. (1984). Overpressure and breathiness in spastic dysphonia. An acoustic (LTAS) and perceptual study. *Acta Otolaryngologica Scandinavia*, *97*, 122-129.

Izdebski, K. (1992). Symptomatology of adductor spasmodic dysphonia: A physiologic model. *Journal of Voice*, *6*, 306-319.

Izdebski, K., Dedo, H. H., & Boyles, L. (1984). Spastic dysphonia. A patient profile of 200 cases. American *Journal of Otolaryngology*, *5*, 7-14.

Izdebski, K. (2007). Clinical Voice Assessment: The Role & Value of the Phonatory Function Studies. In A. Lalwani (Ed.), *Current diagnosis & treatment. Otolaryngology head and neck surgery* (pp. 416-429). New York: McGraw Hill Lange.

Izdebski, K. (2008). Matching and mismatching emotional vocal qualities in radio commercials to influence purchasing decisions. In K. Izdebski (Ed.), *Emotions in the human voice.*

Izdebski, K., & Murry, T. (1980). Glottal waveform variability: A preliminary inquiry. In V. Lawrence (Ed.), *Transcripts from the IXth Symposium Care of Control* (pp. 39-43). New York: The Voice Foundation.

Izdebski, K., Reed, C., Ross, J. C., & Hilsinger, R. L., Jr. (1994). Problems with surgical (TEF) voice restoration in totally laryngectomized patients: A review of 90 cases. *Annals of Otolaryngology-Head and Neck Surgery*, *120*, 840-845.

Izdebski, K., & Shipp, T. (1985). Model of spastic dysphonia. In G. A. Gates (Ed.), *Spastic dysphonia: State of the art 1984* (pp. 44-47). New York: The Voice Foundation.

Izdebski, K., & Ward, R. (1997). Differential diagnosis of ADD-ABDuctor spasmodic dysphonia, vocal tremor and ventricular dysphonia by auditory and phonoscopic observations. In M. Pais Clemente (Ed.), *Voice update, International Congress Series 1997*, 47-60. Amsterdam: Elsevier.

Izdebski, K., & Ward, R. (1997). Glottic physiology after Botox treatment of ADDuctor spasmodic dysphonia, ABDuctor spasmodic dysphonia and vocal tremor. In M. Pais Clemente (Ed.), *Voice update, International Congress Series 1997*, 131-146. Amsterdam: Elsevier.

Kotby, M. N., Titze, I. R., Saleh, M. M., & Berry, D. A. (1993). Fundamental frequency stability in functional dysphonia. *Acta Otolaryngologica*, *113*(3), 439-444.

Krischke, S., Weigelt, S., Hoppe, U., Kollner, V., Klotz, M., Eysholdt, U., et al. (2005). Quality of life in dysphonic patients. *Journal of Voice*, *19*(1), 132-137.

Laukkanen, A.-M., Bjornkner, E., & Sundberg, J. (2006). Throaty voice quality: Subglottal pressure, voice source, and formant characteristics. *Journal of Voice*, *20*(1), 25-37.

Laver, J. (1980). *The phonetic description of voice quality.* Cambridge, UK: Cambridge University Press.

McGurk, H., & MacDonald, J. (1976). Hearing lips and seeing voices. *Nature*, *264*(5588), 746-748s.

Nolan, F. (1983). *The phonetic basis of speaker recognition.* Cambridge, UK: Cambridge University Press.

Provine, R. P. (2001). *Laughter: A scientific investigation.* New York: Penguin Books.

Scherer, K. R., Banse, R., & Wallbott, H. G. (2001). Emotion inferences from vocal expression correlate across language and cultures. *Journal of Cross-Cultural Psychology*, *32*(1), 76-92.

Shipp, T., & Izdebski, K. (1981). Current evidence for the existence of laryngeal macrotremor and microtremor. *Journal of Forensic Science*, *26*, 501-505.

Sulter, A., Schutte, H., & Miller, D. (1996). Standardized laryngeal videostroboscopic rating: Differences in normal glottal closure between untrained and trained male and female subjects, and effects of varying sound intensity, fundamental frequency and age. *Journal of Voice*, *10*, 175-189.

Von Doersten, P. G., Izdebski, K., Ross, J. C., & Cruz, R. M. (1992). Ventricular dysphonia: A profile of 40 cases. *Laryngoscope*, *102*, 1296-1301.

CHAPTER 9

Perception of Emotion in Impaired Facial and Vocal Expression

Ingrid Verduyckt and Dominique Morsomme

Abstract

This chapter tries to give a short overview of the main currents in contemporary theories of emotional expression. First, we attempt to draw a brief outline of how emotions are defined as compared to other affective states. Second, we try to give a short picture of the different views concerning the relationship between emotional expressions and experienced emotions, as well as the role of those expressions in human interactions. Third, the vocal and facial modes of emotion expressions are detailed. Fourth, we focus on how emotional expressions can be affected by different diseases, such as Parkinson's disease, Steinert's disease, and Moebius syndrome, at the vocal and the facial level. The impact of these impairments is considered in the light of the conclusions about the function of emotional expressions in society today. We conclude with a reflection about the therapy possibilities in reeducation of impaired emotional expressions.

Definition, Origin, and Function of Emotion

There is no doubt that emotions and emotional expressions are an essential part of our life. Less obvious, though, is that emotions are central to more than just our affective life.

> Decision making and problem solving behaviors, presumed to be strictly material and rational, are also influenced by our emotional condition. Emotions influence our perception of the world, the way we express ourselves, and our intellectual reasoning and the learning processes already at a very young age (Luminet, 2002).

Although it is common in daily life to speak about emotions, either self-experienced or the ones perceived in others, it is not an easy thing to exactly define what an emotion is. What is for instance the difference between emotions and other affective states such as moods, attitudes, and interpersonal stances or affectively colored personality traits such as hostility or kindness? Scherer, who has mainly studied vocal expression, has suggested that the different affective states should be differentiated according to their intensity, their duration and rapidity of state change, the degree to which they focus on eliciting events, and the extent to which appraisal has been part of the elicitation (Scherer, 2003). The degree of synchronization of organismic subsystems (cognitive appraisal, physiological arousal, motoric system, subjective feeling, and motivational system) and their impact on behavior is also taken into account. Considering those parameters, it appears that emotions are a distinctive category of affective state. They are of a greater intensity but of shorter duration and they change more rapidly. They are characterized by highly synchronized subsystems and influence open behavior, and they are focused on eliciting events as well as based on cognitive appraisal. This conception is in line with Ekman's suggestion of the characteristics of emotions (Ekman, 1992a; 1999). Besides the criteria mentioned by Scherer, Ekman adds unbidden occurrence as another characteristic. He also suggests that emotions are elicited at an abstract level, by automatic appraisal of universals in antecedent events. For example, the loss of a significant person is thought to be a universal antecedent to sadness, although the "significant one" might differ according to the culture. Furthermore, Ekman suggests that the characteristics differentiating emotions from other affective states are also the ones differentiating them from one another.

Ekman stresses the view that our emotions are reactions that were developed in our evolutionary past as a signal and coping system adapted to survival. Though our individual experiences might affect our way to react, it is predominantly our history as a species that has shaped our emotions and made them unique. Emotions are a way of preparing an individual to a specific behavior called forth by the encountered situation. They are accompanied by specific physiological changes that will affect mechanisms such as respiration, phonation, and articulation, enabling the organism to react adequately and leading to facial and vocal changes (Scherer, 2003). One common hypothesis is that the generated vocal and facial expressions will be recognized as the expression of one specific emotion, which implicates the existence of a direct link between experienced and expressed. Emotion expressions are thought to be used as a way to inform conspecifics about a person's internal state emotions (Izard, 1994). The accurate decoding of someone's experienced emotion gives information about the antecedents that most likely provoked that expression and the immediate action to anticipate from that person. Izard illustrates the advantage of precise emotion communication by giving the example of an adult and a juvenile in our evolutionary past, walking through the savannah. The expression of the adult when passing by a stimulus that should be avoided needs to be differentiated according to the nature of the stimulus. Is it a deteriorating carcass, which just shouldn't be approached, or a deadly viper that should be fled? Obviously, in this example, the accurate and precise decoding of the expression is of great value for survival.

The idea that emotional expressions translate a person's inner state is based on a large corpus of studies on recognition of facial and vocal emotion expressions (Elfenbein & Ambady, 2002; Juslin & Laukka, 2003; Russell, 1994; Scherer, 1986; 2003). The results of those studies have shown that humans are capable of perceiving emotions through vocal and facial cues. However, there is an ongoing discussion among emotion theorists as to whether nonverbal emotional expressions are recognized as discrete emotions (Ekman, 1992a; 1992b; 1999), or if they are merely perceived by their localization in a space with two or more dimensions such as valence, arousal, and power and activation (Russell, 1980; Russell & Fehr, 1987). Pollerman (2002), for instance, proposes a unified model of cognition and emotion, based on a three-dimensional affective space of valence, power, and arousal. This framework allows us to establish a continuity from nonemotional to emotional states and processes and reinforces the connection between affect and intelligence.

Also, some authors suggest that the results obtained in many categorical recognition studies of emotion might have been inflated through design procedures (Bachorowski & Owren, 2003; Frank & Stennett, 2001; Russell, 1994). Most often, the stimuli used by the authors have been through a severe preselection and are mostly issued from portrayals of the emotions rather than spontaneous ones. This has led to highly prototypical and intense expressions. Bachorowski and Owren (2003) argue that considering the preselection, much higher recognition scores could be expected. Also, studies using stimuli of moving pictures have yielded a much lower recognition score among the judges (Elfenbein & Ambady, 2002). This is also the case when spontaneous or elicited emotion expressions are used as stimuli. Thus, it seems that pure, spontaneous emotion expressions, directly and unambiguously translating an emotion, might not be that current in daily life. This raises the question of what emotional expressions really are conveying and how they are used in communication.

The idea that our emotional expressions are not necessarily directly linked to our felt emotions is not new. Early Greek and Roman rhetoricians studied vocal and gestural expressions with the aim of using them strategically to touch and convince the audience. They were aware of the possibility of modeling the emotional expressions independently from the experienced emotions (Izard, 1994; Scherer, 2003).

More recently, Scherer accentuates the fact that the expressions of emotion are influenced by our personal past and our adaptation to the social rules of society (Scherer, 1995). He makes a distinction between push and pull effects shaping the acoustic characteristics of vocal expression. Push effects are produced by the physiological changes provoked by the experienced emotion, while pull effects are the result of the influence of external factors such as social display rules, linguistic constraints on the acoustical pattern, or environmental constraints. A noisy room, for instance, would impose a higher vocal intensity level and a slower rhythm, which are also acoustical parameters vital to vocal emotion expression (Juslin & Laukka, 2003; Scherer, 1986). Pollerman (2002) suggests that vocal emotional expressions can have three different semiological statuses: they can be spontaneous indicators, falsely spontaneous indicators, or symbols. The first is a double-faced entity, where the link between the signifier and the signified is naturally given, in accordance with the hypothesis of a direct emotion-expression link. The second is an indicator that is produced on purpose and intended to be perceived as spontaneous. The third is an entity where the link between the signifier and the signified is conventionalized. According to this classification, it is the proportional amount of push and pull effects that will determine which one, or which blend, of semiological status(es) the emotional expression has.

Also, Izard (1994) stipulates that from an evolutionary point of view, it would have been maladaptive not to be able to conceal one's inner state. The ability to modify emotional expressions independently from the felt emotion has probably developed early through phylogeny and studies have shown that already at the age of 4–5 months, changes in emotional expressions due to self-regulation can be observed in children.

Some authors have directed their studies from the point of view that emotional expressions might not be characterized by our inner experienced emotions, but rather by how we want to influence a listener (Bachorowski & Owren, 2003; Russell, Bachorowski, & Fernàndez-Dols, 2003). Emotional expressions are then considered merely as tools used in advanced communication. These tools were developed via socialization processes and social learning, and are used according to individual social context and educational history, as well as according to personal needs and goals. Emotional expressions are instruments, essential for humans to evolve profitably in society.

Studies of nonverbal emotion expression have mainly been conducted with the aim of exploring whether the expression of emotions is perceived categorically, and if that recognition is universal and innate. The question of the universality and innateness of emotion expression is still a matter of discussion and disagreement among emotion theorists. Recently, a meta-analysis of emotion expression studies came to the conclusion that emotion expressions, though to some extent recognized across cultural boundaries, might lose some of their meaning (Elfenbein & Ambady, 2002). The authors make a comparison to differences in linguistic dialects. What seems important to retain from facial and vocal emotion studies is that the emotion a subject attempts to express can be accurately identified by judges of different genders, ages, and cultures. Also, the studies on emotion recognition have given precious information about the nonverbal cues that we use when we decode emotional expressions, specifically regarding both the facial and the vocal channels.

Although it is not entirely clear yet what emotion expressions precisely are and what information we draw out of them, there is no doubt that we commonly use them as a source of information to adapt our behavior.

Facial Cues in Expressions of Emotion

According to Ekman (1992a), there is evidence of a distinct, universal facial expression for anger, fear, enjoyment, sadness, and disgust.

Ekman and Friesen (in Ekman, Friesen, & Ancoli, 1980) have developed the Facial Action Coding System (FACS), a comprehensive, anatomically based system identifying all the possible specific actions of facial muscles, called *action units* (AUs). This coding system has since been used in various studies to map the active muscles in discrete emotion expressions. The FACS coding procedure involves intensity rating of each muscular activation on a five-point intensity scale. It also involves the timing of each action as well as the classification of facial expressions in terms of events. An event is an expression described by its combination of AUs. This coding system has been used in numerous works, with the aim to map the different muscles involved in different emotions, trying to extract the unique combination of muscle contractions contributing to the expression of one specific emotion.

Ekman et al. (1980) examined induced emotions with the FACS and compared the intensity results with the subjective estimation of the subject. The results showed that the intensity of an expressed emotion, measured by the intensity, duration, and frequency of its AUs, correlated to the intensity of the subjective experience of that emotion. For happiness, a raise of the zygomatic major was predictive of the subjective experience of happiness. However, they also found that other facial movements could also occur in moments of self-reported happiness, but the statistical analyses showed no correlations. Also, a raise of the zygomatic major was found in some episodes of self-reports of negative emotions.

Kohler et al. (2003) used the FACS to investigate the specific muscular action in four different emotion expressions of high intensity: happy, sad, angry, and fearful. They used posed and evoked emotion expressions by actors. The FACS ratings showed specific profiles of AUs for the four different emotions. Although some action units are exclusively present or absent in one emotion, several AUs are present in two or more of the emotions. Comparing their results with an earlier study by Gosselin et al. and with the predictions made by Ekman and Friesen (in Kohler et al., 2004), they found unanimous agreement on the occurrence of some AUs specific to the four emotions: cheek raised and lip corner pulled in happiness, eyebrow lowered and lip corner depressed in sadness; eyes wide open, eyebrow lowered, and mouth open in both anger and fear. Still, not all the characteristic AUs found in this study are in complete agreement with Gosselin's findings or Ekman and Friesen's predictions. The authors suggest that the differences might be due to design procedures. It seems that a core of specific, emotion-related AUs exists. However, there seem to be variations within subjects and emotions due to the context. Also, expressions of emotion might differ according to whether they are portrayed or spontaneous. In fact, Ekman (1992a) suggests that some of the muscles involved in natural expressions are difficult or impossible for most people to activate when this emotion is not felt (Ekman, 1992b). The posed expression of joy, for instance, can be differentiated from the spontaneous expression with regard to the "Duchenne smile," that is, the inward pulling of the skin surrounding the eyes by the contraction of the orbicularis oculi, pars lateralis muscle. The lack of this contraction makes a smile look fake or unfelt.

Vocal Cues in Expressions of Emotion

The vocal expressions of emotion have not been as widely studied as their facial counterparts. The vocal channel is complex to study due to the fact that it is the bearer of information, not only regarding emotions, but also language. The vocal expression of emotion is produced by the same apparatus that is used to produce speech. The same acoustical parameters that are used to express emotions are also used to convey linguistic and pragmatic cues (Scherer, 1981). The initial emotional expression can thus be shaped by the use of specific linguistic cues and also by facial expressions affecting the shape of the vocal tract, as for example a smile (Bachorowski & Owren, 2003). Many of the physiological changes called forth by an emotion will affect the voice by changing respiration pattern, tension in the laryngeal musculature, and facial mimicry (Juslin & Laukka, 2003). It is not easy to isolate the vocalizations specific to emotions.

A recent meta-analysis of vocal emotional expression studies comes to the conclusion that vocal cues can be used to accurately infer a person's emotional state (Juslin & Laukka, 2003). The same criticism directed towards the studies of facial emotional expression is reiterated. However, it still seems undeniable that the voice bears emotional cues. Still, though human judges have had little difficulties in the studies reviewed to correctly recognize the emotions joy, anger, sadness, fear, and love/tenderness, establishing the distinct acoustical patterns specific to each of those emotions has proven more difficult. The acoustic cues most often studied and supposed to convey emotional information are voice quality, intensity, pitch, and timing, i.e., articulation rate. Indeed, Juslin and Laukka's meta-analysis shows a correlation between the specific emotions and the acoustical changes regarding these parameters. Speech rate, high frequency energy, fundamental frequency (F_0), intensity variability, and intensity were increased in anger, happiness, and fear but decreased in sadness and tenderness. These characteristic patterns are, although consistent, not sufficiently distinct to explain how the emotions can be specifically and accurately identified. Other, finer acoustical cues need to be examined. Few studies to this day have investigated other specific acoustical cues in a regular manner. Still, the sparse data available suggest that microstructural irregularities with respect to frequency, intensity, and duration are associated with the negative emotions anger, fear, and sadness, while the voice of happiness and tenderness is more regular. Some data also suggest that the attack of the voice plays a role in characterizing the expressed emotion, at least in musical expression. Fast tone attacks seem to be used in anger and happiness, while slow tone attacks are used in sadness and tenderness. It also seems that imprecise articulation is associated to sadness, whereas the contrary is associated with anger. According to Scherer (1986), the primary difficulty with isolating the determining acoustical parameters is their variability in time and within the same emotion. Also, different persons might use those cues differently. Some might specially use variations in intensity to differentiate the emotions, while others might rely more on timing cues. This was the case in a study by Whiteside (1999). Two actors were asked to depict different emotions. When portraying sadness, only one of them used a decreased articulation rate to exemplify it. It is also obvious that there are individual differences in encoding ability (Banse & Scherer, 1996). As Juslin and Laukka (2003) express it, neither cue is necessary nor sufficient to express one specific emotion, but the larger the number of cues utilized, the more reliable the communication.

Perception of Emotion Expressions through Different Channels

It has been observed that the different emotions are not perceived equally well through the facial or the vocal channel.

In studies on the vocal channel, sadness and anger are most often best recognized (Banse & Scherer, 1996; Juslin & Laukka 2001; 2003; Scherer, 1995), followed by fear and joy, while in studies of facial expressions (Elfenbein & Ambady, 2002), joy indisputably yields the highest recognition scores. Elfenbein and Ambady also find in their meta-analysis that joy is less well recognized in the voice than the face, and anger is less well perceived in the face than the voice. The differences linked to the respective channels are sometimes tentatively explained by their phylogenetic background. Disgust, for instance, is not recognized as well in the vocal as in the facial channel (Ekman, 1992a; Russell, 1994) suggesting that the facial expression of disgust is derived from the mouth's movement of rejection when tasting bad or noncomestible food. The sight of that movement of rejection is thought to have served as a signal to conspecifics not to eat the food. The visual signal was of greater importance than any vocalization. Thus, the difficulty of recognizing disgust by voice could be connected to the fact that it wasn't functionally necessary for survival (Banse & Scherer, 1996).

Few studies have investigated the recognition of emotional expressions from the vocal and the facial channel jointly. Also, few have attempted to compare the efficacy of each channel to convey emotional cues using the same stimuli. A study by Wallbott and Scherer (1986) suggested that the visual mode is superior to the audio mode in conveying emotional cues. In that study, the judges were required to recognize emotion expressions in a standard sentence spoken by actors. The emotions were anger, joy, fear, surprise, and sadness, and the recognition rate was examined according to three modes: visual, audio, and audiovisual. The authors came to the conclusion that the visual and the audiovisual modes were superior for the recognition of emotion expression as compared to the auditive mode only. In a study conducted by Morsomme, Verduyckt, Jamart, and Remacle (2007), judges had to categorize and rate the intensity of an actor's and a myotonic patient's emotional expression. The audiovisual mode was found to yield the best categorization scores as compared to both the visual and the auditive mode and also yielded higher intensity ratings. There was no significant difference between the visual or the facial mode only. Other authors have found the superior mode to depend on the situation and the expressed emotion (Berman, Schulman, & Marwit, 1976; Hess, Scherer, & Kappas, 1988). It seems clear that situations where both the visual and auditive cues are available simultaneously improve the emotional perception. However, little is known yet about the interaction of the visual and the auditive mode. Ekman (1992a), for instance, suggests that it is the interaction of vocal and facial cues that makes it possible to accurately differentiate positive emotions such as amusement, joy, and satisfaction. The findings to this day, although sparse, suggest that the two channels do not convey redundant information; rather, they have specific functions that are still to be defined (Elfenbein & Ambady, 2002).

Emotional Expressions and Disease

As we have seen, the emotion expression is not only a way of conveying one's experienced emotion; it is also a highly refined tool, used to regulate interactions with other human beings. The importance of emotional expressions in our life lets us thus conceive the implications of impaired decoding or encoding. The literature has mainly looked at difficulties in the decoding of emotional expressions in patients with, for example, psychiatric disorders or the effects of a stroke (Pell, 2002; Kohler et al., 2003). Different tests have been designed to evaluate the ability of those patients to understand emotional expressions through vocal or facial cues (Pell, 2002). Fewer studies have looked at the other side of the coin, namely patients with difficulties in expressing emotive content through nonverbal cues, not because of a lack of felt emotions, but because of motor or tonus difficulties.

One of the possible answers to why the literature has so few reports on expressive difficulties in emotional communication might be that the diseases affecting the facial or vocal expression (such as for instance Parkinson's, facial palsies, Moebius sequence, dystonias, anarthrias, right hemisphere strokes) are accompanied by symptoms of greater priority to the patients. The patients affected by those diseases often experience feeding difficulties, overall motor difficulties, and language impairment. The impaired emotive communication might be seen as a fairly small concern compared to all other difficulties, and thus not addressed on first hand.

Not being able to convey a nonverbal message in adequacy with the verbal content or with the intended emotion can, however, be of great worry and a source of misunderstanding. Ekman et al. (1980) suggest that facial expressions of emotion might have consequences both interpersonally and intrapersonally. On an interpersonal level, they affect other persons' reactions or behaviors, which will in turn affect the subject's own experience of the emotion. On an intrapersonal level, the facial mimicry might influence the subjective experience of the emotion. Accordingly, having an impairment in moving facial muscles could not only affect the person's possibility of adequately communicating to others, but it might also affect his or her experience of the emotion.

In diseases such as Parkinson's and Steinert's or Moebius syndrome, the linguistic value of an utterance, pragmatic cues, and the emotional content indicated by phonetical variables as well as facial emotional expressions are susceptible to getting lost. This can lead to impaired social relationships and communication breakdowns. Consider, for instance, how you would perceive the degree of veracity in someone telling you, "I'm so happy," with a low intensity of voice and a falling tone at the end of the utterance and with a stiff face. Ekman (1992a) underlines the importance of emotional expression in the development and regulation of interpersonal relationships. He mentions their involvement in the formation of attachments and in the regulation, acceleration, or deceleration of aggression. He also speaks about the case of a patient with Moebius syndrome reporting a great difficulty in maintaining or developing relationships, and of stroke patients with prosodic difficulties having severe interpersonal difficulties (Ekman, 1992a; 1999). Impaired social relationships are also a common observation among patients with Parkinson's disease (Pell, Cheang, & Leonard, 2005).

Parkinson's Disease (PD)

A study investigating the expressive ability of 21 patients with Parkinson's disease reported substantial difficulties in those patients in rendering linguistic prosodic and emotive vocal cues (Pell et al., 2005). The patients were matched with healthy controls and both groups' utterances were judged by naïve adults as to the linguistic and emotive message. The recognition rate for the four tested emotions (joy, anger, fear, and sadness) was significantly lower for the Parkinsonians. Similar results were obtained for the linguistic cues. Regarding the emotions, sadness is the only emotion expression as easily identified in both groups. The vocal characteristics of sadness [lower intensity, slower tempo, less variation in fundamental frequency and intensity, as well as less precise articulation (Juslin & Laukka, 2003)] converge with the motor difficulties provoked by the disease. Joy, anger, and fear demand a greater energy, mean intensity, and variations in F_0 and intensity range. Regarding the linguistic judgment, the raters had difficulties identifying interrogative statements in the Parkinsonians, but not declarative. In fact, the prosody of interrogation demands a rising tone at the end of the sentence, thus requiring more energy and precise adjustment in the end of the utterance. The declarative mode uses a descending tone and the voice organ thus can relax at the end of the utterance. The authors suggest that the expressive difficulties observed in this study are due to a nigrostriatal degeneration of the motor pathways rather than changes in cognition or moods. In a recent investigation of the same patients' comprehension of prosodic meaning, the authors found reduced abilities to identify emotional prosody in the Parkinsonians (in Pell et al., 2005). However, they suggest that the source of the comprehensive and expressive difficulties might be dissociated.

Simon, Smith, Pasqualini, Reddy, and Wood (2003) investigated the capacity of emotional expression in 19 Parkinsonians as compared to healthy controls. They analyzed three types of facial expressions. First, spontaneous emotional expressions were elicited through different situations (watching amusing video clips or having a conversation). The video clips were watched alone, together with the experimenter, or with the spouse. The conversation was held with the spouse or with a stranger. Second, posed expressions of six emotions were requested. Third, specific facial expressions were produced according to verbal descriptions about which part of the face to move. The expressivity was rated by judges with subjective rating scales and correlated to self-evaluation questionnaires answered by the subjects themselves. Also, the expression was objectively measured with the Facial Action Coding System. Overall, the Parkinsonians' results showed less intensive expressivity both in the spontaneous and posed conditions. The conversation condition with a stranger increased the intensity of their expression. Also, in that situation, their self-evaluation showed a higher grade of amusement. In fact, there was a relationship between the judges' rating of facial expressivity and the Parkinsonians' self-rating of emotions. The feeling-expression link thus seems to be preserved in Parkinsonians. The posed expressions of emotions were rated lower by the judges according to both quality and intensity. The smile was especially difficult to identify and often perceived as false or unfelt by the raters. Surprise and disgust were also clearly difficult.

Posed emotions and spontaneous emotions are traditionally thought to originate from different systems. The cortical motor system is believed to control posed emotions, whereas the extrapyramidal motor system is thought to control spontaneous emotions. The impaired expression of both posed and spontaneous emotions in the group of Parkinsonians suggests that their cortical motor system is affected, although this system is traditionally believed to be unaffected by the disease. However, an alternative explanation given by the authors is that different strategies are used for posing emotions, some of them implicating the extrapyramidal motor system. The patients might have used those strategies to elicit their posed emotions.

The Parkinsonians' self-evaluation of their own expressivity, as compared to what is normal for them and what is normal for the average person, showed that they did not judge themselves to be less expressive than the controls. This indicates that they might not be conscious of their expressive difficulties. McNamara and Durso (2003) have discussed the possibility that Parkinsonians might be unaware of their deficit in pragmatic skills, preventing them from compensating or readjusting themselves. Their study compared expert raters' judgment on the pragmatic skills of Parkinsonians and of healthy subjects. The evaluation was done by watching the video recording of a conversation between the subject and the clinician. Open questions were asked to the subjects, to induce casual conversation. The scores of the Parkinsonians were lower for most pragmatic skills: conversational appropriateness, prosodic, gestures, and facial expression. The authors differentiate the origin of the difficulties by attributing the facial and prosodic impairment to motor control and the difficulty with conversational appropriateness to the brain dysfunction associated with PD.

The Parkinsonians in this study were also asked to rate their pragmatic skills on an auto evaluation scale. The spouses also rated the pragmatic skills of their affected partners with the same scale. The comparison of the results indicated a lack of awareness of the pragmatic difficulty in the patients. However, the same analysis was not conducted in the control group, and the results might need to be interpreted with care.

Steinert's Disease

Steinert's disease is a hereditary myotonic atrophy. It is characterized by a slowness and a difficulty in relaxing the muscles during voluntary movements. It is not accompanied by pain but is accentuated by cold and fatigue. The severity of the disease is variable from one individual to the other and ranges from a minimal functional impairment to an inability to walk. Observed symptoms are repeated infections of the respiratory system, a perturbation of the cardiovascular apparatus (particularly the heart), and ocular symptoms such as cataracts. The central nervous system and the endocrine system are also often impaired. The disease touches various muscles and particularly the ones of the hand, the mouth, and the tongue. This yields chewing and swallowing difficulties as well as vocal difficulties. The voice is monotone and nasal. The mouth is often slightly opened and the cheeks are hollow.

In a study by Morsomme et al. (2007), the vocal and facial emotion expression of a patient with Steinert's disease was compared to an actor's. The patient's complaint, besides an action myotony increasing with cold, swallowing problems, and a general fatigue, was his difficulty in adopting a facial mimicry reflecting his oral message. This is impairing his professional occupation, where he is often leading meetings. The facial mimicry of the patient is affected by the muscular rigidity caused by his myotonic dystrophy. On the vocal level, articulation difficulties and a characteristic hyponasality are observed. In order to establish the origin of the deficit of emotion expression in the patient, it was important to isolate the different channels of emotion expression according to the three modes: audio, visual, and audiovisual.

The tasks of the two subjects included reading a neutral content text with four different emotions: joy, anger, sadness, and fear, and with a neutral expression. The two subjects were recorded during the task and the recordings were then judged by adult and adolescent raters regarding the category of the expressed emotion and the intensity of the expression.

The results showed that the actor obtained higher ratings than the patient in the gradation of the intensity. As for the categorical choice, there was no significant difference between the subjects, except for the visual mode. The judges had difficulties identifying the expressed emotions on the sole basis of the patient's facial mimicry. That corroborates the authors' hypothesis that the patient's deficit would impair the judges' ability to correctly identify the emotion. It also objectivated the patient's self-reported difficulty in adopting a facial mimicry that reflects his intended message. The low intensity scores yielded by the patient as compared to the actor also suggest a certain difficulty for him to clearly express his emotions, on both the facial and vocal level.

In this study, the patient's emotions were still quite well identified by the judges, although, in the visual mode, not as well as the actor's expressions. However, some of the judges' reflections during the rating situation made it obvious that the patient's expressions were conveying something else than only emotional content. Comments like, "Oh, he doesn't enjoy this at all," "He must be depressed," "He doesn't care the slightest bit," "He only does this because he has to," or "He is ill" were heard among the judges. Those comments touch a dimension that is not rendered by the categorical choice of emotion, although the intensity judgment might mirror it a bit. Four of the adult judges and all the adolescents were naïve judges in the sense that they had no experience with multiplehandicaps. Their comments also suggested that they were convinced of the lack of enthusiasm in the patient, though he was still capable of decoding the emotions he intended to depict. This is suggesting that before making the requested emotional judgment, the naïve raters reacted to the unusual expression. Not being aware of the disease, they might have interpreted it in terms of motivation, moods, or personality traits. The other adult judges were people with clinical experience of multi-handicap and didn't express those kinds of reflections. They realized quickly that the patient had an impairment and could probably adjust their judgment according to that. The judges' answers to the tasks of the study are probably influenced by their preceding cognitive treatment.

The study allowed the patient's impairment to be objectified in conveying an emotive message through both the vocal and the facial level. The findings are in agreement with the complaint of the patient, which in turn is supported by his wife. In a testimony where she reports her observations about the difficulties encountered in affective communication both with her husband and with two of their affected children, she emphasizes two main difficulties. The first one is, especially in her children, the facial hypotonia, leading to an open mouth, and the ptosis of the eyelids. This facial expression gives the wrong impression of inattention, or even worse, of mental debility. She feels her children are incapable of communicating empathy through their facial expression. They thus have to constantly readjust their verbal message in order to clearly express themselves. The second difficulty is the voice problem. She describes the voice of her husband, and more specifically of her children, as nasal, monotone, and low in intensity. Their vocal quality does not maintain the attention of the listener and makes it difficult for them to take part in a lively discussion. Also, she observes that the constant demands for clarification from the listener lead to a disinvestment in verbal communication and a withdrawal from social interactions. She underlines the fact that communicating requires constant efforts from her husband and children.

Moebius Syndrome

Moebius syndrome is also a disease where emotional expression is impaired. The primary symptom of this disease is a congenital uni- or bilateral-facial paralysis. It is mainly the facial channel that is impaired, especially the smile. Ekman (1992a; 1999) related the case of a patient with Moebius syndrome (MS) who underlined the difficulties in conveying emotions adequately. Recently, a multidisciplinary study related the orofacial difficulties associated to MS (Sjögreen, Andersson-Norinder, & Jacobsson, 2001). The 25 subjects in the study all had impairment in their facial expression. Several patients had developed compensatory ways of communicating emotions, mostly vocally. This study requests more research on what can be done to improve facial expressions, acknowledging the communication difficulties created by this incapacity.

Conclusion

As we have seen, multiple factors influence affective communication; therefore, studies on emotion are difficult to carry out. It is not easy to embrace all the different facets of emotion, and it is equally difficult to isolate separate dimensions. There is, to this date, no unified model of emotion and emotion expression. Different authors support different positions regarding the nature of emotion and emotion expression, as well as its function. Considering the disparity and unevenness of the field, we find it even more imperative for the authors to take interest in the subject. In fact, affective communication might be looked upon as a detail when compared to far more vital functions, and thus it is not attended to. However, impairment on the emotive level does in fact affect the patient's identity, not only as an emotional being, but also as a communicating being.

The studies reported in this chapter contribute to give a framework to the study of impaired emotion expressions and we have tried to investigate possible directions in reeducation. In fact, there is a demand from the patients and their close relations to ease their suffering. The patient participating in the study of Morsomme et al. (2007), for instance, expresses his dismay towards the small existing knowledge about concrete and practical support for his condition.

Studies have shown that emotional content is expressed and perceived through various channels and that the use of these different channels might differ according to the situation, the subject, or the emotive content (Banse & Scherer, 1996; Elfenbein & Ambady, 2002). Also, it has been observed that different subjects can use different cues to express the same emotion (Whiteside, 1999). Those results are interesting from a reeducational perspective. They indicate that though one channel or some parameters in one channel are affected, it might still be possible for the patient to compensate. A detailed analysis of the patient's communication, specifically oriented on the emotive content, might allow the patient and the therapist to elaborate a different communication strategy where the patient could rely on, or compensate with, parameters that were not used before.

Following the results of a study of patients with Parkinson's disease (McNamara & Durso, 2003; Simons et al., 2003), which suggests a lack of self-awareness in these patients, the authors propose that the first step in a reeducation centered on emotive communication must be to direct patients' attention on their difficulties. Indeed, adopting compensatory ways of expressing emotions is of interest for the patient only if he realizes the decreased quality of his emotional expressions and its consequences on social interactions. Also, the observation that the patient's expressiveness is increased when in interaction with a stranger leads the authors to suggest that a reeducation oriented on the interaction partner might be of interest (Simons et al., 2003). Higher expressivity in the spouses or in the clinician during reeducation might yield more expressions from the patient.

Indeed, the communication process involves the interaction of at least two partners. The outcome and the content of this interaction are dependent on the contribution of all partners. Thus, it seems logical that reeducation has to involve not only the patient but also his communication partners. At the very least, observation of the patient in a natural communicating situation seems to be essential. This would allow the clinician to accurately focus on the difficulties actually encountered.

We would like to end this chapter by repeating the words of Luminet (2002), saying that "Emotions influence our perception of the world, the way we express ourselves, and our intellectual reasoning and the learning processes already at a very young age." We feel that this statement reflects the central position of emotion in our lives and should encourage the clinician to give proper value to a patient's or his partner's complaint on the emotive level.

Bibliography

Bachorowski, J.-A., & Owren, M. J. (2003). Production and perception of affect-related vocal acoustics. *Annals of the New York Academy of Sciences, 1000*, 144-165.

Banse, R., & Scherer, K. R. (1996). Acoustic profiles in vocal emotion expression. *Journal of Personality and Social Psychology, 70*(3), 614-636.

Berman, H. J., Shulman, A. D., & Marwit, S. J. (1976). Comparison of multidimensional decoding of affect from audio, video and audiovideo recordings. *Sociometry, 39*(1), 83-89.

Ekman, P. (1992). An argument for basic emotions. *Cognition and Emotion, 6*(3-4), 169-200.

Ekman, P. (1992). Facial expression and emotion. *American Psychologist, 48*(4), 384-392.

Ekman, P. (1999). Facial expressions. In T. Dalgleish & M. Power (Eds.), *Handbook of cognition and emotion* (pp. 301-320). Sussex, UK: John Wiley & Sons.

Ekman, P., Friesen, W. V., & Ancoli, S. (1980). Facial signs of emotional experience. *Journal of Personality and Social Psychology, 39*(6), 1125-1134.

Ekman, P., Friesen, W. V., O'Sullivan, M., & Scherer, K. R. (1980). Relative importance of face, body, and speech in judgments of personality and affect. *Journal of Personality and Social Psychology, 38*, 270-277.

Elfenbein, H. A., & Ambady, N. (2002). On the universality and cultural specificity of emotion recognition: A meta-analysis. *Psychological Bulletin, 128*(2), 203-235.

Frank, M. G., & Stennett, J. (2001). The forced-choice paradigm and the perception of facial expressions of emotion. *Journal of Personality and Social Psychology, 80*(1), 75-85.

Hess, U., Scherer, K. R., & Kappas, A. (1988). Multichannel communication of emotion: Synthetic signal production. In K. R. Scherer (Ed.), *Facets of emotion: Recent research* (pp. 161-249). Hillsdale, NJ: Erlbaum.

Izard, C. E. (1994). Innate and universal facial expressions: Evidence from developmental and cross-cultural research. *Psychological Bulletin, 115*(2), 288-299.

Juslin, P. N., & Laukka, P. (2001). Impact of intended emotion intensity on cue utilisation and decoding accuracy in vocal expression of emotion. *Emotion, 1*(4), 381-412.

Juslin, P. N., & Laukka, P. (2003). Communication of emotions in vocal expression and music performance: Different channels, same code? *Psychological Bulletin, 129*(5), 770-814.

Kohler, C. G., Turner, T., Stolar, N. M., Bilker, W. B., Brensinger, C. M., Gur, R. E., et al. (2003). Differences in facial expressions of four universal emotions. *Psychiatry Research, 128*, 235-244.

Luminet O. (2002). Psychologie des émotions. Confrontation et évitement. Editions De Boeck Université. Bruxelles, Belgium.

McNamara, P., & Durso, R. (2003). Pragmatic communication skills in patients with Parkinson's disease. *Brain and Language, 84*, 414-423.

Morsomme, D., Verduyckt, I., Jamart, J., & Remacle, M. (2007). *Perceptual differences between adults and adolescents regarding vocal emotional and facial cues in a patient affected with Steinert disease and a professional actor.* Manuscript submitted for publication.

Pell, M. D. (2002). Evaluation of nonverbal emotion in face and voice: Some preliminary findings on a new battery of tests. *Brain and Cognition, 48*, 499-504.

Pell, M. D., Cheang, H. S., & Leonard, C. L. (in press). The impact of Parkinson's disease on vocal-prosodic communication from the perspective of listeners. *Brain and Language.*

Pollerman, B. (2002, April). A place for prosody in a unified model of cognition and emotion. In Speech Prosody 2002, Université de Aix-en-Provence, 17-22, 2003 (p. 17).

Russell, J. A. (1980). A circumplex model of affect. *Journal of Personality and Social Psychology, 39*(6), 1161-1178.

Russell, J. A. (1994). Is there universal recognition of emotion from facial expression? A review of the cross-cultural studies. *Psychological Bulletin, 115*(1), 102-141

Russell, J. A., Bachorowski, J.-A., & Fernàndez-Dols, J.-M. (2003). Facial and vocal expressions of emotion. *Annual Review of Psychology, 54*, 329-349.

Russell, J. A., & Fehr, B. (1987). Relativity in the perception of emotion in facial expressions. *Journal of Experimental Psychology General, 3*, 223-237.

Scherer, K. R. (1981). Speech and emotional states. In J. Darby (Ed.), *Speech evaluation in psychiatry* (pp. 189-220). New York: Grune & Stratton.

Scherer, K. R. (1986). Vocal affect expression: A review and a model for future research. *Psychological Bulletin, 99*(2), 143-165.

Scherer, K. R. (1995). Expression of emotion in voice and music. *Journal of Voice, 9*(3), 235-248.

Scherer, K. R. (2003). Vocal communication of emotion: A review of research paradigms. *Speech Communication, 40*, 227-256.

Simons, G., Pasqualini, M. C. S, Reddy, V., & Wood, J. (2003). Emotional and nonemotional facial expressions in people with Parkinson's disease. *Journal of the International Neuropsychological Society, 10*, 521-535.

Sjögreen, L., Andersson-Norinder, J., & Jacobsson, C. (2001). Development of speech, feeding, eating, and facial expression in Moebius sequence. *International Journal of Pediatric Otorhinolaryngology, 60*, 197-204.

Wallbott, H. G., & Scherer, K. R. (1986). Cues and channels in emotion recognition. *Journal of Personality and Social Psychology, 51*(4), 690-699.

Whiteside, S. P. (1999). Acoustic characteristics of vocal emotions stimulated by actors. *Perceptual and Motor Skills, 89*, 1195-1208.

CHAPTER 10

The Music of Language: The Importance of Prosody and Non-Verbal Communication in the Dyadic Interaction between Infant and Caregiver

Victoria Stevens

Introduction

Music and language are both fundamental means of human expression that have been found in all cultures in some form throughout recorded history. There are many theoretical speculations about the origins and functions of both music and language from fields as diverse as paleontology, cognitive neuroscience, linguistics, anthropology, esthetics, biology, ethnomusicology, and developmental psychology. The area of research reviewed in this chapter concerns published work on how the function of music and language accounts for the particular way mothers, fathers, siblings, or/and other older adults speak and sing to infants between the time of their birth and when they approximately reach 2 years.

This sing-song speech in question is typically characterized by elevated pitch, simplified pitch contours, expanded pitch range, decreased tempo, and repetitive melodic and rhythmic patterns. It is variously known as infant-directed speech, motherese, and baby talk, and emerges seemingly spontaneously and instinctively in caregivers in the presence of small babies and often with animals. Infant-directed speech is accompanied by exaggerated facial expressions, gestures, caresses, rocking, and mutual gazes.

The term typically used to describe the musical elements of vocal communication is prosody, and while prosody continues to play a part in conveying both emotional and semantic meaning in linguistic and nonverbal communication throughout the life span, it is especially important in early development. Prosody, which is nonverbal and often unconscious, is a tool of human expression that communicates emotion and meaning through various musical modalities, and it is ubiquitous across cultures. For example, a study about recognition of musical sounds associated with particular emotions found that 40 Central Australian Aborigines of the Warlbiri tribe had scores that were equal to the scores of university students at the University of South Wales, MIT, and the University of California at Berkeley (Clynes, 1982). In addition, prosody is present in lullabies, rituals, spoken languages, poetry, and songs throughout history.

This contribution will also investigate some of the possible functions prosodic interactions play in early childhood development. I will focus on addressing (a) the communication of emotional feelings and states; the facilitation of attunement and attachment; (b) the creating of the basis for the awareness of the difference between play and reality; (c) the development of affect and self-regulation; and (d) the development of affect synchrony between caregiver and infant. I will argue that both music and language originate from within the human brain and serve the adaptive purpose of facilitating attachment between caregiver and infant through the dyadic, intersubjective regulation of emotions, thereby creating a foundation for semantic language, creative exploratory play, and interactions with others in the social environment and resiliency throughout life.

Finally, it is hypothesized that research involving prosody in infant development reveals that the importance of language, both ontogenetically and phylogenetically, may have more to do with the music of it than our left hemispheric linguistic/semantic bias might have led us to believe. In addition, it is suggested that the importance of the human voice as the vehicle for the communication of emotional meaning has been vastly underestimated in terms of its effect on a developing brain and self as well as on human relationships over time. Providing this hypothesis holds, I propose that it is important for everyone to learn how to read the music of language and the meanings conveyed by voiced emotions, especially for those engaged in either caregiving, therapeutic, or teaching roles.

Prosody

There is no such thing as a disembodied word. Every word we hear is saturated by affective-sensory layers of meaning from the intonation of the speech of the caregiver from the time that the auditory systems become active in the developing fetus. One of our earliest experiences as human beings is feeling the vibrations and hearing the sounds of the mother's heartbeat rhythmically beating at faster and slower tempos, accompanied by the gurgling of digestive and intestinal juices, and above that rhythm section a muted voice or voices are heard through the womb wall coming and going in melodic patterns of sounds and silences. The two predominant sounds heard by the fetus are the pulsations from the womb's main artery and the sound of the mother's voice (Piontelli, 1992). All of this begins to occur around the age of 4 months and is experienced while floating in the amniotic fluid, which also amplifies the internal and external sounds.

Research has shown that shortly after birth, infants turn their heads in the direction of the mother or the father whose voice they heard while in the womb (DeCasper & Fifer, 1980). Therefore, an imprint of the timbre, pitch, and melody of the familiar voice appears to be encoded in the infant, although it is difficult to specify how that early experience affects the developing brain-mind of thc fetus. Once a child is born, these intoned words are experienced within a rich mix of nonlinguistic sounds, facial expressions, gazes, gestures and physical holding, caressing and touching—all of which make up the sensory-motor-affective matrix of our earliest experiences of other human beings, the world, and our nascent self.

Prosody includes vocal rhythm, pitch, melody, tempo, and volume as part of the communication of linguistic and paralinguistic (emotional and attitudinal) information. This prosodic "speech" is characterized by elevated pitch, simplified pitch contours, expanded pitch range, decreased tempo, and repetitiveness that convey meaning by varying stress and pitch irrespective of the words and grammatical construction (Mitchell, Elliott, Barry, Crittenden, & Woodruff, 2003).

Prosody is thought to be processed mainly in the right brain along with other crucial socio-emotional information and body states that are central to the regulation of emotions and the origin of a sense of self (Schore, 2005a). This right brain regulatory capacity is dependent on experience—particularly the experience of attunement and synchrony with a caregiver— and develops primarily nonverbally through playful interactions involving gesture, rhythm, melody, tempo, facial expressions, and movements that form patterns of interactions between the developing child and others. A mother's rhythm, melody, pitch, volume, and tempo are ideally finely tuned to the infant's needs and response; even deaf mothers vocalize to their young deaf infants, although neither can hear the sounds (Sieratzki & Wolf, 1996).

Researchers in the field of infant development and linguistics state that the most essential aspects of prosody occur during the preverbal period of infancy and that music is instrumental to the development of language in that the ordering of pitched sounds made by the human voice is the first thing we learn when acquiring a language (Papousek, 1996). It has also been claimed that it is difficult to discern which sounds made by infants are premusical and which are prelinguistic and that this lack of clear distinction continues throughout the language and music acquisition processes. Starting at around 2½ years, they begin to separate out into language as the means of communicating semantic content and meaning, with music and prosody continuing to represent and express emotional content and meaning throughout the lifespan (Steinke, Cuddy, & Holden, 1997).

The Intersubjective Musical Matrix

Bargiel (2005) states that most developmental researchers believe that we are born with a biological predisposition for musical skills, even though some theorists disagree with this (Pinker, 1997). However, the accumulating data emerging from observations of infant-caregiver interactions indicate that this is true. For example, Trehub (2001) has shown the following:

1. Babies can distinguish a change in the melodic contour even when a distraction or delay of 15 seconds separates the original melody from the melody of comparison.
2. Babies can distinguish changing intervals in a brief melody that conforms to the musical conventions of their culture.
3. A 9-month-old baby is capable of detecting an out-of-tune note in a scale at unequal intervals (e.g., tonal scales or ancient scales compared to scales through tones).

Some findings from auditory infant developmental research include the following: (a) newborns listen and turn their heads to pick up the tones and expressive quality of voices and music (Custodero & Fenichel, 2002; Trevarthen & Malloch, 2002); (b) infants can distinguish sounds of speech in different languages, apparently attending to the interpersonal and emotional message (Brazelton, 1993; Brazelton & Cramer, 1991); (c) other persons, such as the father or a sibling, can be recognized on the basis of their voices, but there is an innate preference for the pitch of a female voice; (d) infants have an ability to distinguish sounds of musical instruments or differences in the rhythm and prosody of speech and song, harmony, and intonation with fine discrimination; (e) infants can quickly learn simple, repeating forms of musical or poetic "narrative" (Custodero & Fenichel, 2002; Papousek, 1996); (f) babies move to music from birth, and may engage with the rhythm of a parent's speech by both vocal and gestural replies (Papousek, 1996; Trevarthen & Malloch, 2002); (g) 5-month old infants can discriminate between the smallest intervals used in Western music—semitones (Olsho, 1984); 8- to 11-month-old infants can perceive and remember melodic contour (Trehub, Bull, & Thorpe, 1984); and (h) infants have been shown to be able to tell the difference between two songs they have never heard before—one that was "normal" and one that was a digitally altered version—and when hearing the "mistakes" in the song the infants showed a surprised response (Trehub, 1989).

It has been even suggested that there is a "musical code" in the infant-caregiver dyadic interaction. It is postulated that both partners in the dyad are attuned to very subtle shifts that include a myriad of acoustic features, such as vocal timbre, tempo, and volume variations and negotiate and share a flexible musical pulse, constantly adapting their tempo, intensity, motion, shape, and the contour of their sounds, movements, and gestures. This is apparently for both the purpose of finding a "fit" and to communicate with one another (Bunt & Pavlicevic, 2001).

Trevarthen (1993), in his studies of maternal-infant protoconversations, states that prosodic elements are coordinated with facial expressions, eye-to-eye messages, and tactile and body gestures to create a multilayered sensory-affective matrix of visual and prosodic signals that produce instant emotional effects. This matrix is comprised of and facilitates a complex and fluid series of interactions between the infant-caregiver pair, with each influencing and nonverbally cueing the other. The ongoing interactive synchrony, characterized by nonverbal emotional rapport and empathy, create patterns of experience, which when repeated and elaborated over time, become encoded with meaning. These nonverbal, patterned, affective-sensory clusters of meaning provide the early presymbolic mental representations that form the foundation for the development of the cognitive and symbolic complexity of language and abstract thought.

Stern's (1985; 1995 contributions in the area of interpersonal infant development emphasize further the importance of "temporal feeling shapes" that emerge continuously out of these early interactions between infant and caregiver. What is experienced by the infant subjectively as a feeling is a complex amalgam of patterns of interactions shaped by rhythm, volume, tone, and tempo, which can be stored and recalled and which help to structure and give coherence to the developing self as it evolves in time.

Infant-Directed Speech or Motherese

Motherese is the name given to the prosodic sing-song way of speaking or singing that is a universal characteristic in caregivers when they are responding to and caring for their infants. Throughout the world, mothers speak in melodious tones to infants who cannot understand what they say. They also sing a great deal, using a special genre of music with common features across cultures, such as simple pitch contours, repetition, and narrow pitch range. For example, nonmusically trained listeners can distinguish foreign lullabies from nonlullabies matched on culture of origin and tempo (Trehub, 2003). Infants are interested in the speech of the caregiver, but seem to be much more interested in maternal singing. It appears that the music in speech seems to underlie its attractiveness to prelinguistic infants. This is particularly true of the exaggerated elements in the prosody. Trehub (2003) states intriguingly that hearing as well as deaf infants prefer the gestural patterns of infant-directed sign language to those of conventional sign language and that deaf infants babble in a gestural form of prosodic exaggeration before learning conventional sign language in a similar way to how hearing infants learn to speak a language. It is Trehub's view that what is of primary importance for the developing child is emotional expressiveness, regardless of the modality utilized for the expression.

(More specifics on vocalization and deafness are found in Chapter 12 of this volume: Editor.)

Reissland & Snow (1996) argue that the prosody of the mother's speech can help the infant learn about different pragmatic and social situations. Their results support the claim that the prosodic elements of the parental speech, especially pitch, can cue the infant to the cognitive and social distinctions between different situations. Specifically, they claim that the contrasts in pitch characteristic of infant- or child-directed language introduce the child to the difference between ordinary and play situations. Their research indicates that mothers use pitch cues to distinguish play from reality, even before the infants are able to actively participate in pretend play, suggesting that their pitch cues are not merely in *response* to the child's expression of play behaviors, but may *anticipate* and *support* the child's understanding of the concept of imaginative play. They also suggest that intonation key may be used in the earliest developmental stages to alert the infant to an activity or situation that is different or out of the ordinary.

The results of Reissland and Snow (1996) indicate that when mothers talked to their 11-month-old, a change in pitch height was the feature that mothers used most consistently to prosodically mark the difference between play and reality. This analysis of mothers' responses to infant sounds shows the importance of a responsive and highly interactive social environment for the developing child. This view challenges the view of human vocal learning that has emphasized the signals sent from the infants as having more importance than the responses of the caregivers who receive those responses. By emphasizing the importance of the meaning-making function of the parental receiver of the child's communications, this research makes an important contribution to our understanding of emotional and language development.

Other studies have confirmed that pitch is the most important aspect of prosody that mothers use to mark different pragmatic and social situations. According to Fernald (1989), the melodies or intonations of maternal utterances convey affective meaning to prelinguistic infants. This emotive quality differs when the mother's emotional availability is decreased. For example, mildly depressed mothers use motherese less frequently and respond more slowly to infant vocalizations than do nondepressed mothers (Bettes, 1988). It has been hypothesized that maternal singing tranquilizes the nervous system, as does caregiver proximity (Milligan et al., 2003). There is evidence, moreover, that maternal singing leads to more sustained reductions of infant arousal than does maternal speech. Thus, mothers' sensitive use of singing may affect infants' sense of security and early socialization in general.

Stressed premature and low birth weight newborns, whose bodies are often in pain, are calmed in the hospital ICU by quiet speech and touch, and by music or song (Custodero & Fenichel, 2002), and this experience helps to improve weight gain and earlier hospital discharge. (Application of sensory therapy to free emotions in adult patients and in children who suffer psychiatric deprivation including stupor is discussed in this volume in Chapter 16: Editor).

In a variant of motherese, Trehub (2001) describes parental singing as higher-pitched, slower, and possessing a greater vocal emotional quality than regular singing that is not addressed to a baby; it is found not only in the mother, but in the father and in preschool-age children who sing to their little brother or sister.

Parents, excited by an infant's sounds and gestures, respond instinctively with lively affectionate behaviors called *intuitive parenting* (Papousek, 1996). Infants prefer motherese from the first month (Fernald, 1989). Expressive or emotive speech is used whenever persons of any age are engaged in shared activity with heightened excitement and affection. The parent and infant look at each other's faces and answer each other's gestures, body movements, and vocalizations—taking turns in mutual attuned play by responding to the rhythms and patterns of each other's emotional expressions.

Most human mothers show a preference for cradling their infant on the left side, and this tendency seems to show up early in girls while cradling dolls, but not in boys, and while it is natural for women, it is not for men. This appears to be independent of handedness and is cross-cultural (Manning et al., 1997; Sieratzki & Wolf, 1996). Left-cradling seems to offer a number of practical advantages including facilitating the flow of emotional prosodic and visual cues and communications from the mother into the infant's left ear and eye—thereby being processed in the right hemisphere—and the infant's responses back to the mother also being processed in the mother's right hemisphere (Schore, 2005b). The role of the right hemisphere is crucial in relation to the early nonverbal affect-laden interactions between mothers and infants, and left-cradling appears to offer the optimal physical placement for right hemispheric dominance in early interactions.

Listening experiments with neonates and adults have shown differences in accuracy and speed of response to left-ear and right-ear stimuli, which supports the hemispheric differences for the semantic and prosodic elements of language; the right ear is better at recognizing the structural aspects of speech; the left ear is better at recognizing music and the melodic aspects of language, particularly affective intonation (Sieratzki & Wolf, 1996).

The cross-cultural ubiquity of left-cradling of infants and the unique prosody of a mother speaking and singing to an infant exemplifies the right hemisphere's dominance over early mother-infant communication. As Sieratzki and Wolf say, "The lullaby will not sound the same and will not feel the same with the baby on the other side" (1996, p. 1748).

It is clear that infant-directed speech has many purposes for the ongoing emotional, neural, and linguistic development of children. Fernald & Mazzie (1991) have outlined four developmental stages of infant-directed speech that highlight different purposes as the infant grows from newborn to the age of about 2½: in newborns, the main purpose of infant-directed speech is to provide an auditory stimulus that helps to engage and maintain the child's attention, help with orientation, and elicit responses; overlapping this first stage and continuing on as the infant is a bit older, the main function is the utilization of the vocal prosodic speech to soothe and to regulate and modulate arousal and affective states; in the third stage, prosody becomes the means of communicating the feelings and signaling the intentions of the caregiver; and finally, as children begin to use and understand words, patterns of intonation facilitate the development and use of language itself.

Affect Regulation and Attachment

Interpersonal neurobiology and regulation theory emphasize the fact that psychobiological attunement, interactive resonance, and the mutual synchronization and entrainment of psychological rhythms are fundamental processes that mediate attachment bond formation, and attachment can be defined as the interactive regulation of biological synchrony between organisms through dyadic regulation of emotion (Schore, 2003b; 2005a).

Attachment theory as put forward by Bowlby (1981 and Ainsworth (1974) assumes the existence of a biological predisposition in the baby to transmit signals and cues, and a biological predisposition in the parent to respond to those signals, all within the context of a process of regulation of the affect of the infant through the parent as intermediary and interactive regulator.

As Schore discusses the links between attachment theory, nonverbal communication, and brain development, he says that the infant actively communicates its subjective psychobiological states to the caregiver in intersubjective protoconversations of coordinated visual-facial, tactile-gestural, and auditory-prosodic mutual signaling (Schore, 2001a). The dyadic implicit processing of these nonverbal attachment communications of facial expression, posture, and tone of voice are the product of the operations of the infant's right hemisphere interacting with the mother's right hemisphere. This hemisphere is dominant not only for emotional communication but also for imprinting, the learning mechanism that underlies attachment. Attachment experiences are emotionally encoded and stored in the infant's rapidly developing right brain, creating internal working models that include strategies of affect regulation that act at implicit nonconscious levels.

Lester, Hoffman, and Brazelton (1985) state that synchrony and attunement develop as a result of repetitive sequences of rhythmic patterns over time as each partner learns the timing and structure of the other and modifies his or her behavior to fit that timing and structure. The primary caregiver thus facilitates the infant's information processing by adjusting the mode, amount, variability, and timing of visual and auditory prosodic stimulation to its actual temperamental-physiological abilities. These mutually attuned synchronized interactions are fundamental to the ongoing affective development of the infant (Schore, 2003b).

Due to technical advances, researchers today are able to identify that the human maternal response to an infant's cry—a fundamental behavior of the attachment dynamic—is accompanied by an activation of the mother's right brain, and that engrams related to emotional voices are more strongly imprinted into the infant's early maturing, more active right hemisphere (Lorberbaum et al, 2002).

Research then suggests that what is happening here is that the infant's right hemisphere, which is dominant for the child's processing of visual and prosodic emotional information, is psychobiologically attuned to the output of the mother's right hemisphere, which is involved in the expression and processing of emotional information and in spontaneous and nonverbal communication. The orbital prefrontal cortex is especially expanded in the right cortex. This prefrontal region comes to act in the capacity of an executive control function for the entire right cortex, the hemisphere that modulates affect, nonverbal communication, and unconscious processes.

Contrary to the common idea that the left hemisphere is uniquely specialized for all language functions, it is now well established that the right and not left hemisphere is dominant not only for prosody, but the processing of emotional words, the detection of one's first name, humor, laughter, social discourse, and metaphor (Schore, 2005b). Therefore, the musical, rhythmic, and emotional attunement of the caregiver to the infant's shifting emotional states of being create patterns of interaction that are stored mainly in the right hemisphere and that will facilitate the development of attachment and self-regulatory capacities, which will be important for the expression and understanding of emotional language throughout life.

The right hemisphere can now be seen as having a "nonverbal affect lexicon," a vocabulary for nonverbal affective signals, such as facial expressions, gestures, and prosody (Schore, 2005b).

Emotional perception in music appears quite early on and is very likely innate. Kitamura and Burnham (1998) have demonstrated that babies respond more to the affective qualities of parental language than to its linguistic characteristics, and they present three developmental hypotheses regarding the function of motherese: to engage and maintain the attention of the baby; to permit emotional communication and socialization; and to facilitate language acquisition.

Trehub (2001) discovered that infants who had a more elevated cortisol level (an indicator of the intensity of stress) displayed a lower rate of cortisol after listening to parental singing, while infants with a lower rate of cortisol displayed a higher rate. This finding supports the hypothesis that parental singing and prosodic speech play an important part in affect regulation of the infant through dyadic musical interaction. Schore (1994) posits that parental singing permits a gradual increase in the tolerance of affective tension including the tolerance of intense positive affective states, all serving the purpose of enhancing the closeness of the mother-child attachment.

It is clear that in the discussion thus far the emphasis has been on the "good-enough mother" (Winnicott, 1960) who is able to pay attention to the infant, empathically attune to the infant's emotional states, and respond in a synchronized, playful, rhythmic manner prosodically in terms of tone, volume, pitch, melody, and tempo, as well as in gesture, touch, facial expressions, and movements. It has been stated that if these kinds of interactions occur over time there is a foundation that is created that includes a sense of secure attachment, a coherent sense of self, and emotional self-regulation, all of which remain as a substrate through the child's lifetime and contribute to the child's resilience, empathic capacities, and the ability to tolerate frustration and have a reflective self.

If, however, the early interactions are characterized by overstimulation, understimulation, or misattuned asynchronous responses on the part of the caregiver, this can create the experience of affect dysregulation on the part of the infant, which will have a negative effect on the developing attachment bond and therefore on the infant's experience of security, with perhaps serious consequences for the developing child.

Conclusion

Prosody is a crucial tool for the communication of emotion through the music of language. As music is considered to be significant forms of feeling and the tonal analogue to our emotional life (Langer, 1953), prosodic elements in verbal communication are the vehicles for the expression of emotions through sounds and language. Prosody is thought to be processed mainly in the right hemisphere and plays a crucial role in the development of a child as part of the emotionally laden, nonverbal interactions between mother and infant that include infant-directed speech, laughter, song, rhyming, and play. When the prosodic elements of pitch, tempo, loudness, and rhythm are part of an attuned, synchronous, fluid interplay, they become essential elements in the development of emotional regulation, attachment, and security in the developing infant.

References

Ainsworth, M. D. S. (1974). Mother-infant interaction and the development of competence. In K. Connolly & J. Bruner (Eds.), *The growth of confidence* (pp. 97-118). New York: Academic Press.

Bargiel, M. (2005). Lullabies and play songs: Theoretical considerations for an early attachment music therapy intervention through parental singing for developmentally at-risk infants. In *Voices: A world forum for music therapy*. Retrieved September 5, 2005, from http://www.voices.no/mainissues/mi40004000143.html

Beebe, B., & Lachman, F. M. (2002) *Infant research and adult treatment: Co-constructing interactions*. Hillsdale, NJ: The Analytic Press.

Benowitz, L. I., Bear, D. M., Rosenthal, R., Mesulam, M.-M., Zaidel, E., & Sperry, R. W. (1983). Hemispheric specialization in nonverbal communication. *Cortex*, *19*, 5-11.

Bettes, B.A. (1988). Maternal depression and motherese: Temporal and intonational features. *Child Development*, *59*, 1089-1096.

Blonder, L. X., Bowers, D., & Heilman, K. M. (1991). The role of the right hemisphere in emotional communication. *Brain*, *114*, 1115-1127.

Bourne, V. J., & Todd, B. K. (2004). When left means right: An explanation of the left cradling bias in terms of right hemisphere specializations. *Developmental Science*, *7*, 19-24.

Bowlby, J. (1981). *Attachment and loss. Vol. 3: Loss, sadness, and depression*. New York: Basic Books.

Brazelton, T. B. (1993). *Touchpoints: Your child's emotional and behavioral development*. New York: Viking.

Brazelton, T. B., & Cramer, B. G. (1991). *The earliest relationship: Parents infants and the drama of early attachment*. London: Karnac Books.

Bunt, L., & Pavlicevic, M. (2001). Music and emotions: Perspectives from music therapy. In P. N. Juslin & J. A. Sloboda (Eds.), *Music and emotion: Theory and research* (pp. 181-201). New York: Oxford University Press.

Carpenter, M., Nagell, K., & Tomasello, M. (1998). Social cognition, joint attention, and communicative competence from 9 to 15 months of age. *Monographs of the Society for Research in Child Development*, *63*.

Chavajay, P., & Rogoff, B. (1999). Cultural variation in management of attention by children and their caregivers. *Developmental Psychology*, *35*(4), 1079-1090.

Clynes, M. (1982). *Music, mind and brain*. New York: Plenum Press.

Cross, I. (1999). Music, development and evolution. In Suk Won Yi (Ed.), *Music, mind and science* (pp. 10-39). Seoul, South Korea: Seoul National University Press.

Custodero, L., & Fenichel, E. (Eds.). (2002, September). The musical lives of babies and families. *Zero to Three*, *23*(1), 1-9.

DeCasper, A. J., & Fifer, W. P. (1980). Of human bonding: Newborns prefer their mother's voice. *Science*, *208*, 1174-1176.

Eve, R. (2004). Rhythm in interaction. *Academic Publications* [Electronic version]. Retrieved August 16, 2005, from http://www.shse.u-hyogo.ac.jp

Fernald, A. (1989). Intonation and communicative interest in mother's speech to infants: Is the melody the message? *Child Development*, *60*, 1497-1510.

Fernald, A., & Mazzie, C. (1991). Prosody in speech to children: Prelinguistic and linguistic functions. *Annals of Child Development, 8*, 43-80.

George, M. S., Parekh, P. I., Rosinsky, N., Ketter, T. A., Kimbrell, T. A., Heilman, K. M., et al. (1996). Understanding emotional prosody activates right hemispheric regions. *Archives of Neurololgy, 53*, 665-670.

Goldstein, M., & West, M. (1999). Consistent responses of human mothers to prelinguistic infants: The effect of prelinguistic repertoire size. *Journal of Comparative Psychology, 113*(1), 52-58.

Hobson, P. (2002). *The cradle of thought: Exploring the origins of thinking*. London: Macmillan.

Hubley, P., & Trevarthen, C. (1979). Sharing a task in infancy. In I. Uzgiris (Ed.), *New directions for child development: Vol. 4: Social interaction during infancy* (pp. 57-80). San Francisco: Jossey-Bass.

Kitamura, C., & Burnham, D. (1998). The infant's responses to maternal vocal affect. In C. Rovee-Collier, L. P. Lipsitt, & H. Haynes (Eds.), *Advances in infancy research* (Vol. 12, pp. 221-236). Stanford, CT: Ablex.

Langer, S. (1953). *Feeling and form: A theory of art.* New York: Scribner's Sons.

Lattner, S., Meyer, M. E., & Friederici, A. D. (2005). Voice perception: Sex, pitch, and the right hemisphere. *Human Brain Mapping, 24*, 11-20.

LeDoux, J. (1996). *The emotional brain.* New York: Simon & Schuster.

Lester, B. M., Hoffman, J., & Brazelton, T. B. (1985). The rhythmic structure of mother-infant interaction in term and preterm infants. *Child Development, 56*, 15-27.

Loewy, J. (2004). Integrating music, language and the voice in music therapy. *Voices: A World Forum for Music Therapy*. Retrieved June 16, 2005, from http://www.Voices.No/mainissues/mi40004000140.html

Lorberbaum, J. P., Newman, J. D., Horwitz, A. R., Dubno, J. R., Lydiard, R. B., Hamner, M. B., et al. (2002). A potential role for thalamocingulate circuitry in human maternal behavior. *Biological Psychiatry, 51*, 431-445.

Manning, J. T., Trivers, R. L., Thornhill, R., Singh, D., Denman, J., Eklo, M. H., et al. (1997). Ear asymmetry and left-side cradling. *Evolution and Human Behavior, 18*, 327-340.

Meyer, M., Alter, K., Friederici, A. D., Lohmann, G., & von Cramon, D. Y. (2002). FMRI reveals brain regions mediating slow prosodic modulations in spoken sentences. *Human Brain Mapping, 17*, 73-88.

Milligan, K., Atkinson, L., Trehub, S., Benoit, D., and Pouton, L. (2003). Maternal attachment and the communication of emotion through song. *Infant Behavior & Development, 26*, 1-13.

Mitchell, R. L. C., Elliott, R., Barry, M., Crittenden, A., & Woodruff, P. W. R. (2003). The neural response to emotional prosody, as revealed by functional magnetic resonance imaging. *Neuropsychologia, 41*, 1410-1421.

Nishihara, K., Horiuchi, S., Eto, H., & Uchida, S. (2002). The development of infants' circadian rest-activity rhythm and mother's rhythm. *Physiology and Behavior, 77*, 91-98.

Olsho, L. W. (1984). Infant frequency discrimination. *Infant Behavior and Development, 7*, 27-35.

Papousek, M. (1996). Intuitive parenting: A hidden source of musical stimulation in infancy. In I. Deliège & J. Sloboda (Eds.), *Musical beginnings: Origins and development of musical competence* (pp. 88-112). Oxford, UK: Oxford University Press.

Peretz, I. (2001). Listen to the brain: A biological perspective on musical emotions. In P. N. Juslin & J. A. Sloboda (Eds.), *Music and emotion: Theory and research* (pp. 105-134). New York: Oxford University Press.

Petitto, L. A., Holowka, S., Sergio, L. E., & Ostry, D. (2002). Language rhythms and baby hand movements. *Nature, 413*, 35-36.

Pinker, S. (1997). *How the mind works*. New York: W. W. Norton.

Piontelli, A. (1992). *From fetus to child: An observational and psychoanalytic study.* London: Tavistock/Routledge.

Pipp, S., & Harmon, R. J. (1987). Attachment as regulation: A commentary. *Child Development, 58*, 648-652.

Ranote, S., Elliott, R., Abel, K. M., Mitchell, R., Deakin, J. F. W., & Appleby, L. (2004). The neural basis of maternal responsiveness to infants: An fMRI study. *NeuroReport, 15*, 1825-1829.

Reissland, N., & Snow, D. (1996). Maternal pitch height in ordinary and play situations. *Journal of Child Language, 23*, 269-278.

Ross, E. D., Thompson, R. D., & Yenkosky, J. (1997). Lateralization of affective prosody in brain and the callosal integration of hemispheric language functions. *Brain and Language, 56*, 27-54.

Schore, A. N. (1994). *Affect regulation and the origin of the self.* Mahweh, NJ: Erlbaum.

Schore, A. N. (2001). The effects of a secure attachment relationship on right brain development, affect regulation, and infant mental health. *Infant Mental Health Journal, 22*, 7-66.

Schore, A. N. (2001). The Seventh Annual John Bowlby Memorial Lecture: Minds in the making: Attachment, the self-organizing brain, and developmentally-oriented psychoanalytic psychotherapy. *British Journal of Psychotherapy, 17*, 299-328.

Schore, A. N. (2003a). *Affect dysregulation and disorders of the self.* New York: W. W. Norton.

Schore, A. N. (2003b). *Affect regulation and the repair of the self.* New York: W. W. Norton.

Schore, A. N. (2005). Attachment, affect regulation, and the developing right brain: Linking developmental neuroscience to pediatrics. *Pediatrics in Review, 26*, 204-211.

Schore, A. N. (in press). A neuropsychoanalytic commentary on "Body rhythms and the unconscious: Toward an expanding of clinical attention." *Psychoanalytic Dialogues.*

Sieratzki, J. S., & Wolf, B. (1996). Why do mothers cradle babies on their left? *The Lancet, 347*, 1746-1748.

Sloboda, J. (1989). *The musical mind: The cognitive psychology of music*. New York: Oxford University Press.

Sotillo, M., Carretie, L., Hinojosa, J. A., Tapia, M., Mercado, F., Lopez-Martin, S., et al. (2005). Neural activity associated with metaphor comprehension: Spatial analysis. *Neuroscience Letters, 373*, 5-9.

Spencer, P. E., & Meadow-Orlans, K. P. (1996). Play, language, and maternal responsiveness: A longitudinal study of deaf and hearing infants. *Child Development, 67*(6), 3176-3191.

Steinke, W. R., Cuddy, L. L., & Holden, R. R. (1997). Dissociation of musical tonality and pitch memory from nonmusical cognitive abilities. *Canadian Journal of Experimental Psychology, 51*(4), 316-334.

Stern, D. N. (1995). *The motherhood constellation*. New York: Basic Books.

Stern, D. N. (2000). *The interpersonal world of the infant: A view from psychoanalysis and development psychology* (2nd ed.). New York: Basic Books.

Stroufe, L. A. (1996). *Emotional development: The organisation of emotional life in the early years*. Cambridge, UK: Cambridge University Press.

Trehub, S. E. (1989). Infant's perception of rhythm: Categorization of auditory sequences by temporal structure. *Canadian Journal of Psychology, 43*, 217-229.

Trehub, S. E. (2001). Psychological predispositions in infancy. *Annals of New York Academy of the Sciences, 930*, 3-6.

Trehub, S. E. (2003, July). The developmental origins of musicality. *Nature Neuroscience, 6*(7), 669-673.

Trehub, S. E., Bull, D., & Thorpe, L. A. (1984). Infant's perceptions of melodies: The role of melodic contour. *Child Development, 55*, 821-830.

Trehub, S., Schellenberg, E., & Hill, D. (1997). The origins of music perception and cognition: A developmental perspective. In I. DeLiege & J. A. Sloboda (Eds.), *Perception and cognition of music* (pp. 103-128). Hove, UK: Psychology Press.

Trehub, S. E., & Trainor, L. (1998). Singing to infants: Lullabies and play. In C. Rovee-Collier, L. P. Lipsitt, & H. Hayne (Eds.), *Advances in infancy research* (Vol. 12, pp. 43-77). Stanford, CT: Ablex.

Trevarthen, C. (1990). Growth and education of the hemispheres. In C. Trevarthen (Ed.), *Brain circuits and functions of the mind* (pp. 334-363). Cambridge, UK: Cambridge University Press.

Trevarthen, C. (1993). The function of emotions in early infant communication and development. In J. Nadel & L. Camaioni (Eds.), *New perspectives in early communicative development* (pp. 48-81). London: Routledge.

Trevarthen, C. (1999). Musicality and the intrinsic motive pulse: Evidence from human psychobiology and infant communication. *Musicae Scientiae*, Special issue, 1999-2000, 155-215.

Trevarthen, C. (2001). Intrinsic motives for companionship in understanding: Their origin, development and significance for infant mental health. *International Journal of Infant Mental Health, 22*(1-2), 95-131.

Trevarthan, C., Barr, I., Dunlop, A. W., Gjersoe, N., Maurice, H., & Stephan, C. (2003). Supporting a young child's needs for care and affection, shared meaning and social place. Review of childcare and development of children ages 0-3: Research evidence and implications for out-of-home provisions. *Scottish Executive*, Insight Series No. 6, ISSN 1478-8788.

Trevarthen, C., & Malloch, S. (2002, September). Musicality and music before three: Human vitality and invention shared with pride. *Zero to Three, 23*(1), 10-18.

Weintraub, S., & Mesulam, M. M. (1981). Disturbances of prosody. A right-hemisphere contribution to language. *Archives of Neurology, 38*, 742-744.

Winnicott, D. W. (1960). The theory of parent-infant relationship. In *The maturational processes and the facilitating environment* (pp 37-55). New York: International Universities Press.

CHAPTER 11

Psychobiological Framework of Stress and Voice

A Psychobiological Framework for Studying Psychological Stress and Its Relation to Voice Disorders

Maria Dietrich and Katherine Verdolini Abbott

It is the Zeitgeist to acknowledge that the mind and the body are one. In fact, it is well established that psychological stress[1] may affect health. However, few data are available about the relationship between stress and voice disorders. This chapter will outline key psychobiological mechanisms that may influence a relationship between stress and voice, and implications for research.

General Overview of Stress Mechanisms and Pathways

Life and job stresses are increasingly pervasive and can have physical and economic consequences (Stavroula, Griffiths, & Cox, 2003). In response to this situation, national efforts have increased to research the mind-body relationship as well as treatment and prevention programs that may shed some light on the issue (National Institutes of Health, 1999). Efforts in this direction have been accompanied by an exponential increase in research over the last 2 decades in health psychology investigating the physiological effects of stress on well-being (Cohen & Herbert, 1996). Much recent research has seen a shift away from a traditional biomedical model towards a biopsychosocial model of health and disease in behavioral medicine (Lovallo, 2005).

[1]In the remainder of this chapter, stress will refer to psychological stress.

Given national mandates around mind-body research, the personal and societal importance of addressing the effects of stress on health, and existing groundwork linking stress to health outcomes, the formal extension of mind-body research to the voice domain is both timely and warranted. In this chapter, a general psychobiological framework for studying stress and its relationship to voice and voice disorders is proposed here exemplified by the case of muscle tension dysphonia (MTD). A schematic of the framework is shown in Figure 11-1, which describes the relation between stress and laryngeal behavior. Descriptively, environmental variables interact with person variables to shape the appraisal of a situation. In turn, an individual may *perceive* stress that generally co-occurs with negative emotions and cognitions. Concurrently, an organized psychobiological response is initiated composed of neural autonomic, neuroendocrine, and behavioral responses. Participation of the immune system may also be invoked. Predictions from this model would say that physiological changes in the larynx are anticipated primarily as driven by the autonomic nervous system (ANS) and that increased laryngeal tension is part of the stress response. Further, a central mechanism that may bridge the gap between an acute and a chronic laryngeal disturbance could be delayed recovery. Consequently, a nonorganic voice disorder such as MTD may ensue (laryngeal muscular inhibition) as well as selected organic voice disorders (e.g., phonotrauma, laryngeal muscular activation) depending on individual stress reaction patterns. Thus, as seen for other tissues, stress is proposed to invoke an intertwined psychological, emotional, cognitive, physiological, immunological, and behavioral cascade of events that may affect the larynx.

Psychological Mechanisms in Stress

Although numerous definitions of *stress* have been proposed, approaches usually center on a "process in which environmental demands tax or exceed the adaptive capacity of an organism, resulting in psychological and biological changes that may place persons at risk for disease" (Cohen, Kessler, & Underwood Gordon, 1995, p. 3). However, it is less clear what stress in fact is; for example, is stress basically synonymous with anxiety? This section will address the concept of stress in terms of issues that need to be considered and integrated.

Stressors can be characterized in many different ways (Dickerson & Kemeny, 2004). Table 11-1 categorizes types of stress according to somewhat artificial distinctions distinguishing the time frame, setting, and type of stressor. Among stressor types identified within this model, psychosocial stressors that involve a motivated (active) performance task (e.g., public speaking) under social-evaluative threat in an uncontrollable situation (e.g., time constraint) have been found to be most effective in eliciting a cardiovascular, endocrine, and subjective stress response in the laboratory (Dickerson & Kemeny, 2004).

Stress cannot be adequately discussed without reference to emotion, because stress and emotion are inevitably linked. However, research on the psychology of emotion and research on stress are often dissociated. Complicating matters, many

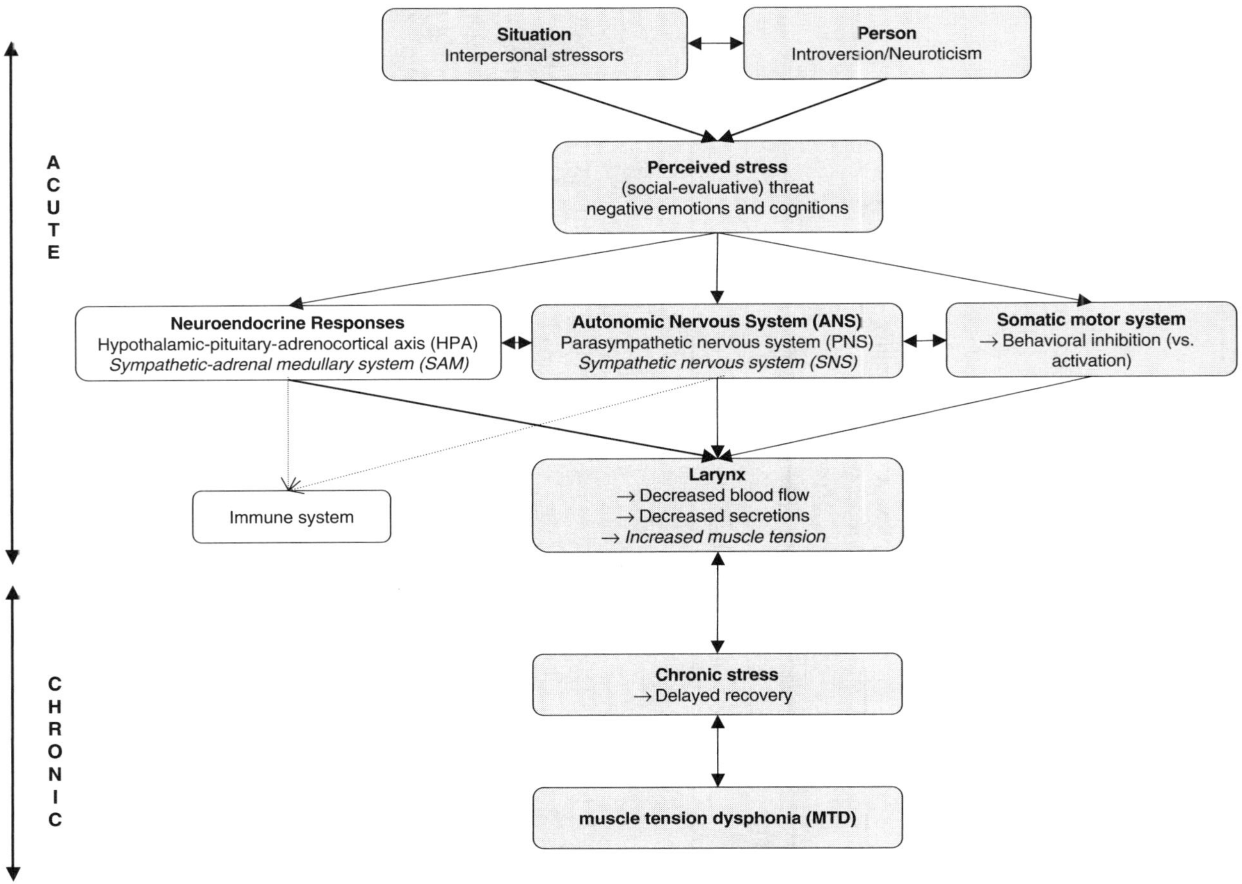

Figure 11–1. Psychobiological pathways that may be implicated in the relation between stress and voice disorders. For simplicity, most arrows are unidirectional; however, bidirectional pathways and feedback loops are conceptually not excluded.

Table 11–1. Categorization of stressors along the dimensions of time, setting, and type

Stressor Dimension		Examples
Time	Acute	Public speaking
	Chronic	Caregiving
Setting	Laboratory	Mental arithmetic
	Naturalistic	Daily hassles, work-family conflicts
Type	Physical	Exercise
	Psychological	Public speaking/verbal interaction tasks; Cognitive tasks: Stroop color-word interference task, mental arithmetic, mirror star tracing Public speaking/cognitive task combination; Emotion induction; Noise exposure.
	Physical-psychological	Cold pressor task
	Biological	Caffeine

unanswered questions exist about emotion itself and, thus, understanding of the relation between emotion and stress is particularly challenging. Three widely debated issues have been emphasized relative to emotion: (a) categorization of emotions, (b) the relationship between emotion and cognition, and (c) the specificity of the emotional response (Juslin & Scherer, in press).

Relative to the categorization of emotion, prominent theories on emotion emphasize (a) a *basic emotions* approach, which proposes a limited universal set of discrete emotions (Ekman, 1999; Izard, 1993, following Darwin, 1872/1998, Tomkins, 1962); (b) a dimensional *circumplex model of emotion* according to which valence (pleasance) and activation (arousal) are seen as converging continua (Larsen & Diener, 1992; Russell, 1980); and (c), *component process theory*, which specifically focuses on the vocal expression of emotion and predicts specific vocal changes based on the physiological effects of particular appraisal outcomes (Scherer, 1986). With regard to the emotion-stress link, from an evolutionary point of view, the prototypical fight-or-flight stress response has been noted to elicit anxiety, fear, and anger (Lovallo, 2005) and Darwin was the first to address additionally vocal expression from an evolutionary point of view (Darwin, 1872/1998). However, a comment has also been that stress is usually measured as a one-dimensional construct, although one could argue that stress could come in different variants as modulated by emotions (Juslin & Scherer, in press). Thus, one could propose the relevance of distinguishing "anger stress" versus "fear stress," for example (Juslin & Scherer, in press). In fact, research has not yet systematically investigated the range or quality of emotions involved in stress responses. A multidimensional space might integrate stress and emotion more adequately considering the different dimensions of stress as outlined in Table 11-1. An exception is Social Self-Preservation Theory, which proposes that shame may be an important affective mediator of social-evaluative threat relative to physiological parameters sometimes manifesting in stress reactions (Dickerson, Gruenewald, & Kemeny, 2004).

Relative to the relation between emotion and cognition, there is continuing debate about the nature of the link. From the point of view of appraisal theory, stress is highly governed by cognition including operations involving (a) primary appraisal, in which a situation is evaluated as threat or challenge, thus evoking various emotions, and (b) secondary appraisal, where the availability of emotional coping responses is evaluated (emotion-focused coping versus problem-focused coping) (Lazarus & Folkman, 1984). Within this theory, the specific appraisal of human interactions determines the specific subsequent emotion. However, appraisal theory has been criticized for its dependence on cognitive processes (Zajonc, 1984). The criticism is based on some research pointing to a primacy of *affect* (independence of emotion from cognition) for a subset of emotions, at least (e.g., fear; Zajonc, 1984).

Relative to the specificity of the emotional response, debate has centered on the pattern of the physiological response to emotion as well as to stress: Does emotion-specific physiological patterning exist—as might be the case for basic emotions—or is emotional arousal instead nonspecific (Scherer, 2000)? This question will be pursued in the next section that provides background about physiological responses to stress.

Physiological Pathways in Stress

As part of the larger peripheral nervous system, the ANS is a largely involuntary, visceral sensory and motor system contrasting with the voluntary, somatic motor system (Iversen, Iversen, & Saper, 2000). The ANS regulates smooth muscles (skin, blood vessels), cardiac muscle, and exocrine glands and mediates visceral reflexes (ocular, cardiovascular, glandular, gastrointestinal, urogenital). Two divisions of the ANS are recognized: the sympathetic nervous system (SNS) and the parasympathetic nervous system (PNS). The SNS is primarily involved in the *fight-or-flight* response in which sympathetic motor fibers respond quickly and in a highly coordinated fashion in order to activate the body. Sympathetic neurons initially run together with spinal nerves, then project to the ganglia of the sympathetic chains, and travel in spinal nerves to the target organs. The exception are postganglionic neurons, which leave the superior cervical ganglion, where sympathetic fibers travel along branches of the carotid arteries to targets in the head. The response of that chain involves a general adaptive arousal reaction resulting in an integrated set of cardiovascular, autonomic, and neuroendocrine changes. At the most basic level, changes include increased heart rate and increased force of heart contraction, vasoconstriction in selected parts of the body, and inhibition to most glands. In contrast, the PNS supports *resting and digesting* under normal conditions. Parasympathetic neurons originate in the brainstem (cranial nerves III, VII, IX, and X) or sacral spinal cord. Most parasympathetic nerve fibers project via the vagal nerve. A high vagal tone maintains normal function in the heart, esophagus, and respiratory and gastrointestinal systems (Iversen et al., 2000).

At a molecular level, sympathetic postganglionic nerve fibers use the neurotransmitter norepinephrine at the neuroeffector junction (Iversen et al., 2000). Norepinephrine generally enhances the rate and force of contraction of target muscles, leads to vasoconstriction, and decreases glandular secretions. Secretions are rendered viscous both by their paucity and by vasoconstriction. Cardiovascular effects, such as increases in blood pressure and heart rate, are common. For example, blood pressure increases due to increased cardiac output and peripheral resistance. On the other hand, parasympathetic postganglionic nerve fibers use the neurotransmitter acetylcholine. Acetylcholine slows the heart rate, leads to vasodilation, and promotes normal glandular secretions or even copious, watery saliva associated with local vasodilation (Iversen et al., 2000).

Neural autonomic responses in stress are accompanied by endocrine responses (Lovallo, 2005). Key systems for stress hormone secretion are the sympathetic-adrenal medullary system (SAM) and the hypothalamic-pituitary-adrenocortical axis (HPA) (Kemeny, 2003). Sympathetic preganglionic nerve fibers to the adrenal medulla induce the release of epinephrine and to a lesser extent norepinephrine into the general circulation (SAM) (Kemeny, 2003). Especially epinephrine reinforces the actions of sympathetic neuromuscular transmission (Iversen et al., 2000). Another hormonal response under stress is mediated by the hypothalamus (Lovallo, 2005). Stimulation of the HPA system releases cortisol into the bloodstream, which potentiates the activities of the SNS. Glucocorticoids (e.g., cortisol) and catecholamines (e.g., epinephrine and norepinephrine) both promote the mobilization of fuel stores (glucose and fat) to meet metabolic demands in physical activity. Cortisol initially has an immune system enhancing function, but in the long run it is immunosuppressive (Lovallo, 2005).

In sum, a stress response involves several levels of physiological regulation (Lovallo, 2005). Both branches of the ANS are tonically active and have often, but not always, opposing effects (Iversen et al., 2000). Balance between the SNS and PNS is key as it contributes to physical homeostasis in the face of demanding external conditions. The ANS also acts in concordance with the somatic motor system in an integrated way to regulate behavior and to maintain ecological homeostasis (Iversen et al., 2000; Lovallo, 2005). More centrally, the hypothalamus plays a crucial role, because it controls the endocrine system at a general level, and thus basically controls the ANS (Lovallo, 2005). Ultimately, the hypothalamus integrates autonomic function with more complex endocrine, prefrontal, and behavioral responses and metabolic needs (Iversen et al., 2000; Lovallo, 2005).

A great deal of discussion in the current literature concerns the nonspecificity versus specificity of physiological stress patterns (Kemeny, 2003). Previous literature emphasized a stereotyped (nonspecific) physiological response to all stressors. This *generality model* has been assumed in much stress research. However, increasing evidence suggests that specific stressful conditions and their associated cognitive appraisals can elicit qualitatively distinct emotional and physiological responses (*stressor-physiology specificity perspective;* Kemeny, 2003). For instance, the quality of cardiovascular reactivity can be different depending on whether a situation is perceived as threatening or as merely challenging. Challenge is associated with increases in sympathetic arousal (increased cardiac performance) coupled with reduced or unchanged peripheral resistance to blood flow, which would parallel changes observed with metabolically demanding aerobic exercise. Threat is also associated with increased cardiac performance. However, in contrast to the *challenging* situation, perceived threat is associated with *increased* peripheral resistance, leading to an increase in blood pressure (Kemeny, 2003).

Generally speaking, the SNS has an effect on (a) muscle tone (increased), (b) glandular secretions (decreased), and (c) blood flow (decreased) in response to a stressor. A range of regulatory systems is involved in the stress response including neural autonomic, neuroendocrine, and cardiovascular systems—which in turn influence respiratory functioning—and metabolic processes in which catecholamines and cortisol are the primary stress mediators (Lovallo, 2005).

Immunological Pathways in Stress

Psychoneuroimmunology (PNI) provides an alternative approach to neural autonomic and hormonal models for examining the effects of stress on health. PNI investigates how immunological pathways may mediate a relationship between stress and health (Glaser, 2005). There are sufficient data to conclude that stress-induced alterations of immune function mediate actual health changes by way of stress-induced dysregulation of pro-inflammatory cytokines (Kiecolt-Glaser, McGuire, Robles, & Glaser, 2002). The strongest evidence thus far has been provided around relationships (a) between stress and infectious disease (e.g., upper respiratory infection), by showing that stress can increase susceptibility to such disease (Cohen, Tyrrell, & Smith, 1991), and (b) stress and wound healing, by showing that stress can delay healing (Kiecolt-Glaser, Page, Marucha, MacCallum, & Glaser, 1998). However, the clinical significance of stress-induced immune changes is still debated for other diseases (Cohen & Rabin, 1998).

Stress and Disease

An important question is how stress may be detrimental to health if physiological reactions to stressful situations are indeed adaptive responses to stress. The concept of *allostatic load* may be useful in this regard. This concept extends the notion of *chronic stress* by referring to the overload of physiological adaptations but also to the potential underactivity of biological systems (McEwen & Stellar, 1993). Four types of allostatic load responses are described as illustrated in Figure 11-2 (McEwen, 1998): (1) repeated physiological activations from stressors; (2) lack of habituation or diminished physiological response to repeated stressors; (3) delayed recovery from a single-event stressor; and (4) physiological underactivity to a single-event stressor resulting in hyperactivity of other physiological systems as a compensatory response.

Further, individuals are differentially vulnerable to stress and may differ at one or several levels of the stress response including appraisal and emotion, hypothalamic and brainstem activation, and peripheral responses (Lovallo, 2005).

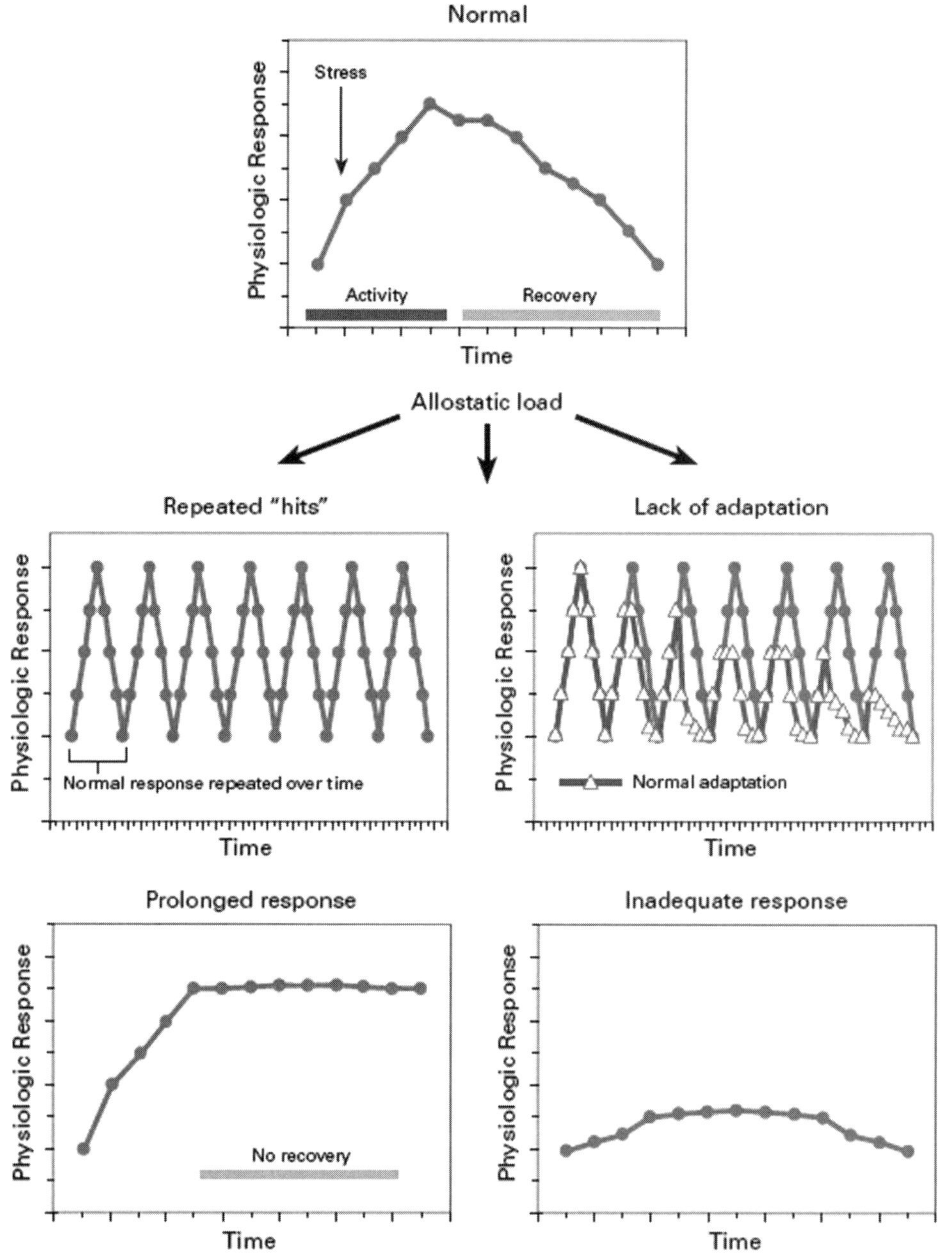

Figure 11–2. Four types of allostatic load. The top panel illustrates the normal allostatic response, in which a response is initiated by a stressor, sustained for an appropriate interval, and then turned off. The remaining panels illustrate four conditions that lead to allostatic load: repeated "hits" from multiple stressors; lack of adaptation; prolonged response due to delayed shutdown; and inadequate response that leads to compensatory hyperactivity of other mediators (e.g., inadequate secretion of glucocorticoids, resulting in increased concentrations of cytokines that are normally counterregulated by glucocorticoids). Figure drawn by Dr. Firdaus Dhabhar, Rockefeller University. Reprinted by permission from "Protective and Damaging Effects of Stress Mediators," by B. S. McEwen, 1998, *The New England Journal of Medicine*, *338*, pp. 171–179. Copyright 1998 Massachusetts Medical Society. All rights reserved.

In fact, stress reactivity may affect the personal risk for disease by way of a within-individual stable characteristic in physiological responding to stressors (Cohen & Hamrick, 2003). However, generally researchers continue to debate the required magnitude and type of stress necessary to invoke negative health outcomes (Cohen & Williamson, 1991). In this debate, negative affective states have been identified as a key mechanism linking stress to physical and psychiatric disease (Cohen et al., 1995). Negative emotions play a central role in certain personalities and health behaviors and can be modifiers of health outcomes as described next (Kiecolt-Glaser et al., 2002).

Personality

Personality is conceptualized as a moderator of emotion in that differential predispositions to various emotional states can be generally predicted as a function of personality type (Zelenski & Larsen, 1999). For example, a correlation has been consistently observed between positive affect and extraversion and between negative affect and neuroticism (Gross, Sutton, & Ketelaar, 1998). Moreover, a link between personality, affect, and health is shown by data pointing to personality styles described as passive, negative, withdrawn, unhappy, anxious, dissatisfied, or impulsive, and coping styles characterized by repression, denial, escape-avoidance, or concealment as detrimental to health (Cohen & Herbert, 1996; Kiecolt-Glaser et al., 2002).

Consequently, a crucial question is whether personality determines basal physiology, which in turn influences health. Research comparing personality dimensions and their tonic cardiovascular, neuroendocrine, and immunologic parameters have indeed suggested a contributory role of personality to basal physiology (Miller, Cohen, Rabin, Skoner, & Doyle, 1999). In particular, subjects low in agreeableness and subjects low in extraversion had higher levels of blood pressure and circulating epinephrine than subjects with different characteristics. In fact, strong evidence points to a link between the emotional trait of cynical hostility associated with type A personality and coronary heart disease (Matthews, 1988). Another personality trait that has received considerable attention is neuroticism (Costa & McCrae, 1985). Neuroticism has been consistently linked to an increased number of somatic symptoms and complaints. However, research has failed to demonstrate a consistent link between neuroticism and adverse health outcomes, at least in the case of coronary heart disease (Costa & McCrae, 1985).

Another role for personality in relation to health has been identified by Social Self Preservation Theory, which suggests that stress conditions high in social evaluation may be especially detrimental for individuals with certain characteristics such as social anxiety that would make them more vulnerable in such situations (Dickerson & Kemeny, 2004).

Health Behavior and Treatment Compliance

Stress may have indirect effects on health by way of behavior (Cohen & Herbert, 1996). Common issues in health behaviors include limited physical activity, poor sleep patterns, poor diet, and smoking (Cohen & Herbert, 1996). Stress can also influence bodily perceptions and decision making to seek medical care (Pennebaker, 1983). An individual may be hyperattentive to physical sensations during stress reactions and, in turn, symptoms may be correctly attributed to a stressor or incorrectly labeled as disease (Pennebaker, 1983). Finally, research in the general health psychology literature shows that stress and negative emotions can decrease compliance with a medical or treatment regimen, thereby influencing the course of disease (Anderson, Kiecolt-Glaser, & Glaser, 1994).

Voice Disorders and the Psychobiology of Stress

Stress can be expressed in many different ways. One avenue may involve voice, because voice and emotion appear inextricably linked. Voice is generally considered to be an indicator of overall well-being and can provide considerable insight into the structure and function of parts of our body (Titze, 1995). Figure 11-3 illustrates how voice reflects multiple influences from body and mind. Apart from normal emotional fluctuations revealed in the voice, it has been hypothesized that individuals may also develop a chronic voice disorder due to or precipitated by emotional factors (Roy, 2003). The voice disorder that has most been linked to stress and psychological conflict is muscle tension dysphonia (MTD; Roy, 2003).

As for stress, the discussion about voice disorders requires consideration of the thorny classification problem. According to the *Classification Manual of Voice Disorders—1*, primary MTD (hyperfunctional voice disorders, hypo-

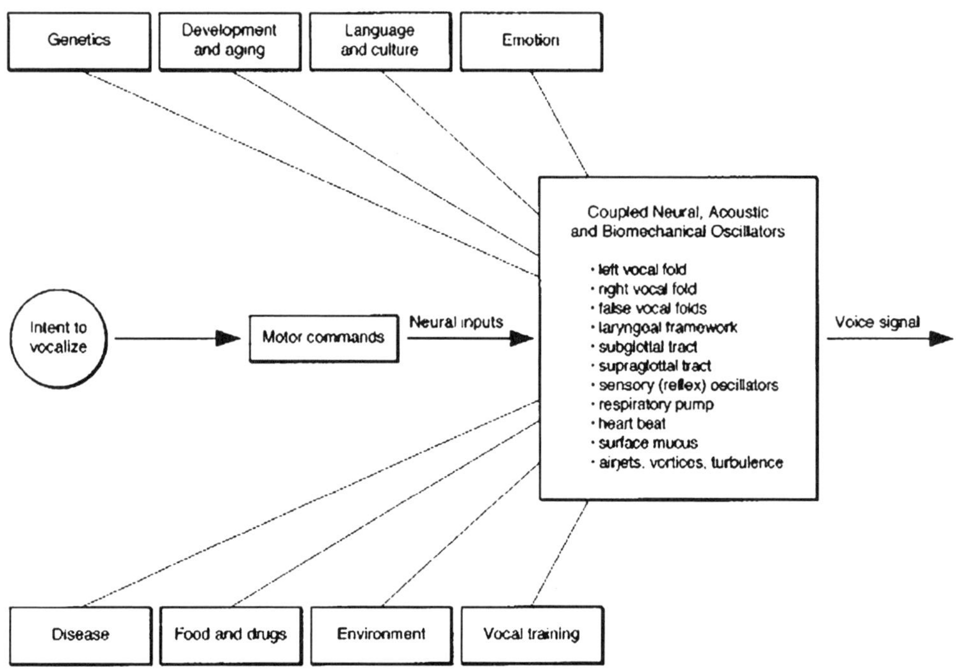

Figure 11–3. A list of biological oscillators involved in voice production and factors that may influence them. Reprinted by permission from *Workshop on Acoustic Voice Analysis: Summary Statement* (p.5), by I. R. Titze, 1995, Iowa City, IA: National Center for Voice and Speech.

adducted hyperfunction) involves a dysphonia without current organic vocal fold pathology or psychogenic or neurologic etiology (Verdolini, Rosen, & Branski, 2005). In that classification system, a voice disorder can only be qualified as *psychogenic* in the verified presence of a psychiatric or psychological disorder satisfying criteria from the *Diagnostic and Statistical Manual of Mental Disorders (DSM-IV)* (Verdolini et al., 2005). However, it is generally thought that unspecified precipitating events, for example those conceptualized as stressors, can be involved as predisposing factors to some pathologies affecting voice, and thus the diagnosis eludes proper categorization as *psychogenic* (Verdolini et al., 2005).

Research efforts to elucidate psychological and psychiatric factors involved in MTD have pointed to the possible contribution of many influences: introversion, neuroticism, emotion-oriented coping, anxiety, depression, inhibition, interpersonal sensitivity, social anxiety, somatic complaints, and stress reactivity (Aronson, Peterson, & Litin, 1966; Deary, Wilson, Carding, & Mackenzie, 2003; Demmink-Geertman & Dejonckere, 2002; Goldman, Hargrave, Hillman, Holmberg, & Gress, 1996; Morrison, Nichol, & Rammage, 1986; Rosen & Murry, 2000; Roy, Bless, & Heisey, 2000). Of relevance for our discussion is the fact that this list of attributes is consistent with those discussed earlier in the chapter with reference to certain persons' vulnerability to negative health outcomes. Further, the concern is that if the combination of stressful life situations and emotional or personality features that contributed to, maintained, or exacerbated the voice disorder remains unaddressed, logically, the risk of a relapse post-voice therapy increases (Nichol, Morrison, & Rammage, 1993; Roy et al., 2000).

Personality and Voice Disorders

Research on links between personality traits and voice has generated a *theory of the dispositional bases of functional dysphonia and vocal nodules* (Roy & Bless, 2000; Roy et al., 2000). In the relevant research, *functional dysphonia* was defined as dysphonia in the absence of vocal fold pathology or neurological abnormalities and *vocal nodules* involved presumed phonotrauma. Within this framework based on biopsychological personality theory, the proposal was made that personality traits may contribute to relatively predictable and conditioned laryngeal responses to certain environmental signals (Roy & Bless, 2000). On average, patients with functional dysphonia were high in introversion and neuroticism. It was hypothesized that in this condition, laryngeal inhibitory responses occur to environmental cues, which in turn increase laryngeal tension resulting in incomplete or disrupted vocalization in the absence of structural changes to the larynx. In contrast, on average, patients with vocal nodules were characterized by extraversion and neuroticism. These patients may be laryngeally overactive in response to environmental cues and engage in extensive voice use. In conclusion, the authors of this research highlighted the complex interplay among personality, voice use patterns, anatomical, and physiological vulnerability and they note that the physiological pathways involved have not yet been examined empirically (Roy & Bless, 2000).

This observation invites new directions in research to investigate the physiological mechanisms involved in psychological factors that may mediate voice production. For instance, the common denominator in the previously described theory is neuroticism. It will be informative to investigate physiological stress reactivity patterns in extroverted and introverted individuals and the specific role of neuroticism in that context.

In addition, results from research on the relation between type A personality, as predominantly seen in males, and speaking style and facial behavior can be informative. Type A personalities are characterized by an aggressive and hostile attitude, including nonverbal facial tension such as teeth-clenching (Chesney, Ekman, Friesen, Black, & Hecker, 1997). Research on speaking style has shown the largest differences between type A and control personalities for syllabic emphasis, voice loudness, voice harshness, hostility, and speaking rate, indicating an increase in all of these factors with type A personality (Chesney et al., 1997). Interestingly, investigations on psychological characteristics of patients with vocal fold granulomas seem to parallel these results (Kiese-Himmel, Pralle, & Kruse, 1998). Thus, future research could incorporate the type A construct as a potential predictor of some voice disorders.

Psychopathology in Voice Disorders

Although stress and anxiety are closely related, stress can be present without concurrent psychological distress such as anxiety and depression (Cohen & Williamson, 1988). However, allostatic load or chronic stress can be conceptualized as a precursor predicting a risk for *future* psychiatric disease (Cohen, Kamarck, & Mermelstein, 1983). More specifically, research has investigated the relation between stress and psychiatric diseases and results have pointed to a stress-induced, biological basis of anxiety and depression, by way of HPA dysregulation (Cohen et al., 1995).

A recent study obliquely related to this notion was conducted on the frequency of perceived stress as compared to anxiety and depression in patients with voice disorders (Dietrich, Verdolini, Gartner-Schmidt, & Rosen, in press). The study aimed to explore (a) the relationship between stress and laryngeal diagnosis, and (b) the relation between stress and anxiety and depression in relation to laryngeal diagnosis. Two hundred eighty-one new patients (65% female) presenting to a voice center completed self-report questionnaires that assess perceived global stress within the preceding 1 month (Perceived Stress Scale-10, PSS-10; Cohen & Williamson, 1988) and anxiety and depression based on symptoms from the preceding week (Hospital Anxiety and Depression Scale, HADS; Zigmond & Snaith, 1983). Findings indicated the following results. About 25% of all patients with MTD (primary and secondary) and vocal fold lesions, about 30% of patients with laryngopharyngeal reflux (LPR), and about 40% of patients with paradoxical vocal fold motion disorder (PVFMD) produced stress scores equal to or greater than one standard deviation above the mean for normative data. Further, fully 50% of all patients with vocal fold lesions, PVFMD, LPR, and primary MTD (as compared to about 30% of patients with secondary MTD), had at least mild anxiety. Only a small number of patients had depression scores indicating at least mild depression: about 15% of patients with primary MTD and PVFMD and 10% of all other patients. In comparison, patients with glottal insufficiency due to paralysis and other causes had significantly lower stress and anxiety scores compared to subjects in other diagnostic categories, and also had the lowest depression scores. In conclusion, primarily elevated anxiety and to a lesser degree stress appeared to co-occur with voice disorders in roughly the following descending order of magnitude of relation: PVFMD, LPR, vocal fold lesions, and MTD (Dietrich et al., in press).

Only one other study of which we are aware investigated the prevalence of *adjustment-related stress*, anxiety, voice use, and somatic complaints in a population of individuals with voice disorders (Schedule of Recent Experiences, SRE; Davis, Eschelman, & McKay, 1988; Goldman et al., 1996). In that study, patients with vocal fold nodules showed no higher stress scores compared to controls, whereas a comparison group composed of individuals with hyperfunctional voice disorders (MTD, vocal fold lesions other than nodules) did show higher stress scores. In addition, both groups showed higher state and trait anxiety scores as compared to healthy controls (Goldman et al., 1996).

Comparing the two studies, the commonalities are elevated anxiety scores for individuals with hyperfunctional voice disorders with and without lesions. Results surrounding stress are weaker and less easily comparable, but research should pursue the relationship between anxiety and stress in voice disorders. The pervasiveness of anxiety and stress in individuals with voice disorders is striking, and possibly may influence the occurrence and maintenance of a *wide range of voice disorders* relevant in clinical practice. However, no causality can be implied at this point, based on the noted cross-sectional studies, and no predictions can be made about risk factors for future voice disorders due to anxiety or stress. Further, the likely bidirectionality between stress and voice disorders on one hand, and voice disorders and stress on the other hand, makes it difficult to disentangle the pathways. For instance, it has been established that voice disorders decrease an individual's quality of life (Smith et al., 1996), and thus may increase stress.

Physiological Pathways in Voice and Stress

Past research around psychological factors involved in certain individuals with voice disorders has focused primarily on personality issues and psychopathology using self-report measures as previously discussed, and on the general importance of stress in professional voice users (Rosen & Sataloff, 1997). New frontiers for investigation include studies around (a) the *specific role of stress* in voice disorders, and (b) the potential *pathways* by which stress may affect voice. Stated differently, no ***physiological or biological*** research exists to date of which we are aware that specifically studies the link between stress and voice disorders using a psychobiological framework incorporating complex stress-emotion-voice interactions. However, recent work has made some forays in that direction. For example, one study looked at the effects of "vocal constitution" (i.e., dynamic range), autonomic reactivity, and state and trait anxiety on vocal endurance in female student teachers without vocal complaints (Schneider et al., in press). Interestingly, autonomic stress reactivity did not predict fundamental frequency changes during actual teaching in the classroom—although it should be noted that other vocal parameters that may be associated with stress, such as voice intensity, were not tracked.

In thinking about the investigation of the relation between stress and voice within a psychobiological framework, it is relevant that the ANS regulates the same functions in the larynx during stress as in the general body. Autonomic innervation of the larynx is generally accepted to regulate laryngeal muscle tone, laryngeal secretions, and laryngeal blood flow (Hisa & Sato, 1991). Thus, hypothetically, stress should alter muscular, glandular, and vascular functions in the larynx with possible interactive effects on laryngeal function (e.g., MTD) and laryngeal structure (e.g., phonotrauma). Further, an evolutionary-driven framework should be relevant for vocal expressions as seen in animal research, according to which hard-wired reflexive vocal responses are triggered under various emotion-stress states (Jürgens, 2002).

Laryngeal Muscle Tension

In patients with MTD, the tangible cause for the dysphonia often appears to be a dysregulated and poorly balanced activity of the intrinsic and extrinsic laryngeal muscles, which is further described as involving widespread dyscoordination among respiratory, phonatory, resonatory, and articulatory gestures (Morrison et al., 1986; Rosen & Sataloff, 1997; Roy, 2003). However, the specific mechanisms of such incoordination remain unclear (Roy, 2003). The increase of muscle tension in the head and neck is generally of concern for voice disorders because of subsequent changes that are assumed to occur in the biomechanical vibratory properties of the vocal folds, which could further generate increased perceived phonatory effort, increased subglottic pressure, increased vocal fold adduction, and in turn increased vocal fold impact stress (Berry et al., 2001; Jiang & Titze, 1994; Morrison & Rammage, 1993; Roy & Bless, 2000).

One approach that has been used to describe differences in head and neck muscle tension between healthy individuals and those with hyperfunction has been surface laryngeal electromyography (S-EMG), which has also been used as a biofeedback tool. Results have shown that patients diagnosed with laryngeal hyperfunction tend to demonstrate greater laryngeal S-EMG activity as compared to controls (Hoãevar-BolteÏar, Janko, & Îargi, 1998; Stemple, Weiler, Whitehead, & Komray, 1980). The only line of research of which we are aware that systematically uses a psychobiological stress reactivity protocol and that has specifically linked stress to muscular activation in voice production was first tested for feasibility using a single-subject design and thereafter was expanded to a pilot study. Results from the single-subject design indicated that speech-induced stress, as verified by cardiovascular activation, increased S-EMG values in several laryngeal strap muscles more than in a distal, lower limb control site (Dietrich, Verdolini, & Barkmeier-Kraemer, 2005). The pilot study provided further valuable insights (Dietrich & Verdolini, 2007). Six female vocally healthy subjects above the norm on introversion and neuroticism and six female vocally healthy subjects above the norm on extraversion and below on neuroticism participated in two sessions of a social-evaluative stress reactivity protocol (Trier Social Stress Test; Kirschbaum, Pirke, & Hellhammer, 1993) that included a baseline rest, stress (public speaking and non-speech mental arithmetic one week apart), and recovery phase as well as non-stressed speech recordings for reference. Results indicated that subjects highest on the trait introversion reacted with more negative emotions and rumination throughout the protocol than subjects who did not exhibit these characteristics. Cardiovascular reactivity was generally correlated with the degree of negative affect experienced. Further, increased *perceived* vocal effort during stress was *only* experienced in selected subjects who ranked highest on introversion. The S-EMG findings are intriguing, because for the extraverts EMG activity increased primarily in the submental muscle group during stress and to a lesser degree in the infrahyoid muscle group. The EMG pattern for the introverted subjects was the reverse. The data may indicate a tendency for counterproductive laryngeal co-contraction and inhibition driven by disproportional activity of the infrahyoid muscles in introverted individuals. In conclusion, stress *may influence vocal perceptions and behaviors.* Importantly, individuals may be differentially vulnerable and at risk for laryngeal muscle tension based on their pattern of stress reactivity. Similar future data for patients with MTD will further enlighten the specific pathways that regulate relations between stress and voice in a theoretically-guided context (Dietrich & Verdolini, 2007).

Laryngeal Secretions

During stress exposures, glandular secretions in general decrease in amount and increase in viscosity (Iversen et al., 2000). Numerous submucosal glands have been found in the human laryngeal, tracheal, and bronchial mucosa (Sato & Hirano, 1998). Given this setup, a decrease in laryngeal secretion amount or a decrease in secretion fluidity due to stress may be an analog to a decrease in local hydration. The relevance is that the hydration literature has indicated that a reduction in either surface or systemic hydration to the vocal folds can increase phonatory threshold pressure (Fisher, Ligon, Sobecks, & Roxe, 2001; Jiang, Verdolini, Aquino, Ng, & Hanson, 2000; Verdolini, Titze, & Fennell, 1994). Also, some evidence indicates an inverse relation between hydration exposures and laryngeal lesions (Verdolini-Marston, Sandage, & Titze, 1994).

Laryngeal Blood Flow

Blood flow is regulated through vasoconstriction and vasodilation as modulated by ANS and endocrine systems (Iversen et al., 2000). With changing physical and emotional states, blood flow is redistributed to various parts of the body including sympathetically mediated vasoconstriction in nonworking muscles and ANS-mediated vasodilation in exercising muscles to meet metabolic demands (Lovallo, 2005). Similarly as for the body in general, vascular supply to the laryngeal tissue can be affected during physical and emotional states. A range of factors is associated with variations in changes in laryngeal blood flow: muscle fiber type, muscle activity level, neurotransmitters, metabolites, tissue integrity, and tissue morphology (Lyon & Barkmeier-Kraemer, 2004). In addition, it has been found that the vascular supply to the lamina propria and vocalis muscle has differential blood distribution properties. Changes in vocal fold vascular supply in particular have been investigated in the context of etiological factors for vocal fold lesions (Lyon & Barkmeier-Kraemer, 2004). Finally, it has been hypothesized that vasoconstriction in the larynx under stress, and thus a decrease in oxygen supply, may underlie vocal fatigue (Švek & Šram, 2001).

Laryngeal Wound Healing

In the context of current knowledge on the link between the immune system and health, immunological research on the laryngeal inflammatory and wound healing system is imperative to optimize treatment approaches and recovery from phonotrauma and other laryngeal disease. Current in vivo, in vitro, and in silico research on inflammatory and wound healing responses in the larynx is advancing our knowledge on key inflammatory mediators and their responses over time to various types of phonotrauma (Branski, Rosen, Verdolini, & Hebda, 2005; Li, Verdolini, Qi, Hebda, & Vodovotz, 2005; Thibeault, Rousseau, Welham, Hirano, & Bless, 2004; Verdolini, Rosen, Grillo, Branski, & Hebda, in preparation). Consequently, this line of research should be extended in the future to investigate the effects of biological stress markers on laryngeal wound healing.

Future Directions

A long-term goal for future investigations is to explore and address the research gap in the voice disorders literature relative to the relation between stress and voice, and relative to possible *biological pathways* by which stress affects voice, by applying a psychobiological framework that has evolutionary validity. Future research should emphasize research methodologies that include *biological markers* of the ANS that allow inferences around underlying mediating mechanisms. Based on the foregoing review, at least six experimental questions can be proposed related to voice disorders research: (1) Can evidence be found that stress-induced physiological changes, as seen by measures of increased muscle tone, decreased secretions, and altered blood flow in the larynx, are mediated by pathways of the ANS? (2) If so, is the magnitude of changes sufficient to be clinically relevant? (3) Do the magnitude and quality of change (stress reactivity) depend (a) on the type of stressor; and (b) on the type of person? (4) Is stress an initiating, maintaining, or exacerbating factor for specific diagnoses affecting voice? (5) Does acute or chronic stress affect the rate and quality of wound healing in the larynx as mediated by immunological dysregulation? (6) Do complementary and alternative medicine approaches aimed at stress reduction have a positive effect on *psychobiological pathways* relevant for laryngeal functioning, and thus on clinical profiles?

Conclusion

Clearly, the signs of the time point towards a concerted effort to advance mind and body research. The proposed psychobiological framework for studying stress and its relationship to voice and voice disorders offers a model for addressing research questions by systematically assessing potential psychobiological pathways linking stress to vocal functioning. The main goal of the chapter was to increase awareness of the complex relationship between stress and health and to highlight the widespread implications of stress on health in the context of voice. The ultimate goal is to further explore the specific role of stress in voice disorders, including the mediating and moderating pathways of acute and chronic stress, to identify and optimize efficacious biologically and psychologically motivated treatment approaches for selected diagnostic categories of voice disorders, and to enhance treatment compliance and long-term treatment efficacy. The future for systematic stress research in the context of voice disorders is promising.

References

Anderson, B. L., Kiecolt-Glaser, J. K., & Glaser, R. (1994). A biobehavioral model of cancer stress and disease course. *American Psychologist*, *49*, 389-404.

Aronson, A. E., Peterson, H. W., & Litin, E. M. (1966). Psychiatric symptomatology in functional dysphonia and aphonia. *Journal of Speech and Hearing Disorders*, *31*, 115-127.

Berry, D. A., Verdolini, K., Montequin, D. W., Hess, M. M., Chan, R. W., & Titze, I. R. (2001). A quantitative output-cost ratio in voice production. *Journal of Speech, Language, and Hearing Research*, *44*, 29-37.

Branski, R. C., Rosen, C. A., Verdolini, K., & Hebda, P. A. (2005). Biochemical markers associated with acute vocal fold wound healing: A rabbit model. *Journal of Voice*, *19*, 283-289.

Chesney, M. A., Ekman, P., Friesen, W. V., Black, G. W., & Hecker, M. H. L. (1997). Type A behavior pattern: Facial behavior and speech components. In P. Ekman & E. L. Rosenberg (Eds.), *What the face reveals: Basic and applied studies of spontaneous expression using the facial action coding system (FACS)* (pp. 453-466). New York: Oxford University Press.

Cohen, S., & Hamrick, N. (2003). Stable individual differences in physiological response to stressors: Implications for stress-elicited changes in immune related health. *Brain, Behavior, and Immunity*, *17*, 407-414.

Cohen, S., & Herbert, T. B. (1996). Health psychology: Psychological factors and physical disease from the perspective of human psychoneuroimmunology. *Annual Reviews Psychology*, *47*, 113-142.

Cohen, S., Kamarck, T., & Mermelstein, R. (1983). A global measure of perceived stress. *Journal of Health and Social Behavior*, *24*, 386-396.

Cohen, S., Kessler, R. C., & Underwood Gordon, L. (1995). Strategies for measuring stress in studies of psychiatric and physical disorders. In S. Cohen, R. C. Kessler, & L. Underwood Gordon (Eds.), *Measuring stress: A guide for health and social scientists* (pp. 3-26). New York: Oxford University Press.

Cohen, S., & Rabin, B. (1998). Psychologic stress, immunity, and cancer. *Journal of the National Cancer Institute*, *90*, 3-4.

Cohen, S., Tyrrell, D. A., & Smith, A. P. (1991). Psychological stress and susceptibility to the common cold. *The New England Journal of Medicine*, *325*, 606-612.

Cohen, S., & Williamson, G. (1988). Perceived stress in a probability sample of the United States. In S. Spacapan & S. Oskamp (Eds.), *The social psychology of health* (pp. 31-67). Newbury Park, CA: Sage.

Cohen, S., & Williamson, G. M. (1991). Stress and infectious disease in humans. *Psychological Bulletin*, *109*, 5-24.

Costa, P. T., Jr., & McCrae, R. R. (1985). Hypochondriasis, neuroticism, and aging. When are somatic complaints unfounded? *American Psychologist*, *40*, 19-28.

Darwin, C. (1998). *The expression of the emotions in man and animals* (3rd ed.). London: Harper-Collins. (Original work published 1872)

Davis, M., Eschelman, E. R., & McKay, M. (1988). *The relaxation and stress reduction handbook*. Oakland, CA: New Harbinger.

Deary, I. J., Wilson, J. A., Carding, P. N., & Mackenzie, K. (2003). The dysphonic voice heard by me, you and it: Differential associations with personality and psychological distress. *Clinical Otolaryngology, 28*, 374-378.

Demmink-Geertman, L., & Dejonckere, P. H. (2002). Nonorganic habitual dysphonia and autonomic dysfunction. *Journal of Voice, 16*, 549-559.

Dickerson, S. S., Gruenewald, T. L., & Kemeny, M. E. (2004). When the social self is threatened: Shame, physiology, and health. *Journal of Personality, 72*, 1191-1216.

Dickerson, S. S., & Kemeny, M. E. (2004). Acute stressors and cortisol responses: A theoretical integration and synthesis of laboratory research. *Psychological Bulletin, 130*, 355-391.

Dietrich, M., & Verdolini, K. (2007, August). *The effects of acute stress on perceived and objective extralaryngeal muscle tension in vocally healthy subjects.* Paper presented at the 7th Pan European Voice Conference (PEVOC7), Groningen, Netherlands.

Dietrich, M., Verdolini, K, & Barkmeier-Kraemer, J. (2005, September). *Physiological changes in the larynx under acute stress: Surface EMG findings.* Paper presented at the 6th Pan European Voice Conference (PEVOC6), London, UK.

Dietrich, M., Verdolini, K., Gartner-Schmidt, J., & Rosen C. A. (in press). The frequency of perceived stress, anxiety, and depression in patients with common pathologies affecting voice. *Journal of Voice*.

Ekman, P. (1999). Basic emotions. In T. Dalgleish & M. Power (Eds.), *Handbook of cognition and emotion* (pp. 45-60). Sussex, UK: John Wiley & Sons.

Fisher, K. V., Ligon, J., Sobecks, J. L., & Roxe, D. M. (2001). Phonatory effects of body fluid removal. *Journal of Speech, Language, and Hearing Research, 44*, 354-367.

Glaser, R. (2005). Stress-associated dysregulation and its importance for human health: A personal history of psychoneuroimmunology. *Brain, Behavior, and Immunity, 19*, 3-11.

Goldman, S. L., Hargrave, J., Hillman, R. E., Holmberg, E., & Gress, C. (1996). Stress, anxiety, somatic complaints, and voice use in women with vocal nodules: Preliminary findings. *American Journal of Speech-Language Pathology, 5*, 44-54.

Gross, J. J., Sutton, S. K., & Ketelaar, T. (1998). Relations between affect and personality: Support for the affect-level and affective-reactivity views. *Personality and Social Psychology Bulletin, 24*, 279-288.

Hisa, Y., & Sato, F. (1991). Autonomic innervation of the canine larynx. In M. Hirano, J. A. Kirchner, & D. M. Bless (Eds.), *Neurolaryngology: Recent advances* (pp. 56-64). San Diego, CA: Singular.

Hoãevar-BolteÏar, I., Janko, M., & Îargi, M. (1998). Role of surface EMG in diagnostics and treatment of muscle tension dysphonia. *Acta Otolaryngologica (Stockholm), 118*, 739-743.

Hsiao, T. Y., Liu, C. M., Hsu, C. J., Lee, S. Y., & Lin, K. N. (2001). Vocal fold abnormalities in laryngeal tension-fatigue syndrome. *Journal of Formos Medical Association, 100*, 837-840.

Iverson, S., Iverson, L., & Saper, C. B. (2000). The autonomic nervous system and the hypothalamus. In E. R. Kandel, J. H. Schwartz, & T. M. Jessell (Eds.), *Principles of neural science* (4th ed., pp. 960-981). New York: McGraw-Hill.

Izard, C. E. (1993). Organizational and motivational functions of discrete emotions. In M. Lewis & J. M. Haviland (Eds.), *Handbook of emotions* (pp. 631-641). New York: Guilford Press.

Jiang, J. J., & Titze, I. R. (1994). Measurement of vocal fold intraglottal pressure and impact stress. *Journal of Voice, 8*, 132-144.

Jiang, J., Verdolini, K., Aquino, B., Ng, J., & Hanson, D. (2000). Effects of dehydration on phonation in excised canine larynges. *Annals of Otology, Rhinology, and Laryngology, 109*, 568-575.

Jürgens, U. (2002). Neural pathways underlying vocal control. *Neuroscience and Biobehavioral Reviews, 26*, 235-258.

Juslin, P. N., & Scherer, K. R. (in press). Vocal expression of affect. In J. A. Coan & J. B. Allen (Eds.), *The handbook of emotion elicitation and assessment*. New York: Oxford University Press.

Kemeny, M. E. (2003). The psychobiology of stress. *Current Directions in Psychological Science, 12*, 124-129.

Kiecolt-Glaser, J. K., McGuire, L., Robles, T. F., & Glaser, R. (2002). Psychoneuroimmunology and psychosomatic medicine: Back to the future. *Psychosomatic Medicine, 64*, 15-28.

Kiecolt-Glaser, J. K., Page, G. G., Marucha, P. T., MacCallum, R. C., & Glaser, R. (1998). Psychological influences on surgical recovery: Perspectives from psychoneuroimmunology. *American Psychologist, 53*, 1209-1218.

Kiese-Himmel, C., Pralle, L., & Kruse, E. (1998). Psychological profiles of patients with laryngeal contact granulomas. *European Archives of Oto-Rhino-Laryngology, 255*, 296-301.

Kirschbaum, C., Pirke, K.-M., & Hellhammer, D. H. (1993). The "Trier Social Stress Test" —A tool for investigating psychobiological stress responses in a laboratory setting. *Neuropsychobiology, 28*, 76-81.

Larsen, R. J., & Diener, E. (1992). Promises and problems with the circumplex model of emotion. In M. S. Clark (Ed.), *Emotion: Review of personality and social psychology* (Vol. 13, pp. 25-59). Newbury Park, CA: Sage.

Lazarus, R. S., & Folkman, S. (1984). *Stress, appraisal, and coping*. New York: Springer.

Li, N. Y. K., Verdolini, K., Qi, M., Hebda, P. A., & Vodovotz, Y. (2005, September) *An agent-based model of acute phonotrauma*. Paper presented at the 4th International Conference on Complexity in Acute Illness, Cologne, Germany.

Lovallo, W. R. (2005). *Stress & health: Biological and psychological interactions* (2nd ed.). Thousand Oaks, CA: Sage.

Lyon, M., & Barkmeier-Kraemer, J. (2004). Vascular supply of the larynx. In C. M. Sapienza & J. Casper (Eds.), *Vocal rehabilitation for medical speech-language pathology* (pp. 69-107). Austin, TX: Pro-Ed.

Matthews, K. A. (1988). CHD and type A behaviors: Update on and alternative to Booth-Kewley and Friedman quantitative review. *Psychological Bulletin, 104*, 373-380.

McEwen, B. S. (1998). Protective and damaging effects of stress mediators. *The New England Journal of Medicine, 338*, 171-179.

McEwen, B., & Stellar, E. (1993). Stress and the individual: Mechanisms leading to disease. *Archives of Internal Medicine, 153*, 2093-2101.

Miller, G. E., Cohen, S., Rabin, B. S., Skoner, D. P., & Doyle, W. J. (1999). Personality and tonic cardiovascular, neuroendocrine, and immune parameters. *Brain, Behavior, and Immunity, 13*, 109-123.

Morrison, M. D., Nichol, H., & Rammage, L. A. (1986). Diagnostic criteria in functional dysphonia. *Laryngoscope, 94*, 1-8.

Morrison, M. D., & Rammage, L. A. (1993). Muscle misuse voice disorders: Description and classification. *Acta Otolaryngologica (Stockholm), 113*, 428-434.

National Institutes of Health. (1999). NIH establishes five mind-body research centers. NIH news release. Retrieved October 22, 2004, from http://www.nih.gov/news/pr/sept99/od-30.htm

Nichol, H., Morrison, M. D., & Rammage, L. A. (1993). Interdisciplinary approach to functional voice disorders: The psychiatrist's role. *Otolaryngology—Head and Neck Surgery, 108*, 643-647.

Pennebaker, J. (1983). *The psychology of physical symptoms*. New York: Springer.

Rosen, C. A., & Murry, T. (2000). Voice handicap index in singers. *Journal of Voice, 14*, 370-377.

Rosen, D. C., & Sataloff, R. T. (1997). *Psychology of voice disorders*. San Diego, CA: Singular.

Roy, N. (2003). Functional dysphonia. *Current Opinion in Otolaryngology & Head and Neck Surgery, 11*, 144-148.

Roy, N., & Bless, D. M. (2000). Personality traits and psychological factors in voice pathology: A foundation for future research. *Journal of Speech, Language, and Hearing Research*, *43*, 737-748.

Roy, N., Bless, D. M., & Heisey, D. (2000). Personality and voice disorders: A superfactor trait analysis. *Journal of Speech, Language, and Hearing Research*, *43*, 749-768.

Russell, J. A. (1980). A circumplex model of affect. *Journal of Personality and Social Psychology*, *39*, 1161-1178.

Sato, K., & Hirano, M. (1998). Age-related changes in the human laryngeal glands. *Annals of Otology, Rhinology, and Laryngology*, *107*, 525-529.

Scherer, K. R. (1986). Vocal affect expression: A review and a model for future research. *Psychological Bulletin*, *99*, 143-165.

Scherer, K. R. (2000). Emotion. In M. Hewstone & W. Stroebe (Eds.), *Introduction to social psychology: A European perspective* (3rd ed., pp. 151-191). Oxford, UK: Blackwell.

Schneider, B., Enne, R., Cecon, M., Diendorfer-Radner, G., Wittels, P., Bigenzahn, W., et al. (in press). Effects of vocal constitution and autonomic stress-related reactivity on vocal endurance in female student teachers. *Journal of Voice*.

Smith, E., Verdolini, K., Gray, S., Nichols, S., Lemke, J., Barkmeier, J., et al. (1996). Effect of voice disorders on quality of life. *Journal of Medical Speech-Language Pathology*, *4*, 223-244.

Stavroula, L., Griffiths, A., & Cox, T. (2003). *Work organisation and stress: Systematic problem approaches for employers, managers and trade union representatives* (Protecting workers' health series; no. 3). Geneva, Switzerland: World Health Organization.

Stemple, J. C., Weiler, E., Whitehead, W., & Komray, R. (1980). Electromyographic biofeedback training with patients exhibiting hyperfunctional voice disorder. *Laryngoscope*, *90*, 471-476.

Švec, J. G., & Šram, F. (2001, August). *Violet-reddening of the vocal folds and the vocal fatigue.* Poster presented at the 25th World Congress of the International Association of Logopedics and Phoniatrics (IALP), Montreal, Canada.

Thibeault, S. L., Rousseau, B., Welham, N. V., Hirano, S., & Bless, D. M. (2004). Hyaluronan levels in acute vocal fold scar. *Laryngoscope*, *114*, 760-764.

Titze, I. R. (1995). *Workshop on acoustic voice analysis: Summary statement.* Iowa City, IA: National Center for Voice and Speech.

Tomkins, S. (1962). *Affect, imagery, and consciousness: Vol. 1. The positive affects.* New York: Springer.

Verdolini, K., Rosen, C. A., & Branski, R. C. (2005). *Classification manual for voice disorders—1.* Mahwah, NJ: Erlbaum.

Verdolini, K., Rosen, C. A., Grillo, E., Branski, R. C., & Hebda, P. A. (in press). *The effect of voice use on inflammatory status in the vocal folds.*

Verdolini, K., Titze, I. R., & Fennell, A. (1994). Dependence of phonatory effort on hydration level. *Journal of Speech and Hearing Research*, *37*, 1001-1007.

Verdolini-Marston, K., Sandage, M., & Titze, I. R. (1994). Effect of hydration treatments on laryngeal nodules and polyps and related voice measures. *Journal of Voice*, *8*, 30-47.

Zajonc, R. B. (1984). On primacy of affect. In K. R. Scherer & P. Ekman (Eds.), *Approaches to emotion* (pp. 261-292). Hillsdale, NJ: Erlbaum.

Zelenski, J. M., & Larsen, R. J. (1999). Susceptibility to affect: A comparison of three personality taxonomies. *Journal of Personality*, *67*, 761-791.

Zigmond, A., & Snaith, R. P. (1983). The hospital anxiety and depression scale. *Acta Psychiatrica Scandinavica*, *67*, 361-370.

CHAPTER 12

The Role of Auditory Feedback in Nonverbal Vocal Behavior of Normally Hearing and Hearing Impaired Infants

Elisabeth Scheiner and Kurt Hammerschmidt

Abstract

Results of a longitudinal study of the preverbal vocalizations of a cohort of normally hearing and profoundly hearing-impaired infants, based mainly on multiparameter acoustic analyses are reported. First, we described and compared their preverbal vocalizations, the emergence of their vocal types, and the developmental changes during the first year of life. Then we focused on how different emotions influence the structure of preverbal vocalizations and if there are differences between both groups of infants and discussed how our results contribute to the ongoing debate on infant emotions. Following this, we integrated our findings into a broader phylogenetic view, and finally, we discussed whether our findings could be useful for diagnostic purposes of early hearing loss.

Our results indicate that the emergence and the acoustic structure of preverbal vocalizations are to a great extent independent of the auditory input and, hence, seem to be essentially predetermined. The basic information of whether an infant feels good or bad is encoded in the structure of its vocalizations. Similar emotional correlates in acoustic structure of vocalizations are also described for other mammalian species, indicating that this kind of emotional encoding is phylogenetically old.

In contrast to the weak emotion-related differences in the acoustic structure of single vocalizations, we found clear differences in the composition of the vocal sequences between normal hearing and hearing-impaired infants. Whereas normal hearing infants showed an improved correspondence between emotion and sequence composition, hearing-impaired infants showed hardly any emotion-related changes in the composition of their vocal sequences. Thus it seems that sequence composition is influenced by auditory learning. However, due to the high variability of infants' vocal production, the analysis of sequence composition seems to be not a practical method for the early diagnosis of hearing impairment.

Introduction

From birth on, nonverbal vocal expressions are pervasive behavioral patterns in infants, which occur in a broad variety of situations. Parents normally pay intense attention to the vocal utterances of infants. Underlying this attention is the assumption that infants' nonverbal vocalizations provide listeners with information about the emotional and physical state of the child. Nevertheless, most studies focus on the development of phonation and articulation with respect to features of mature speech (Locke, 1993; Murai, 1963; Nakazima, 1962; Oller, 1980; Papousek, 1994; Stark, 1980; Tonkova-Yampol'skaya, 1969). As a rule, investigations of speech development exclude so-called "reflexive vocalizations," that is, sounds that can be elicited by specific stimulation, and consequently cannot be said to be arbitrary. Cries, coughs, and hiccups for example are classified as such reflexive vocalizations (Oller, 1980).

In spite of their intuitive relevance, there is only limited knowledge about what kind of information in detail is transmitted via nonverbal vocal utterances. Since Darwin (1872), the voice of humans and animals is seen as an important carrier of emotional signals. Emotions have been explained to be evolved, adaptive mechanisms that facilitate an organism to cope with important events affecting its well-being (Darwin, 1872; Scherer, 1993). Although there is an ongoing debate about the nature of emotions, there is a growing consensus among theorists that emotion needs to be viewed as a multicomponent entity (Frijda, 1986; Lazarus, 1991; Scherer, 1984). In comparison to infants, the vocal expression of emotions in human adults is investigated relatively well. Adults can report their emotions introspectively, they can be asked to express different emotions by will, and they can be asked to judge vocal emotional expressions of other people. In contrast, it is much more difficult to estimate the emotional state of infants. It currently is being discussed to which degree the emotional system of young infants is differentiated compared to that of adults.

Besides their communicative function and their function as potential precursors of spoken language, infant vocalizations are also in focus because of their potential usefulness for the early detection of hearing impairment. Hearing impairment in human infants is relatively widespread [1-2 of 1000 infants internationally (Garvel & Tocci, 1998)]. To develop spoken language despite hearing deficiency, therapeutic interventions are required. It is known that the early start of therapy is one of the decisive factors for its success (Diller, Graser, & Schmalbrock, 2001; Yoshinaga-Itano, Sedey, Coulter, & Mehl, 1999). For early diagnosis and effective therapy it is important to know whether and to what extent the early preverbal vocalizations are influenced by hearing impairment. Therefore, we studied how hearing impairment affects the early preverbal vocalizations and whether this knowledge could lead to an earlier diagnosis and more effective therapy.

In the following, we will focus on a longitudinal study of the preverbal vocalizations of normally hearing and profoundly hearing-impaired infants, based mainly on multiparameter acoustic analyses. First, we will describe and compare their preverbal vocalizations, the emergence of their vocal types, and the developmental changes during the first year of life. Then we will focus on the question of how different emotions influence the structure of preverbal vocalizations and if there are differences between both groups of infants and discuss how our results can contribute to the ongoing debate on infant emotions. Following this, we try to integrate our findings into a broader phylogenetic view. Finally, we will discuss whether our findings could be useful for diagnostic purposes.

Methodological Issues

The study investigated the preverbal vocalizations of seven normally hearing and seven severely hearing-impaired infants during the first year of life (Scheiner, Hammerschmidt, Jürgens, & Zwirner, 2002; 2004; 2006). The infants were recorded regularly in their familiar surrounding in 11 different situations of normal infant life. For each recording, the assumed emotional state of the infants was noted. The emotional state of the infants was judged by their parents, which could use all available sources of information—voice, mimics, body gesture, and contextual information—for their decision. The parents could choose between the terms joy, contentment, interest, surprise, unease, anger, and pain. These emotions were assumed to occur regularly enough without intervention to allow systematic recordings.

Since the preverbal utterances are hardly describable with linguistic methods, we used a multiparameter acoustic analysis to examine the physical structure of the utterances in terms of time, frequency, and energy characteristics. This kind of analysis is also comparable to studies of nonhuman primates (e.g., Fichtel, Hammerschmidt, & Jürgens, 2001;

Fischer, Hammerschmidt, Cheney, & Seyfarth, 2002; Fischer, Hammerschmidt, & Todt, 1995; Gouzoules, Gouzoules, & Marler, 1984; Hammerschmidt & Fischer, 1998; Symmes, Newman, Talmage-Riggs, Katz, & Lieblich, 1979).The advantage of this method is the independence of any structural prerequisites; even simple sounds could be described and classified. Therefore, we digitized the recorded vocalizations and submitted them to a Fast Fourier transformation (FFT). The resulting frequency-time spectra were analyzed using LMA 9.2 (developed by Kurt Hammerschmidt). LMA is a software tool which extracts different sets of acoustic parameters to describe acoustic signals. We defined the vocal types based on the descriptions of infant vocalizations in the literature and the vocal variation we found in our own sample. We established multiparameter limits for every vocal type. In this way, most vocalizations could be assigned to one of 11 vocal types (see below). The few vocalizations that did not fit in this classification were put into a *rest* group.

Vocal Repertoire of Human Infants

As already mentioned, research on infant vocal development has focused almost completely on speech development (Locke, 1993; Oller, 1980; Papousek, 1994). Only little work has been done on the development of nonverbal vocalizations. Following these studies, most authors agree that there are essentially five preverbal stages in the infant's vocal development. In the first stage (0-1 month), infants produce sounds that do not show any systematic contrast between opening and closing of the vocal tract, nor do they make use of the full potential of the vocal cavity as a resonating tube (Oller, 1980). In the second stage (2-3 months), infants start to produce an increasing number of vocalizations with differing modulations. Also, at this age, the first appearance of laughing occurs (Stark, 1980). Typical for the third stage (4-6 months) is the exploration of the vocal tract capacities, called *vocal play* by Stark (1980), in the form of squealing, growling, or yelling sounds, production of noises by blowing air, food, or saliva through oropharyngeal constrictions, and nasal murmurs (Stark, 1980). In the fourth stage (7-10 months), infants begin to produce regular syllables [*reduplicated babbling*, according to Stark (1980); *canonical babbling*, according to Oller (1978; 1980)]. Typical for this period are sequences, like *bababa* or *dadada*. During the fifth stage (11-12 months), infants produce alternating syllables with differing consonantal and vocalic elements [*variegated babbling*, according to Stark (1980); *nonreduplicated babbling*, according to Oller (1980); *play with complex vocal patterns*, according to Papoušek & Papoušek (1981)].

Although the different stages of preverbal utterances are long known, there is a very limited knowledge about structural differences and information content of these vocalizations. The exceptions are cries and babbling. In our study we include all vocalizations produced by the infants during the first year of life. Based on a small number of acoustic variables we could classify 11 expiratory vocal types (Scheiner et al., 2002). The acoustic variables are fundamental frequency (F_0) or the respective lowest dominant frequency band in atonal parts of vocalizations. Further, the amount of harmonic energy and the frequency range, measured as the range from the lowest to the highest frequency above the noise threshold, are recorded. In addition to these frequency parameters, temporal parameters, such as vocal duration and the rhythm of the single units, are used to classify the different vocal types.

Figure 12-1 shows typical examples of the 11 expiratory vocal types. Five vocal types, wail/coo, moan, cry, short cry, and babble, show a predominantly tonal structure, but they can include atonal or chaotic parts, like the middle segment of the coo/wail call in Figure 12-1. Cry and short cry can easily be distinguished by their vocal duration. Moan is also a short vocal type but has a lower F_0 with nearly no modulation. Coo/wail may have similar low F_0 like moan but has a higher modulation. In addition, coo/wail may have some atonal segments. Both vocal types have a relatively small frequency range. Babbling in contrast has a large frequency range and a long vocal duration. It could easily be distinguished from the other vocal types by its characteristic rhythmic structure, which consists of at least one consonant and one vowel. Babbling sounds most speechlike but is meaningless (e.g., Stark, 1980; Oller, 1980).

Laugh is another rhythmic vocalization, made up of alternating noisy and tonal parts, separated by short pauses (see also Kipper & Todt, 2001). Laugh usually appears in positive emotional context; but a structurally similar vocal type may occur in negative emotional contexts. Whoop/squeal is a medium-long vocal type characterized by a prominent frequency modulation and the highest F_0 (Figure 12-1). Groan and hic can be distinguished from the other predominantly noisy vocal types by vocal duration. Hic itself can be distinguished from groans by a smaller frequency range and the typical rhythmic structure. It consists of at least two parts separated by a short amplitude gap. Croak, another mainly atonal vocal type, shows a larger frequency range and a longer vocal duration in comparison to groan and hic. The hearing-impaired infants produced the same vocal types as the normally hearing infants. Additionally, we did not find more vocalizations that did not fit in the classification in the recordings of hearing-impaired infants than in those of normally hearing ones.

Emergence of Vocal Types

From the first recording on, the infants regularly uttered 7 out of the 11 vocal types (coo/wail, moan, cry, short cry, hic, groan, and croak). *Regularly* means that more than 50% of the infants uttered these vocal types per recording session. Whoop/squeal was rare during the entire first year. Laughs could be regularly heard at the age of 24 weeks. Babbling did not appear before the age of 29 weeks (Scheiner et al., 2002).

Both normally hearing and hearing-impaired infants shared the same vocal repertoire. With one exception, we found no differences in the time of emergence of the vocal types between normally hearing and hearing-impaired infants (Figure 12-2). The only exception was the emergence of babbling. Babbling emerged later if at all in the repertoire of hearing-impaired infants. Although all these infants were provided with hearing aids on both ears soon after diagnosis, one hearing-impaired infant never babbled in the first 16 months. Two others of the seven infants babbled only one and three times in the first 20 months, respectively.

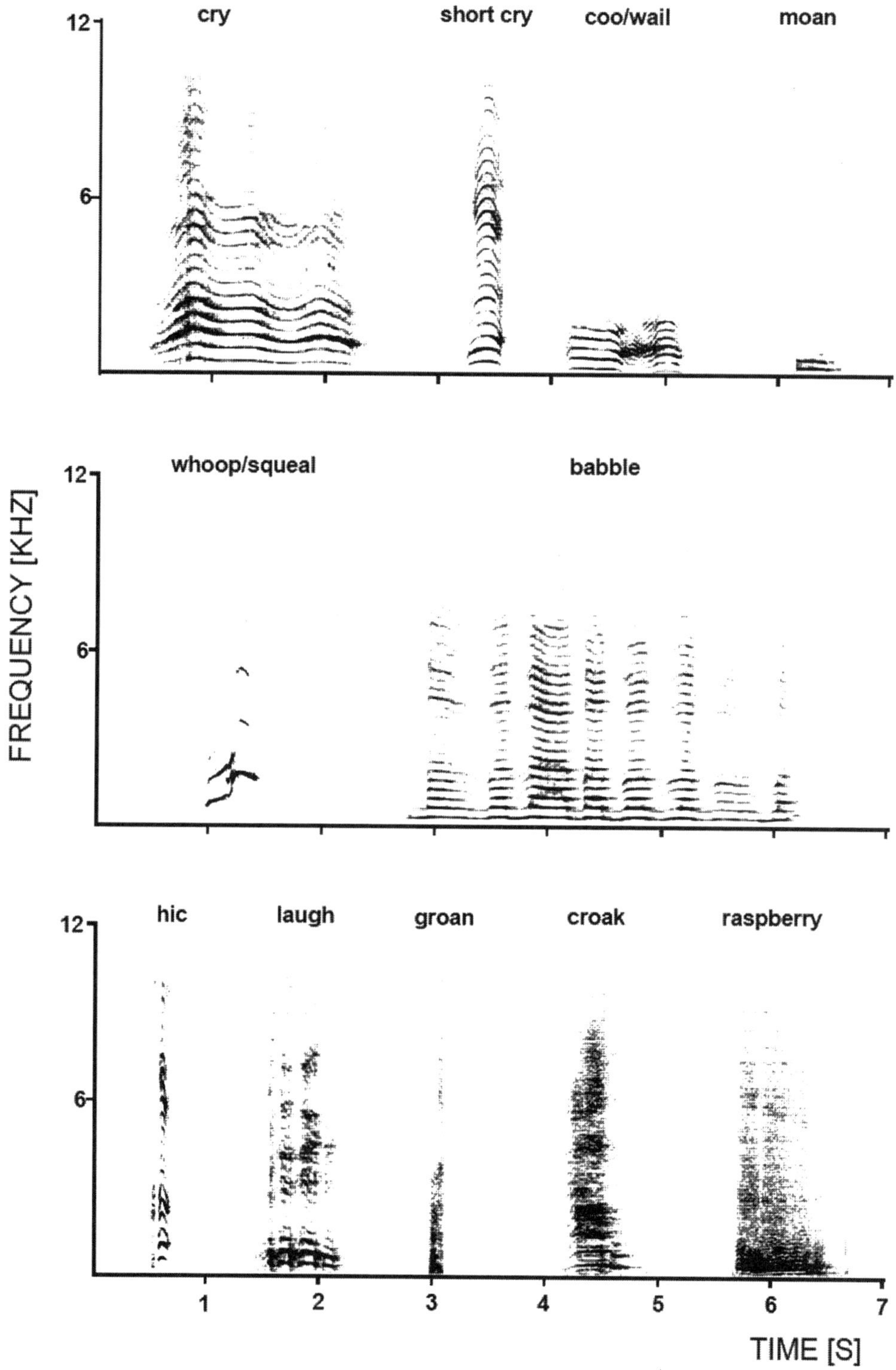

Figure 12–1. Typical frequency-time spectrograms of the 11 vocal types.

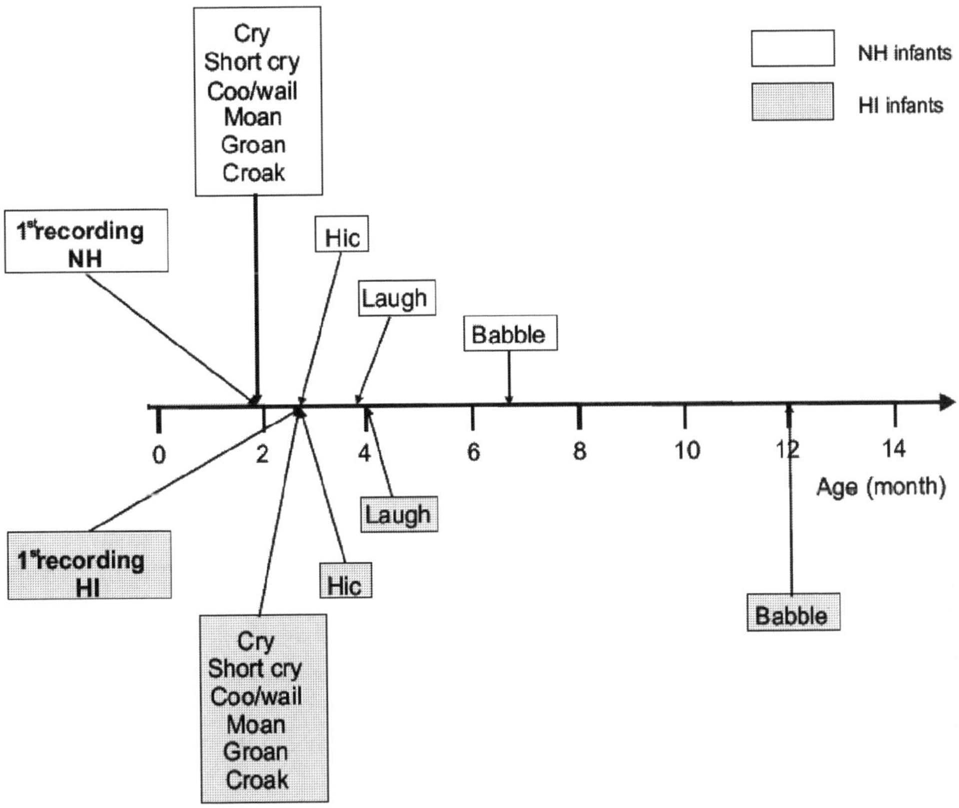

Figure 12–2. Emergence of infant vocalizations separated for normal hearing and hearing-impaired infants. The figure indicates at which age at least half of the infants uttered certain vocalizations. The age of first recording differs slightly for NH and HI infants.

We had two early starters at the age of 6–7 months, but they babbled only at a low rate. The other started to babble at the age of 10 months (Scheiner et al., 2004). These observations are in line with results of other studies (e.g., Eilers & Oller, 1994; Oller, Eilers, & Basinger, 2001; Stark, 1983). Together, these findings show that the majority of preverbal utterances, except babbling, are predetermined and that the production must be to a great extent independent from the auditory input (see also Bloom, D'Odorico, & Beaumont, 1993; Oller, 2000).

In addition, we found nearly no differences in the acoustic structure of the vocal types between normally hearing and hearing-impaired infants (Scheiner et al., 2004). A multivariate statistic analysis of the three most frequent vocalizations (cry, coo/wail, and moan) revealed no significant differences in vocal structure of both groups. Only cries showed some subtle structural differences. Hearing-impaired infants had a slightly higher peak frequency and frequency range than normal hearing infants. In addition, cries of hearing-impaired infants differed in their melody contour. A study done by Möller and Schönweiler (1999) also found some subtle differences. Cries of hearing-impaired infants, in their study, had a longer duration and a more complex melody contour. In contrast to our results, Möller and Schönweiler found a decrease in the energy parameters in the cries of hearing-impaired infants. Möller and Schönweiler did not investigate other vocal types than cries; therefore, we cannot compare our findings regarding the other vocal types. Although our number of infant participants was relatively low and a higher number would lead to an increase of statistical power, it is unlikely that the main result would be changed. If at all, only subtle difference could be expected.

Vocalizations as Expression of Emotions in Adults

There are different ways that emotions could be encoded in nonverbal vocalizations. For instance, different emotional states of the sender could be expressed by different vocal types, such as "cries of pain" and "laughter of joy." Another possibility is that different underlying emotional states influence the acoustic structure of one and the same vocal type in different ways. The influence of emotions on the vocal utterances of human adults has been extensively studied (for reviews, see Van-Bezooyen, 1984; Frick, 1985; Murray & Arnott, 1993; Scherer, 1979). These investigations constitute an important background for studying infant vocalizations. They focus on two major questions: Do listeners identify emotions from vocal cues, and which are the specific acoustic structures encoding specific emotions? The identification of emotions has been studied with sentences spoken by professional actors with different emotions (Banse & Scherer, 1996; Bezooyen, 1984), with single words (Hammerschmidt & Jürgens, 2007; Leinonen, Hiltunen, Linnankoski, & Laakso, 1997), or with natural speech uttered under different levels of stress, like recordings of pilots in crashing airplanes (Ruiz-Miranda, Wells, Golden, & Seidensticker, 1998; Williams & Stevens, 1972). Ratings of the vocalization by listeners showed that they were able to infer vocally expressed emotions significantly better than by chance (Murray & Arnott, 1993; Banse & Scherer, 1996).

However, to assign specific emotions to particular vocalizations seems to be a difficult task. First, the recognition accuracy varies among different emotions. Accuracy, for example, is much higher for hot anger than for disgust (Banse & Scherer, 1996). Second, there is confusion between emotions that share certain properties. For example, hot anger and panic fear are often confused by listeners, because they have a similar intensity, and anxiety and panic fear are often confused because they are of similar quality (Banse & Scherer, 1996). It is also difficult to assign a specific acoustic structure to a specific emotion. For example, anger and fear seem to be characterized by an increase in level and variability of the fundamental frequency, increase in high frequency energy, and range of the fundamental frequency, but joy is characterized by nearly the same acoustic features. Hammerschmidt and Jürgens (2007) showed that an increase in aversion and an increase in intensity of an emotional state are mainly characterized by similar structural changes of the vocalizations uttered by human speakers. This may lead to misinterpretations, especially in cases of single calls or words.

Vocal Expression of Emotions in Normally Hearing Infants

Up to now, studies that focus on the question of to what extent infant vocalizations contain information about different emotional states were done mainly on crying behavior. The results of these studies are controversial. According to Wasz-Höckert et al. (1968), four types of cries can be discriminated: birth, hunger, pain, and pleasure cries. However, Muller et al. (1974) and Murry et al. (1975) reported that mothers were not able to identify the stimulus that elicited crying in their infant. Other authors suggest that infant crying is a graded signal, mirroring a continuum of emotional states reaching from arousal to urgency (Brennan & Kirkland, 1982; Porter, Miller, & Marshall, 1986; Protopapas & Eimas, 1997; Zeskind, Sale, Maio, Huntington, & Weiseman, 1985). Porter et al. (1986), for instance, investigated infant cries during painful circumcision procedures. They found correlations between the acoustic structure of the elicited cries and the degree of intrusiveness of the particular procedure. In the perceptual test, the cries elicited by the most intrusive procedures were judged by adult listeners also to be the most urgent ones.

According to Keller and Schölmerich (1987), parents interpret the vocalizations of even 2-week-old infants as expressions of emotional states and respond in a differentiated way to different vocalizations. There is no general agreement, however, whether infants during their first months of life are able to express specific emotions in their behavior at all (for an overview, see Strongman, 1996). Some authors suggest that, in the first months, the expressive behavior is to a large extent random. This assumption is based on the observation that specific vocal or facial patterns often occur without a specific stimulus preceding them (for an overview, see Camras, 1994). One reason for this low predictability of specific behavior patterns could be a low degree of emotional differentiation in early infanthood. Most authors agree that from the very beginning, there is a differentiation into at least two emotional states: aversive and nonaversive (Giblin, 1981; Izard & Malatesta, 1987; Lewis, 1993; Malatesta-Magai, Izard, & Camras, 1991; Sroufe, 1979). Some authors, however, argue that more than two emotional states can be distinguished (Giblin, 1981; Izard & Malatesta, 1987; Malatesta-Magai et al., 1991). This disagreement about the expression of infant emotions may be partly due to the difficulties in estimating the emotional state of an infant, because we rely on assumptions about the infants' internal state. These assumptions can be strengthened by contextual information (e.g., certain contexts in which specific emotions are probable), or by comparing the facial expressions of infants with the facial expressions of emotions of adults (see Ekman & Oster, 1979; Izard, Huebner, Risser, McGinnes, & Dougherty, 1980). A further possibility to judge the emotional state of infants is to use their parent's ratings (Wasz-Höckert, Lind, Vurenkoski, Patanen, & Valannen, 1968), since in a communication process the receivers of a signal should be able to decode the transmitted information.

In our study (Scheiner et al., 2002; 2004; 2006), we used a combination of parent ratings and contextual information to judge the emotional state of the infants. We tested the four most common vocal types of normally hearing infants, cry, short cry, coo/wail, and moan, with respect to emotion-related differences in acoustic structure. A multivariate GLM procedure testing the differences between vocalizations uttered in positive (contentment and joy) and negative (unease and anger) emotions found significant differences for all four vocal types (cry: HT = 2.08, F = 6.93, $p = 0.008$; coo/wail: HT = 2.55, F = 8.5, $p = 0.004$; moan: HT = 2.49, F = 6.64, $p = 0.015$; short cry: HT = 3.65, F = 12.16, $p = 0.001$). The detailed results of the subsequent univariate tests are given in Table 12-1. In sum, the results indicate that changes from positive to negative emotional states are accompanied by increases in duration, frequency range, and numerous variables describing the pitch of a vocalization. Thus, important information that reflects whether an infant feels good or bad is encoded in the acoustic structure of individual vocal types.

In contrast to the clear differences between positive and negative emotional states, we could not find any differences between single positive emotions (joy and contentment) or single negative emotions (unease and anger). There are several possible reasons for this result. As already mentioned, one reason could be that in young infants the emotional system is not as well differentiated as in older children or adults. A second reason for the failure to separate emotions with

Table 12–1. Differences between vocalizations uttered under positive and negative emotions

Call types	Cry	Short cry	Coo/wail	Moan
Parameter				
Duration	↑*	↑*	↑*	↑*
F_0 median		↑*		
PF tonal mean	↑*		↑*	↑*
PF max location	↑*	↑*	↑	
Pf/F_0 coefficient	↑*			↑*
Range mean	↑	↑*		↑*
Range max	↑	↑*	↑*	

Note. Arrow upward (↑) indicates an increase of the corresponding acoustic variables in negative emotions relative to positive emotions. Arrow downward (↓) indicates a decrease of the corresponding parameter. Parameters marked with an arrow have a p-value below 0.1; p-values below 0.05 are marked in addition with an asterisk. *F_0 mean [Hz]:* fundamental frequency, mean across all time segments of a vocalization; *Pf tonal mean [Hz]:* mean of the frequencies with the highest amplitude in the spectrum across tonal time segments of a vocalization; *Pf max location:* relative position of PF maxima, calculated as a coefficient of sound duration and min location; *Pf/F_0 coefficient:* ratio between peak frequency and fundamental frequency [(PF - F_0)/F_0]; *range mean [Hz]:* difference between highest and lowest frequency in the spectrum, mean across tonal time segments; *range max [Hz]:* maximum difference between the highest and lowest frequency across all time segments of a vocalization.

the same valence might be that not each vocalization uttered in a given emotion is typical for this state. A third reason could be that infants are able to express various emotions, but the parents' ratings are not very reliable. Uncertainty might arise, for instance, from interferences between the parents' own mood or expectations and the infant's behavior, or from incoherence in emotional labeling. To examine the latter possibility, we did a cross-check analysis. We analyzed the same vocalizations, but instead of testing for differences in acoustic structure related to emotional categories, we tested for differences related to the contexts in which the infants were recorded. This analysis produced the same results as the analysis based on the emotional ratings. We found differences in acoustic structure between vocalizations uttered in positive and negative contexts, but no differences between vocalizations uttered in different positive contexts or in different negative contexts. Therefore, it seems unlikely that a mismatch between the parents' emotional estimations and the emotion eliciting context is the main reason for the low discriminability of related emotions in individual vocal types (Scheiner et al., 2002).

Vocal Expression of Emotions in Hearing Impaired Infants

As already mentioned above, we found only subtle differences in acoustic structure between the vocalizations of normally hearing and hearing-impaired infants. Except for babbling, the vocal types of the preverbal repertoire emerge at the same age in both groups. The same is true for the structural differences regarding the emotional state. We found for hearing-impaired infants the same results as for normally hearing infants. While it was again no problem to differentiate vocalizations uttered in positive and negative emotional states, it was impossible to distinguish specific positive or negative emotional states by acoustic structure of the vocalizations. Table 12-2 shows a comparison between the differences regarding hearing ability and emotion. For hearing-impaired infants we found significant differences only in the least meaningful factor and only for one vocal type, the cry. In contrast, differences between positive and negative emotional states were found in several factors (see Table 12-2). In sum, these results indicate that one of the most important functions of infants' vocal signalling, to signal their needs and states to their caregivers (Maestripieri & Call, 1996), is not categorically altered by hearing impairment.

Differences in Call Sequences Related to Emotion and Hearing Ability

So far, we only looked at the acoustic structure of single vocal types. But infants usually do not utter single vocalizations, but streams of vocalizations. Beside the structural differences in single vocalizations, the composition of a vocal sequence might be a source of information about the emotional state and the hearing ability of the infants.

An influence of hearing impairment on the temporal organization of vocal sequences is indicated by the finding of Möller and Schönweiler (1999), who reported that rhythmic patterns in cry bouts and babbling differ between NH and HI

Table 12–2. Differences in vocal structure related to hearing impairment and emotion

		NH/HI	Emotions		
Factors	**Explained variance (%)**	**Cry**	**Coo/wail**	**Moan**	**Cry**
F1: Frequency range, main energy, frequency with the highest amplitude (= peak frequency/PF)	20.3	0.054	—	—	—
F2: Distribution of frequency amplitudes (DFA)	9.8	—	—	—	0.000
F3: Fundamental frequency	9.2	—	0.001	0.001	0.010
F4: Energy in the high frequencies	5.4	—		0.000	0.005
F5: Trend and modulation of PF	5.3	—	0.033	0.000	0.004
F6: Trend and modulation of the first dominant frequency band	3.7	—	0.020	0.000	0.021
F7: Duration, tonality	3.4	—	0.025	0.012	0.000
F8: Location of maximum of DFA or PF	3.4	0.018	—	—	—

Note. A principal component analysis was performed on the 88 original acoustic variables to reduce the number and the correlations between the different acoustic measurements. The first column describes those principal component analysis factors with an explained variance above 3. The second column shows the explained variance. The third column shows the differences between the cries of normally hearing and hearing impaired infants. The fourth to sixth columns show the differences between the four emotions (joy, contentment, unease, and anger) for the call types coo/wail, moan, and cry. The tests for differences between emotions were calculated for normally hearing and hearing impaired infants together. The numbers refer to the *p*-values of the univariate tests (GLM repeated measure, SPSS 10).

infants. According to Möller and Schönweiler the cry bouts of HI infants have "lower" rhythmic frequencies than cry bouts of NH infants. The few studies that investigated the influence of hearing impairment on the succession of specific vocal types yielded inconsistent results. Oller and colleagues (1985) showed that the relative frequency of various vocal types was the same in 1 deaf and 11 normally hearing infants, while Clement and Koopmans-van Beinum (1995) found that HI infants produced some vocal types more often than their hearing peers.

First, our own investigations of the composition of vocal sequences have shown that the influence of the emotional state on vocal sequence composition is not the same in normally hearing and hearing-impaired infants (Scheiner et al., in press). Vocal sequences uttered by normally hearing infants in different emotions differed significantly in their composition. Though the infants produced all vocal types in positive and in negative emotional states, some vocal types were uttered more frequently in positive and others in negative emotional states. It was even possible to find differences between vocal sequences uttered in the two positive emotional states joy and contentment. In hearing-impaired infants, though they were principally able to produce all vocal types that differentiated the emotions in normally hearing ones, there were hardly any emotion-related changes in vocal sequence composition. A second result of the sequence comparison was that normally hearing and hearing-impaired infants' vocal sequences differ in their composition, independent of the emotion (Scheiner et al., 2006).

To sum up, our study revealed that emotions are not only encoded in the acoustic structure of single vocalizations but additionally in the composition of vocal sequences. However, while the encoding of emotions in acoustic structure seems to be to a great extent independent of the auditory input, the composition of vocal sequences seems to be influenced by auditory learning.

Phylogenetic Roots of Emotional Expression

One function of nonverbal vocalizations in humans and nonhuman primates seems to be the communication of the affective state of the signaler. In humans, although they develop speech as an additional way of vocal communication, the nonverbal vocal expression of emotions persists. It is existent in the prosody that underlies speech utterances and in the nonverbal utterances like cries and laughter. Our study showed that different emotional states are encoded in nonverbal vocalizations in two ways. First, the composition of vocal sequences seems to be dependent on auditory input, which indicates that auditory learning takes place. Second, emotion-related changes in acoustic structure are the same in both infant groups (Scheiner et al., 2004; Scheiner et al., 2006). Vocalizations uttered in negative emotional states are mainly characterized by increased pitch manifested in several acoustic parameters, like peak frequency, describing energy distribution in the spectrum.

There are several other studies on nonhuman mammals supporting the view that peak frequency could be an important acoustic variable to communicate a negative emotional state. Schrader & Todt (1998) found a positive correlation between the plasma level of adrenaline and the rate of "squeal-grunts" and a negative correlation between plasma cortisol and normal grunts in domestic pigs (*Sus scrofa*) subjected to stress through social isolation. In comparison to squeal-grunts, grunts exhibit a lower peak frequency. Weary and Fraser (1995) studied the vocalizations of piglets that had been removed from their mothers immediately before suckling. They compared these vocalizations with those recorded from piglets that had been removed from their mothers immediately after suckling, and found that the latter had lower peak frequencies than the former. After a disturbance at their sleeping site, Barbary macaques uttered series of shrill barks. Immediately after the disturbance, these calls had a higher peak frequency than calls uttered at the end of the call series (Fischer et al., 1995).

Similar results were found in a study in which the degree of aversiveness/pleasantness of the concomitant emotional state accompanying a specific vocalization was measured more directly. That study was carried out by Jürgens (1979) in the squirrel monkey (*Saimiri sciureus*). Different calls were elicited by activating specific brain regions responsible for controlling these calls. Activation was carried out by electrical stimulation of stereotactically implanted intracerebral electrodes. The animals were able to switch on and off the vocalizing-eliciting stimulation themselves. In this way, a quantitative measure indicating the degree to which the stimulation was avoided or sought could be obtained. With this method, the aversive or pleasant quality of the affective state underlying the production of specific calls could be determined. A subsequent acoustic analysis of the vocalizations elicited in this study revealed that the calls expressing different degrees of aversion differ in their acoustic structure (Fichtel et al., 2001). Here again, more aversive calls showed higher pitch (characterized by peak frequency, distribution of frequency amplitudes, and dominant frequency), higher frequency range, and a higher amount of nonharmonic energy. Out of the numerous pitch-related parameters, peak frequency seemed to be the most important acoustic variable, because this variable was the only one which differed in all call categories in relation to the degree of aversion. Moreover, a playback study on squirrel monkeys indicated that subtle shifts in the peak frequency were perceptually salient to the listeners (Fichtel & Hammerschmidt, 2003). The same principles have been found in general alarm calls of red-fronted lemurs (*Eulemur fulvus rufus*) (Fichtel & Hammerschmidt, 2002).

The fundamental nature of aversive or pleasant states suggests that their behavioral expressions might be phylogenetically ancient, and possibly so old that related species share common acoustic features in the vocal expression of these states. Our findings in normally hearing and hearing-impaired infants support the view that the vocal expression of emotion in humans has deep-reaching phylogenetic roots (see also Jürgens, 2003; Hammerschmidt & Fischer, in press).

Analyzing Preverbal Vocalizations for Diagnostic Purposes

Several studies investigate the influence of hearing impairment on the preverbal vocalizations of human infants (e.g., Locke, 1993; Murai, 1963; Nakazima, 1962; Oller, 1980; Papousek, 1994; Tonkova-Yampol'skaya, 1969). Until now the only clear evidence was that babbling, which sets in between 7 and 10 months of age in normally hearing infants, is affected by an auditory deficiency. In hearing impaired infants, canonical babbling appears later than in normally hearing infants or does not appear at all. In addition, the phonemic inventory in babbling as well as its temporal structure also differs between hearing impaired and normally hearing infants (Eilers & Oller, 1994; Kent, Osberger, Netsell, & Hustedde, 1987; Oller, 2000; Oller, Eilers, Bull, & Carney, 1985; Papousek, 1994; Stoel-Gammon, 1988; Stoel-Gammon & Otomo, 1986).

This study revealed that in the first year of life the vocal production of hearing-impaired infants is in many aspects very similar to the vocal production of normally hearing infants. Both infant groups shared the same vocal repertoire, most of their call types emerged at the same age, there were only minor differences in the acoustic structure of normally hearing and hearing-impaired infants' vocalizations, and hearing-impaired infants were equally able to encode their general emotional state in the structure of their calls as their normally hearing peers. These findings may explain why parents often recognize the hearing deficiency of their infants relatively late. Additionally, they imply that probably neither acoustic analysis nor the inspection of call sequences is a practicable diagnostic method. Though we found differences in sequence composition, the inspection of call sequences seems to be too labor-intensive to provide a practicable diagnostic tool. Due to the high intra- and intersession variability of infant vocalizations, the differences between normally hearing and hearing-impaired infants' vocal sequences will hardly be detectable by a small sample of vocal series. Furthermore, parents will probably not be able to report whether the relevant call types are uttered more or less often in specific emotional contexts, or if there is an increased or decreased rate of specific call types uttered by their infant compared with a certain standard. The only exception to this general statement concerns the onset of babbling. As a study of Oller et al. (2001) showed, it is not complicated to inform parents what babbling sounds like, and that they should pay attention to whether babbling is uttered or not. Thus, information on the onset of canonical babbling obtained from parents can be used as a reliable tool for risk assessment of hearing impairment in infants aged 6–12 months (Oller et al., 2001).

Summary

The results of this study indicate that the emergence and the acoustic structure of preverbal vocalizations are to a great extent independent of the auditory input and, hence, seem to be essentially predetermined. The basic information of whether an infant feels good or bad is encoded in the structure of its vocalizations. This kind of emotional expression is apparently inherent. Similar emotional correlates in acoustic structure of vocalizations are also described for other mammalian species, indicating that this kind of emotional encoding is phylogenetically old.

In contrast to the weak emotion-related differences in the acoustic structure of single vocalizations, we found clear differences in the composition of the vocal sequences between normal hearing and hearing-impaired infants. Whereas normal hearing infants showed an improved correspondence between emotion and sequence composition, hearing-impaired infants showed hardly any emotion-related changes in the composition of their vocal sequences. Thus it seems that sequence composition is influenced by auditory learning. However, due to the high variability of infants' vocal production, the analysis of sequence composition seems to be not a practicable method for the early diagnosis of hearing impairment.

Outlook

One question which remains open is to which extent the emotion-related differences in acoustic structure are indeed salient for adult listeners. To answer this question it is necessary to take up the perceptual perspective, and test possible receivers of the infant vocal signals. Pilot studies with adult raters showed that it is difficult to judge correctly whether infant vocalizations presented singly were uttered in positive or negative emotional states. Systematic recognition tests with different vocal types presented as single stimuli have still to be done. In these tests, first natural vocalizations could be used, and second the acoustic structure of vocalizations could be artificially altered according to the structural differences that change with positive and negative emotional states in our study.

First pilot tests also showed that recognition accuracy for the valence of the emotional state increased when infant vocalizations were not presented singly, but embedded in their natural vocal sequence. This could be the result of two separate mechanisms. First, in a vocal sequence the information encoded in the acoustic structure of single vocalizations is presented in a redundant way. This probably facilitates recognition. Second, the composition of the vocal sequence may contain additional information about the emotional state of the sender. Our results support this possibility. However, only the sequence composition of normally hearing infants correlates with the emotional state. This indicates that emotion-related sequence composition is dependent on auditory learning. At what exact age and in which way infants learn to produce their vocalizations in specific combinations is still unclear and requires further investigation.

A detailed examination of the ontogeny of sequence composition could possibly also lead to more knowledge about the development of different emotions in infants. We found that in normally hearing infants, not only positive and negative emotional states but also the two positive emotional states joy and contentment could be discriminated by the composition of the respective vocal sequences. We do not know if the differences in the composition of vocal sequence uttered in different emotions of the same valence (e.g., joy and contentment) emerge at the same age as differences in composition of vocal sequences uttered in positive and negative emotions. To explore this could help to enlighten the time course of emotional differentiation in infants.

Acknowledgements. We are indebted to all the physicians who helped us to contact the families participating in the study and grateful to the parents and children for their cooperation and patience during the data acquisition. We are thankful to Uwe Jürgens and Petra Zwirner who initiated and supported the study. Many thanks also to Claudia Fichtel and Julia Fischer for their helpful comments on the manuscript. Part of this research was supported by the Deutsche Forschungsgemeinschaft (Grant ZW 42/21).

References

Banse, R., & Scherer, K. R. (1996). Acoustic profiles in vocal emotion expression. *Journal of Personality and Social Psychology, 70*, 614-636.

Bloom, K., D'Odorico, L., & Beaumont, S. L. (1993). Adult preferences for syllabic vocalizations: Generalizations to parity and native language. *Infant Behavior and Development, 16*, 109-120.

Brennan, M., & Kirkland, J. (1982). Classification of infant cries using descriptive scales. *Infant Behaviour and Development, 5*, 341-346.

Camras, L. A. (1994). Two aspects of emotional development: Expression and elicitation. In P. Ekman & R. J. Davidson (Eds.), *The nature of emotion* (pp. 347-351). New York: Oxford University Press.

Clement, C. J., & Koopmans-van Beinum, F. J. (1995). Influence of lack of auditory feedback: Vocalizations of deaf and hearing infants compared. *Proceedings of the Institute of Phonetic Sciences Amsterdam*, 19, 25-37).

Darwin, C. R. (1872). *The expression of emotions in man and animals*. London: John Murray.

Diller, G., Graser, P., & Schmalbrock, C. (2001). Early natural auditory-verbal education with profound hearing impairments in the Federal Republic of Germany: Results of a 4 year study. *International Journal of Pediatric Otorhinolaryngology, 60*, 219-226.

Eilers, R. E., & Oller, D. K. (1994). Infant vocalizations and the early diagnosis of severe hearing impairment. *The Journal of Pediatrics, 124*, 199-203.

Ekman, P., & Oster, H. (1979). Facial expressions of emotions. *Annual Review of Psychology, 30*, 527-554.

Fichtel, C., & Hammerschmidt, K. (2002). Responses of redfronted lemurs to experimentally modified alarm calls: Evidence for urgency-based changes in call structure. *Ethology, 108*, 763-777.

Fichtel, C., & Hammerschmidt, K. (2003). Responses of squirrel monkeys to their experimentally modified mobbing calls. *Journal of the Acoustical Society of America, 113*, 2927-2932.

Fichtel, C., Hammerschmidt, K., & Jürgens, U. (2001). On the vocal expression of emotion. A multiparametric analysis of different states of aversion in the squirrel monkey. *Behaviour, 138*, 97-116.

Fischer, J., Hammerschmidt, K., Cheney, D. L., & Seyfarth, R. M. (2002). Acoustic features of male baboon loud calls: Influences of context, age, and individuality. *Journal of the Acoustical Society of America, 111*, 1465-1474.

Fischer, J., Hammerschmidt, K., & Todt, D. (1995). Factors affecting acoustic variation in Barbary macaque (*Macaca sylvanus*) disturbance calls. *Ethology, 101*, 51-66.

Frick, R. W. (1985). Communicating emotion: The role of prosodic features. *Psychological Bulletin, 97*, 412-429.

Frijda, N. H. (1986). *The emotions*. Cambridge, UK: Cambridge University Press.

Garvel, J. S., & Tocci, L. L. (1998). Setting the stage of universal hearing screening. In L. G. Spivak (Ed.), *Universal newborn hearing screening* (pp. 1-27). New York: Thieme.

Giblin, P. T. (1981). Affective development in children: An equilibrium model. *General Psychology Monographs, 103*, 3-30.

Gouzoules, S., Gouzoules, H., & Marler, P. (1984). Rhesus monkey (*Macaca mulatta*) screams: Representational signalling in the recruitment of agonistic aid. *Animal Behaviour, 32*, 193.

Hammerschmidt, K., & Fischer, J. (1998). The vocal repertoire of Barbary macaques: A quantitative analysis of a graded signal system. *Ethology, 104*, 203-216.

Hammerschmidt, K., & Fischer, J. (in press). Constraints in primate vocal production. In D. K. Oller & U. Griebel (Eds.), *The evolution of communicative creativity: From fixed signals to contextual flexibility*. Cambridge, MA: MIT Press.

Hammerschmidt, K. & Jürgens, U. (2007). Acoustical correlates of affective prosody. *Journal of Voice, 21*, 531-540.

Izard, C. E., Huebner, R. R., Risser, D., McGinnes, G. C., & Dougherty, L. M. (1980). The young infant's ability to express discrete emotion expressions. *Developmental Psychology, 16*, 132-140.

Izard, C. E., & Malatesta, C. (1987). Perspectives on emotional development: I. Differential emotions theory of early emotional development. In J. D. Osofsky (Ed.), *Handbook of infant development* (pp. 494-554). New York: Wiley.

Jürgens, U. (1979). Vocalization as an emotional indicator. A neuroethological study in the squirrel monkey. *Behaviour, 69,* 88-117.

Jürgens, U. (2003). Zum stimmlichen Ausdruck emotionaler Zustände. Eine vergleichend verhaltens- und neurobiologische Untersuchung. *Sprache Stimme Gehör, 27,* 71-74.

Keller, H., & Schölmerich, A. (1987). Infant vocalizations and parental reactions during the first 4 months of life. *Developmental Psychology, 23,* 62-67.

Kent, R. D., Osberger, M. J., Netsell, R., & Hustedde, C. G. (1987). Phonetic development in identical twins differing in auditory function. *Journal of Speech and Hearing Disorders, 52,* 64-75.

Kipper, S., & Todt, D. (2001). Variation of sound parameters affects the evaluation of human laughter. *Behaviour, 138,* 1161-1178.

Lazarus, R. S. (1991). *Emotion and adaptation.* New York: Oxford University Press.

Leinonen, L., Hiltunen, T., Linnankoski, I., & Laakso, M.-L. (1997). Expression of emotional-motivational connotations with a one-word utterance. *Journal of the Acoustical Society of America, 102,* 1853-1863.

Lewis, M. (1993). Self-conscious emotions: Embarrassment, pride, shame and guilt. In M. Lewis & J. M. Haviland (Eds.), *Handbook of emotions* (pp. 563-574). New York: The Guilford Press.

Locke, J. L. (1993). *The child's path to spoken language.* Cambridge, MA: Harvard University Press.

Maestripieri, D., & Call, J. (1996). Mother-infant communication in primates. *Advances in the Study of Behavior, 25,* 631-642.

Malatesta-Magai, C., Izard, C. E., & Camras, L. (1991). Conceptualizing early infant affect: Emotions as fact, fiction or artefact? In K. T. Strongman (Ed.), *International review of studies of emotion* (pp. 1-36). Chichester, UK: Wiley.

Möller, S., & Schönweiler, R. (1999). Analysis of infant cries for the early detection of hearing impairment. *Speech Communication, 28,* 175-193.

Muller, E., Hollien, H., & Murry, T. (1974). Perceptual responses to infant crying: Identification of cry types. *Journal of Child Language, 1,* 89-95.

Murai, J.-I. (1963). The sounds of infants. *Studia Phonologica, 3,* 17-43.

Murray, I. R., & Arnott, J. L. (1993). Toward the simulation of emotion in synthetic speech: A review of the literature on human vocal emotion. *Journal of the Acoustical Society of America, 93,* 1097-1108.

Murry, T., Hollien, H., & Muller, E. (1975). Perceptual responses to infant crying: Maternal recognition and sex judgements. *Journal of Child Language, 2,* 199-204.

Nakazima, S. (1962). A comparative study of the speech developments of Japanese and American English in childhood: 1. A comparison of the developments of voices at the prelinguistic period. *Studia Phonologica, 2,* 27-54.

Oller, D. K. (1978). Infant vocalization and the development of speech. *Allied Health and Behavioral Sciences, 1,* 523-549.

Oller, D. K. (1980). The emergence of the sounds of speech in infancy. In G. H. Yeni-Komshian, J. F. Kavanagh, & C. A. Ferguson (Eds.), *Child phonology* (pp. 93-112). New York: Academic Press.

Oller, D. K. (2000). *The emergence of the speech capacity.* Mahwah, NJ: Lawrence Erlbaum Associates.

Oller, D. K., Eilers, R. E., & Basinger, D. (2001). Intuitive identification of infant vocal sounds by parents. *Developmental Science, 4,* 49-60.

Oller, D. K., Eilers, R. E., Bull, D. H., & Carney, A. E. (1985). Prespeech vocalizations of a deaf infant: A comparison with normal metaphonological development. *Journal of Speech and Hearing Research, 28,* 47-63.

Papousek, M. (1994). *Vom ersten Schrei zum ersten Wort: Anfänge der Sprachentwicklung in der vorsprachlichen Kommunikation.* Bern, Switzerland: Verlag Hans Huber.

Papousek, M., & Papousek, H. (1981). Musical elements in the infant's vocalization: Their significance for communication, cognition and creativity. In L. P. Lipsitt (Ed.), *Advances in infant research* (pp. 163-224). New York: Ablex.

Porter, F. L., Miller, R. H., & Marshall, R. E. (1986). Neonatal pain cries: Effect of circumcision on acoustic features and perceived urgency. *Child Development, 57*, 790-802.

Protopapas, A., & Eimas, P. D. (1997). Perceptual differences in infant cries revealed by modifications of acoustic features. *Journal of the Acoustical Society of America, 102*, 3723-3734.

Ruiz-Miranda, C. R., Wells, S. A., Golden, R., & Seidensticker, J. (1998). Vocalizations and other behavioral responses of male cheetahs (*Acinonyx jubatus*) during experimental separation and reunion trials. *Zoo Biology, 17*, 1-16.

Scheiner, E., Hammerschmidt, K., Jürgens, U., & Zwirner, P. (2002). Acoustic analyses of developmental changes and emotional expression in the preverbal vocalizations of infants. *Journal of Voice, 16*, 509-529.

Scheiner, E., Hammerschmidt, K., Jürgens, U., & Zwirner, P. (2004). The influence of hearing impairment on the preverbal vocalizations of infants. *Folia Phoniatrica et Logopaedica, 56*, 27-40.

Scheiner, E., Hammerschmidt, K., Jürgens, U. & Zwirner, P. (2006). Vocal expression of emotions in normally hearing and hearing-impaired infants. *Journal of Voice, 20*, 585-604.

Scherer, K. R. (1979). Nonlinguistic vocal indicators of emotion and psychopathology. In C. E. Izard (Ed.), *Emotions in personality and psychopathology* (pp. 495-527). New York: Plenum.

Scherer, K. R. (1984). On the nature and function of emotion: A component process approach. In K. R. Scherer & P. Ekman (Eds.), *Approaches to emotion* (pp. 293-318). Hillsdale, NJ: Erlbaum.

Scherer, K. R. (1993). Neuroscience projections to current debates in emotion psychology. *Cognition and Emotion, 7*, 1-41.

Schrader, L., & Todt, D. (1998). Vocal quality is correlated with levels of stress hormones in domestic pigs. *Ethology, 104*, 859-876.

Sroufe, L. A. (1979). Socioemotional development. In J. D. Osofsky (Ed.), *Handbook of infant development* (pp. 462-518). New York: Wiley.

Stark, R. E. (1980). Stages of speech development in the first year of life. In G. H. Yeni-Komshian, J. F. Kavanagh, & C. A. Ferguson (Eds.), *Child phonology* (pp. 73-92). New York: Academic Press.

Stark, R. E. (1983). Phonatory development in young normally hearing and hearing-impaired children. In I. Hochberg (Ed.), *Speech of the hearing impaired: Research, training and personnel preparation* (pp. 251-266). Baltimore: University Park Press.

Stoel-Gammon, C. (1988). Prelinguistic vocalizations of hearing-impaired and normally hearing subjects: A comparison of consonantal inventories. *Journal of Speech and Hearing Disorders, 53*, 302-315.

Stoel-Gammon, C., & Otomo, K. (1986). Babbling development of hearing-impaired and normal hearing subjects. *Journal of Speech and Hearing Disorders, 51*, 33-41.

Strongman, K. T. (1996). *The psychology of emotion. Theories of emotion in perspective.* Chicester, UK: John Wiley & Sons.

Symmes, D., Newman, J. D., Talmage-Riggs, G., Katz, A., & Lieblich A. K.. (1979). Individuality and stability of isolation peeps in squirrel monkeys. *Animal Behaviour, 27*, 1142.

Tonkova-Yampol'skaya, R. V. (1969). Development of speech intonation in infants during the first two years of life. *Soviet Psychology, 7*, 48-54.

Van-Bezooyen, R. (1984). *Characteristics and recognizability of vocal expressions of emotion.* Dordrecht, Netherlands. Foris.

Wasz-Höckert, O., Lind, J., Vurenkoski, V., Patanen, T., & Valannen, E. (1968). *The infant cry. A spectrographic and auditory analysis.London, UK*: Spastics International Medical Publications.

Weary, D. M., & Fraser, D. (1995). Calling by domestic piglets: Reliable signals of need? *Animal Behaviour*, *50*, 1047-1055.

Williams, C. E. & Stevens, K. N. (1972). Emotions and speech: Some acoustical correlates. *Journal of the Acoustical Society of America*, *52*, 1238-1250.

Yoshinaga-Itano, C., Sedey, A. L., Coulter, D. K., & Mehl, A. L. (1999). Language of early- and later-identified children with hearing loss. *Pediatrics*, *102*, 1161-1171.

Zeskind, P. S., Sale, J., Maio, M. L., Huntington, L., & Weiseman, J. R. (1985). Adult perceptions of pain and hunger cries: A synchrony of arousal. *Child Development*, *56*, 549-554.

CHAPTER 13

The Vocal Dance of Seduction: From Being Anyone to Being Someone

Luigi Anolli

Seduction as a Sequential Interactive Game

In the mammal kingdom, courtship is a universal device aimed at mating and procreating offspring, in order to guarantee the survival of the species over time. In species where the females have a manifest estrus, courtship is a specific interactive routine that takes place only during this period. In contrast, in those species where the females have a latent (or cryptic) estrus, courtship is a behavior distributed over a longer period of time. Based on this difference, we may distinguish between courtship and seduction. The former is more tactical and of limited duration, with the specific aim of having sexual intercourse; the latter is a psychological strategy with the aim of creating and maintaining an intimate relationship over time.

Seduction may be defined as a strategic sequence of moves and countermoves, in which the primary target is to attract another person and create a fascinating and absorbing tie with him or her, with the ultimate objective of forming an intimate relationship. According to the biosocial model of Kendrick & Trost (1987), seductive interaction consists of a timed sequence of signals and behaviors, characterized by progressively increasing involvement, along a series of unfolding "steps" (Givens, 1978).

The starting point of the "seductive game" is the recognition and identification of a potential partner, based on appeal and attraction (first phase). The seducer then attempts to make contact with the partner by adopting specific and contingent strategies of exhibition to capture his or her interest (second phase). Subsequently, the seductive game progresses into mutual recognition and attraction, where the aim is to create an intimate relationship between the partners, via a gradual reduction of their degree of uncertainty (third phase). Recognition then develops through a relatively lengthy process of mutual appraisal, focused on the beliefs and disbeliefs system, affective sensitivity, emotional patterns, social competence, interests and values profiles, and so on, of the two partners. The outcome of this process is the definition of a common relational platform, with shared goals and ideals (fourth phase). Finally, the main outcome of seduction is that the partners continue to provide each other with a long-lasting bond (fifth phase). The whole sequence of the seductive process is shown in Figure 13-1.

In humans, gender stereotypes are most prominent with regard to the role played by social position and physical attractiveness in the seduction game. Women place a higher value on men's socioeconomic status, success, wealth, fame, and the like, than on their physical attractiveness. Conversely, men attribute a higher value to women's physical attractiveness, health, and youth than to their social status (Buss & Schmitt, 1993). Men are also more inclined to have multiple short-term mates, and are less discriminate in their selection than women (Buss, 1992). In contrast, women are more interested in lasting bonds and are more selective than men (Buss & Schmitt, 1993).

In folk psychology, the man is considered to be the initiator of seductive interaction, and the woman, the gatekeeper of sexual activity. In actual fact, the inverse seems more likely. In the early moments, during the attention getting (soliciting interest) and recognition (acknowledging interest) phases of seduction, the initial moves of making nonverbal contact are performed more frequently by females than by males (Moore, 1985). Females attract attention by displaying subtle nonverbal cues like primping (tidying their clothes without any noticeable necessity), coy smile (a smile fol-

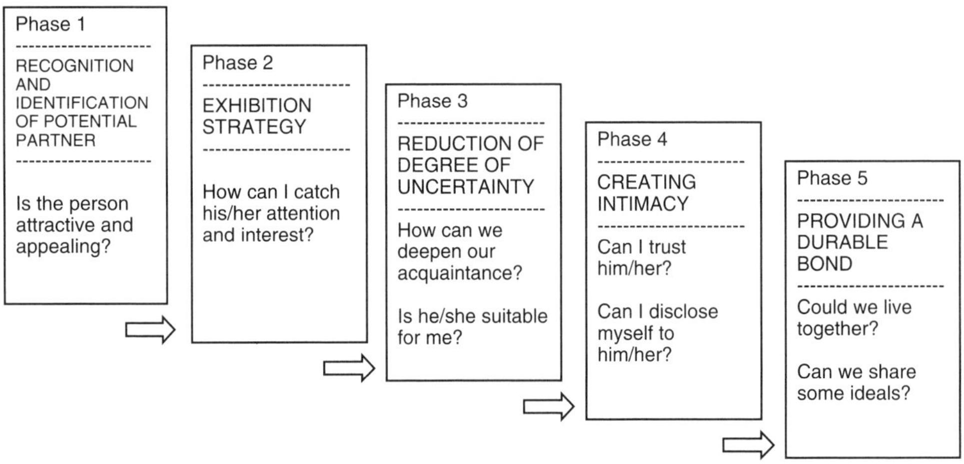

Figure 13–1. The sequence of seduction phases.

lowed immediately by turning away and lowering the head), looking "through" (looking at the other person, followed by immediate aversion of gaze), short glance (eye contact lasting under 3 seconds) (Eibl-Eibesfeldt, 1995; Grammer, Kruck, Juette, & Fink, 2000), as well as wearing revealing, sheer, or tight clothing (Grammer, Renninger, & Fischer, 2004). Such cues are very important, as males are hesitant to approach a female in the absence of any nonverbal signals of interest. It is likely that they make the first verbal conversation-initiation move with an unacquainted woman only if they have received suitable nonverbal cues from the female (Grammer et al., 2000).

The Exhibition Paradox in Seduction

In particular in the first two phases, seductive interaction is distinguished by a "dance" of mutual moves and countermoves that are stereotyped in a basic way by conventional standards, and that lay the basis for an approach between the two parties. Specifically, the seducer's first goal is to come out and "*change status*: from being anyone to being someone" (Baudrillard, 1979, p. 27). They must draw attention to themselves with the aim of being desired and chosen.

Seduction can be likened to an advertisement, a picture of oneself, or an electoral campaign. It entails an "appearance strategy," capable of combining information about oneself with skill in "sensual involvement" (Baudrillard, 1979). This type of exhibition is a powerful relational strategy because it requires direct involvement of the self. It encompasses a strong, albeit implicit, declaration of willingness to embark on an adventure, as well as the taking on of a commitment and relational responsibility towards the potential partner (Dindia, 2000). For this reason, the exhibition, being a global exposition of self, is associated with a condition of self-vulnerability.

Once contact between the partners has been initiated, the phase of mutual approach ensues. This experience may take different paths. As the Latin etymology of the verb *seducere* (composed of *sed* "separation" and *ducere* "to lead," which in German comes out as *Verführung*) suggests, the word *seduction* has taken on contrasting meanings throughout the centuries. One, basically negative, meaning is to "to lead astray" or "to deviate," therefore to trick the other person in some way. In literature, from the classical tragedies through romanticism, seduction was considered to be an inexorable force of fate, a trap that was capable of leading the individual onto the wrong path. In this scenario, the seducer was seen as a hunter, cold and Machiavellian in his or her tactics, while the seduced party was considered as prey and victim to his or her feelings. Another, quite different, meaning of seduction is "to be led along." He or she who is seduced is attracted and led quite simply somewhere else, into a totally private world. In this experience, the partners make one another feel of exclusive and absolute importance.

In both meanings, the idea of separation is prevalent. Attaining such an outcome is not a simple undertaking. A complex process of negotiation and accommodation is inevitably required, given the intrinsic asymmetry between the male and female partners for biological, psychological, and cultural reasons. On the one hand, exhibition is an imperative need, as without it, it is impossible to change status and signal one's interest to a potential partner; in order to seduce another, individuals must expose themselves and let themselves go. On the other hand, the "coming out" move is risky, as the seducer does not know whether his or she interest will be reciprocated by the other. Since he or she is deeply involved during the early stage of the seduction process, he or she cannot risk a plain refusal from the potential partner. If this were to occur, his or her self-image would be seriously damaged, with a consequent significant lowering of self-esteem. Therefore, the seductive exhibition should not exceed the limits given by social and cultural standards. Furthermore, it should not be so extreme as to intrude on the other's privacy and subjectivity (Anolli & Ciceri, 2002).

These conditions lead to the *exhibition paradox* in the seduction process. The signaling of interest should be clear without being explicit, detectable without being evident. The seducer should make his or her attention and attraction noticeable to the partner, while at the same time denying them. This requires the ability to say something without saying it, in order to leave the responsibility of interpreting the move to the potential partner. "Saying a little and intriguing, but not saying too much too explicitly" seems to be a winning tactic in this communicative process. In order to reach this target, it is very effective for the seducer to "dilute" statements and nonverbal cues.

It is a matter of degree and shading, as the seductive interaction swings constantly like a pendulum. If the signaling of interest is too weak, it may not reach the potential partner; conversely, if it too strong, it may be rejected. For this reason, nonverbal signals are called on very frequently in the playing out of the seductive process, as they are more ambiguous and fuzzy at semantic and relational levels. In the case of a refusal, the seducer may always think and say that the receiver was mistaken in his or her interpretation and mind reading.

Therefore, the exhibition is carried out within a relatively narrow psychological space that is defined, on the one hand, by the desire of attracting the potential partner and, on the other hand, by the need to respect freedom and privacy in order to obtain the object of desire. Any false move in this relational "corridor" could risk compromising the continuation of the seduction interaction in a serious, or even definitive, way.

In some circumstances, an effective indirect seduction strategy consists of putting on an exhibition of vulnerability in order to get the potential partner to lower his or her resistance, thereby increasing the degree of intimacy. In this strategy, the seducer displays submissive and somewhat childlike behavior in search of help and care. He or she conveys the need to be looked after, in a similar way to that found in the mother-child relationship. These signals of subordination and request for mothering by the seducer encourage the partner to approach and take care of the other (Hass, 1970).

Seduction, Deception, and Unpredictability

Generally, in Western culture, socially constructed gender stereotypes imply that men take the initiative in initial mixed-sex encounters more often than women (Bruch, Giordano, & Pearl, 1986).

Such stereotypes support the asymmetric investment theory, according to which women, having the higher investment in their offspring, have more to lose from making a poor choice of mate than do men (Trivers, 1972).

In the seductive game, both partners are compelled to enhance and stress their good qualities and strong points, as well as to conceal their defects and mask their limitations in order to be attractive. The goal is to become the other person's object of sexual desire. As an outcome, each partner tries during the courtship to appear better than he or she actually is. In fact, the communication of enticement has much in common with deceptive communication.

In particular, following the asymmetric investment hypothesis, women need to avoid male deception, which may be the outcome of male-male competition and female mate selection standards. As a matter of fact, men report that they try to deceive women with status symbols, whereas women are more likely to deceive by enhancing their physical appearance (Buss, 1992).

Men's deception is more often aimed at attaining a short-term sexual relationship, while women are more interested in learning and evaluating the men's mating intentions—whether short- or long-term. Usually, this evaluation takes place without male awareness. In consequence, men are likely to believe that it was them, rather than the women, who initiated and managed the seductive interaction. In reality, the inverse is more likely, as already stated.

Due to the conflict generated by simultaneous demands for advertising and deception, two potential partners who meet for the first time find themselves in a delicate situation. On the one hand, interest in the other person should be displayed to communicate approachability, whereas, on the other hand, overt signaling may generate suspicion in the potential partner of a higher likelihood of deception.

Within this framework, initial opposite-sex encounters are distinguished by ambiguity and implicitness, as both partners are inclined to hide their intentions and are aware of the need to reveal information about possible commitment in a gradual manner. Their intentions should be communicated without being openly revealed. Exhibition does not entail total exposition, so as to avoid the risk of a potential refusal. In this game, men are usually more inclined to perceive women in a sexualized way than vice versa (Abbey, Cozzarelli, McLaughlin, & Harnish, 1987). As a trend, men overestimate female sexual interest, while women underestimate male sexual interest (Edmonson & Conger, 1985).

A specific communicative strategy pursued in the opening phase of the seductive game consists of adopting unpredictable behavior. In standard conditions, humans, as well as animals, need to live in a predictable environment, where players can foresee the behavior and movements of other relevant conspecifics. Predictability is connected with a feeling of confidence in the reliability of their knowledge and with a sense of control over the environment. Conversely, unpredictability creates a high degree of uncertainty, and is therefore useful in detecting the concealed intentions of the potential partner.

However, the condition of uncertainty only applies in the early phases of the seductive interaction. If the partners choose to continue in their mutual interest, they must reduce uncertainty and disclose themselves to one another. The reduction of uncertainty is one of the most evident signals of mutual attraction and seduction. To reach this growing intimacy, the partners encourage each other to reveal themselves gradually through a progressive and selective exchange of information about personal history. This process of self-disclosure entails narrating one's life to the other. The sharing of mutual experiences enables a gradual reduction in the degree of uncertainty between the partners, and limits the risk of their becoming vulnerable too early in the seductive interaction (Derlega, Metts, Petronio, & Margulis, 1993; Dindia 1994).

Nonverbal Behavior in Seductive Interaction

Given its complex nature, seductive interaction is profoundly shaped by nonverbal communication. In general, human nonverbal behavior is a continuously changing process, composed of multisignal and multichannel units that are strictly context bound. In particular, it has a relational meaning, capable of defining, maintaining, and sustaining the relationship between partners.

Unlike persuasion, seduction has not only to convince the partner but also to attract him or her. Moreover, the seducer must be able to act in an implicit and intriguing way, because seduction requires an attentive and sensitive process of negotiation in approaching and attracting the other person. Nonverbal cues enable the seducer to invade the other's territory and, at the same time, to signal and reassure him or her that it is not an invasion. On the one hand, nonverbal communication must be effective in attracting the potential partner, and, on the other, it must foster the synchronization of mutual biopsychological rhythms.

Using an anecdotal approach, Argyle (1988) found different nonverbal signs of attraction and interest displayed by both potential partners during the first steps of seductive interaction: high level of mutual gaze, touch, general arousal, increase in body movements, smiling, erect and open body posture, proximity, and high pitch in voice. In particular, movements and gestures, especially when produced in rhythmical patterns, seem to function as advertisers and attractants.

Grammer (1990, 1992) identified a list of nonverbal cues by filming first encounters between opposite-sex strangers in a standardized laboratory setting. In addition to body movements, gazing appears to be closely related to mutual interest during the beginning of such encounters. The dilation of the pupils is a clear signal of attraction and a specific physiological cue of interest (Morris, 1997). In general, the greater the tendency to exchange glances and prolong the period of eye contact, the greater the likelihood that there will be a reduction in interpersonal distance between partners (Anolli & Ciceri, 2002).

Those who look more during interaction are perceived as attentive and interesting, and mutual gaze creates a feeling of mutual attraction and intimacy. In particular, females spend more time gazing than males (Fehr & Exline, 1987), and prefer males who look at them for longer periods (Kleinke, Bustos, Meeker, & Staneski, 1973). Moreover, they rely more heavily on visual feedback than do men (Cupach & Metts, 1994). Men also look more at females when interest has been enhanced (Kleck & Rubinstein, 1975).

It is worth pointing out that gaze may function as a cue of involvement in both sexes. Obviously, these behaviors change significantly according to the cultural framework. For instance, Japanese women gaze at their partner less often but for longer compared to German women. Also, mutual gaze lasts longer between Japanese than between German, partners (Grammer, Honda, Juette, & Schmitt, 1999).

Smile is another basic cue in seductive interaction. In particular, the disguised shy smile (the aforementioned coy smile) is a recurrent cue, used more often by women (Andersen, 1985; Coker & Burgoon, 1987). Smiling means proximity, accommodation, as well as availability. This nonverbal signal often occurs with nodding, which creates a sensation of attention and interest. In general, Eastern women, especially Japanese women, display a regular nodding movement in seductive interaction (Grammer et al., 1999).

Furthermore, in Western cultures, personal space reduction, leaning back or forward, crossing and uncrossing legs, and opening arms are further nonverbal cues that communicate interest and attraction by orienting the body toward the potential partner (Morris, 1971, 1997). [Incidentally, crossing legs is culturally forbidden for Japanese women as such behavior is considered to be obscene (Grammer et al., 1999)]. Similarly, when men feel engaged in the seductive process with a woman, they exhibit more space-maximization movements (e.g., stretching the arms, extending the legs), display open-body positions more frequently, and increase their automanipulatory behaviors (Buss, 1992; Renninger, Wade, & Grammer, 2004).

Interestingly, the meaning and relevance of such nonverbal signals in the seductive interaction increase when they are communicated in rhythmical patterns shared by both partners. Synchronization of movements seems to be an important factor of success in seduction, as it enhances the evaluation of satisfaction and mutual understanding (Grammer, Kruck, & Magnusson, 1998).

The Voice of Seduction

Perceptual Evaluation of Voice in Seductive Interaction

As is well known, voice plays a basic role in the seduction process. Already in Latin literature, P. Ovidius Naso (Ovid) in *Ars amatoria* speaks about the relevance of a soft voice in seduction. Within the scientific domain, the few studies carried out to date on the voice of seduction have been based on the subjective perception of voice during the seductive interaction (Berry, 1990; Givens, 1978; Köppel, Montagne-Miller, O'Hair, & Cody, 1993; Montepare & Zebrowitz-McArthur, 1987; Zuckerman, Hodgins, & Miyake, 1990).

In general, according to these studies, the voice of seduction is characterized by less power and more warmth, signaling the willingness of the parties to go on getting to know each other. Montepare and Zebrowitz-McArthur (1987) defined this vocal feature as "babyish." As regards gender, a seductive male voice is associated with strength and power, whereas a seductive female voice is characterized by warmth, affection, and kindness. To produce this kind of voice, the seducer increases pitch and lowers intensity in a similar way to adults when speaking to babies.

The vocal profile may be used to distinguish the nature of the ongoing interaction between interlocutors. During a friendly interaction, voice pitch is neutral, laughs are not frequent, and there are several silent pauses, whereas in the seductive process there is a noticeable increase in the number of laughs and hence interpersonal warmth, speech is more animated, and the number of silences decreases (Köppel et al., 1993). In an intimate relationship, voice pitch is low, speech is fluent, and there are fewer silent pauses and more laughs.

The aforementioned studies highlighted the relevance of the voice in the seductive game but were limited to the perceptual analysis of voice only. Moreover, they did not consider the temporal sequence of the progressive approach in creating an intimate relationship. In the research carried out by Anolli and Ciceri (2002), the suprasegmental features of the male voice during a seductive interaction were analyzed by comparison with the properties of neutral speech. Moreover, the suprasegmental differences between successful seducers (those who were able to arrange a subsequent date with the partner) and unsuccessful ones (those who failed in this target) were examined. The research concerned only the male voice, since in a Mediterranean culture, although the sex role of women has changed greatly over recent decades, women may still be reluctant to engage in seductive performance in a public (and experimental) situation.

The Experiment

The experiment was designed to simulate a first opposite-sex encounter between strangers. Forty university students (between the ages of 20 and 27) were recruited to take part. In a preliminary phase, it was ascertained that they were neither married nor engaged in a stable relationship. They also did not know each other. Participants then consented to participate in the experiment and were randomly paired off. The man was considered as the "seducer" and the woman as the "seducee." In the start phase, they were told that the experimental situation concerned the formation of the first impression of a person whom they had not previously known, as well as the initial process of mutual acquaintance.

The protocol for the research was in line with the Ethical Principles of Psychologists and Code of Conduct (12/01/92) of the American Psychological Association. It received official institutional approval. Informed consent was provided by all participants, who, at the end of the follow-up meeting, were fully debriefed on the nature and results of the research.

The experiment consisted of four phases. In the first phase (*observation and attractiveness evaluation*), a research assistant led the woman into a room for an informal conversation. The conversation was filmed without the awareness of the female participant, while her potential male partner observed it in real time on a monitor in another room. At the end of this phase, which lasted about 5 minutes, the man completed an assessment questionnaire (Questionnaire Interest, entitled only A to avoid bias). The assessment inventory consisted of seven items, including the woman's physical traits, her beauty, her voice, her way of moving, and her overall degree of attractiveness. These features are considered essential to arouse attraction in men (Grammer, 1990; Taylor, Hoy, & Haley, 1996). Each item was rated on a scale of 1 to 20. If the average score was 10 or more, the experiment proceeded; if not, the man and woman were dismissed.

Nineteen couples got through this phase, and went on with the experimental situation to the end.

In the second phase of the experiment (*meeting and seductive interaction*), the assistant gave the man the task of arranging a subsequent meeting with the woman. He was told he could use whatever seductive manner he thought would be most effective in reaching this aim. In the course of the interaction, the male participant was to say to the woman, "I would like to see you again" (target utterance). In this phase, the woman participant was still not aware of the goal of the experimental situation.

The man and woman participants were then brought together in a third room, where they had to carry out some activities suggested by the assistant via written notes. The activities were designed to progressively enhance their level of mutual interaction. First, they were invited to choose pictures that gave an account of some campus experiences; then they were asked to comment on photographs of film/TV stars taken from gossip magazines; finally, they were encouraged to talk about how young people spend their spare time, especially in the evening. During this conversation, the couple was alone. The interaction, which lasted for an average of 31 min 40 s (*SD* = 5 min 35 s), was fully recorded on an audio-recorder.

In the third phase of the experiment (*final feedback*), the male and female participants filled in the questionnaire Performance (called Questionnaire B) and the questionnaire Availability (called Questionnaire C), respectively. Questionnaire B, filled in by the man, consisted of 15 items to investigate possible changes in his evaluation of the woman's attractiveness during the interaction, as well as to ascertain the sequence of the seductive moves he had played (Givens, 1978; Kendrick & Trost, 1987). Questionnaire C, filled in by the woman, consisted of 15 items to assess her interest in the man with whom she had been paired and to verify her availability for a subsequent meeting (Dindia, 1994; Duck, 1998). At the end of this phase, participants were separately informed of the aim of the research, and asked for their consent.

The fourth phase (*follow-up*) took place about 1 month later when the assistant met separately with each participant to verify his or her recall of the experimental situation. During this conversation, the assistant was able to pick up information about which couples had actually met again after the experiment. Nine couples out of 19 had met again spontaneously, at least once during the 1-month follow-up period. The male participants from those couples that had freely met again were classified as "successful seducers," whereas the others were considered to have been "unsuccessful seducers."

From the digital recording of each man's speech a set of vocal data was extracted for acoustic analysis. The stream of speech was carefully edited to eliminate all acoustic signals such as sighs, coughs, laughs, as well as any noises (Walbott, 1984). Each data set was divided into (a) the baseline speech (extracted from the male speech during the first phase in a neutral situation), (b) the target utterance (the standard phrase, "I would like to see you again"), and (c) seductive speech (composed of three speech units corresponding to each of the three periods of the seductive interaction—Speech Unit A, the early initial period; Speech Unit B, the middle period; Speech Unit C, the final period—the mean duration for Unit A was 24.65 s, *SD*

= 3.66; for Unit B, M = 26.57 s, SD = 4.76; and for Unit C, M = 31.83, SD = 5.4).

Each vocal data set was analyzed with CSL (Computerized Speech Lab, model 4300 B, software version 5.X, Kay Elemetrics Corp.) for 11 acoustic parameters regarding time (rate of articulation), pitch (fundamental frequency, F_0), and energy (intensity in dB). For both pitch and energy, the mean, range (gamma +, gamma –), and standard deviation were calculated.

Furthermore, the vocal data were subjected to a participant-by-participant analysis, to determine the vocal profiles of the male seducers (Ekman, O'Sullivan, Friesen, & Scherer, 1991). This analysis only took into consideration variations between each individual participant's own speech samples. In this way, each participant effectively acted as statistical control for himself. Thus, different categories of participants were identified from the analysis of the variations from the respective baseline values. The analysis consisted of (a) quantification of the differential values of each participant (i.e., the differences between the raw values of the seductive speech units and the raw values of the baseline speech); (b) calculation of the differential threshold for the definition of the vocal profile categories (the differential threshold value was equal to or greater than twice the standard error); and (c) the definition of the vocal profile categories as "participants +" (those who had positive differences equal to or greater than twice the threshold value), "participants –" (those who had negative differences equal to or greater than twice the threshold value), or "participants =" (those who showed positive or negative differences lower than twice the standard error). Based on this analysis, several further categories were identified for the vocal profiles (high-pitched, low-pitched, variable, monotone, and intermediate voice for pitch; loud, soft, variable, stable, and intermediate voice for energy; fast, slow, and intermediate rate of articulation).

Main Vocal Features of Seduction

As general result, the voice of seduction in the standard utterance was characterized by a high modulate pitch (F_0 = 156.32), loud speech (dB = 58.23), and a fast rate of articulation (M = 8.97 syllables/s). Generally, when inviting the partner to meet him again, the potential seducer spoke at a higher pitch, higher intensity, and accelerated rate of articulation, compared to his standard speech.

More interestingly, the temporal disposition of the vocal profiles in three periods (beginning, middle, and end) of the experimental situation revealed the richness of vocal variations in the seductive behavior of the male participants. At the very beginning, most participants (57.89%) spoke in a higher voice than they did in baseline speech, whereas only a minority (15.79%) lowered the pitch. In any case, all participants tended to modulate their pitch in a variable way. Conversely, in the middle period, there was a drop in the percentage of participants who spoke at a high pitch (26.32%) compared to those who spoke at a low or intermediate pitch. During this period, the voice became more monotonous. In the final period, an increase in the trend shown in the middle period was observed: participants spoke to the partner with a low and monotone (whispered) pitch.

As regards voice intensity, initially most participants (52.63%) spoke at a high volume intensity with a loud and variable voice, whereas only a minority (21.05%) spoke in a low-intensity voice. In the middle period, the vocal condition was reversed and most participants (57.89%) spoke at a low volume, using a variable soft voice. In the last period, most of the participants spoke consistently at a lower volume.

With regard to speed (rate of articulation), in the first period only a very small minority (5.26%) spoke slowly, while most participants (94.74%) spoke at a medium or fast rate. In the middle period, there was an increase in the number of participants who spoke slowly (21.05%). Conversely, in the last period, the number of participants who spoke quickly increased (52.63%),

In sum, during the seductive interaction, the male partners produced a high level of vocal variations, as revealed by the participant-by-participant analysis. At the very beginning of the interaction, most of participants spoke louder and at a higher pitch than their standard. In the middle and at the end of the interaction, their voices became progressively lower and softer. Conversely, the rate of articulation increased constantly during the seductive process, even more so at the end.

The Voice of Successful and Unsuccessful Seducers

The follow-up data enabled the "efficacy" of the seductive strategies used by male participants during the experimental situation to be tested. On the basis of this efficacy, it was possible to distinguish between successful and unsuccessful seducers, as outlined above. As shown in Figure 13-2, the differences between the vocal cues employed by successful and unsuccessful seducers during the seductive interaction were general and marked.

As regards pitch, at the very beginning, most of the successful seducers spoke at a high pitch and none used a low pitch, whereas more than half of those unsuccessful spoke at a low or medium pitch. In the middle of the interaction, the percentage of successful seducers who spoke at a high pitch dropped compared with the previous period, while only 14.29% of them spoke at a low pitch. Conversely, more than 90% of the unsuccessful seducers spoke at a low or medium pitch in the middle of the interaction. This trend continued into the last period for the unsuccessful seducers, while the successful seducers changed their voice, lowering further their pitch.

As far as intensity is concerned, at the start of the interaction, successful seducers spoke in a loud voice, whereas only 41.67% of unsuccessful ones spoke loudly, and 25% spoke at a low volume. In the middle of the interaction, the successful seducers reduced the intensity of their voice (only 14.29% went on speaking in a loud voice, while 42.86% spoke in a soft voice). Among the unsuccessful seducers, a greater percentage lowered the volume of their voice in the middle of the interaction. In the last period, this trend was consolidated by the unsuccessful seducers (75% of them used a low-intensity voice), while the successful ones spoke at a medium intensity.

With regard to the rate of articulation, most of the successful seducers spoke quickly and none spoke slowly at the beginning of the interaction. Conversely, only one third of unsuccessful seducers spoke quickly. In the middle of the interaction, successful seducers markedly

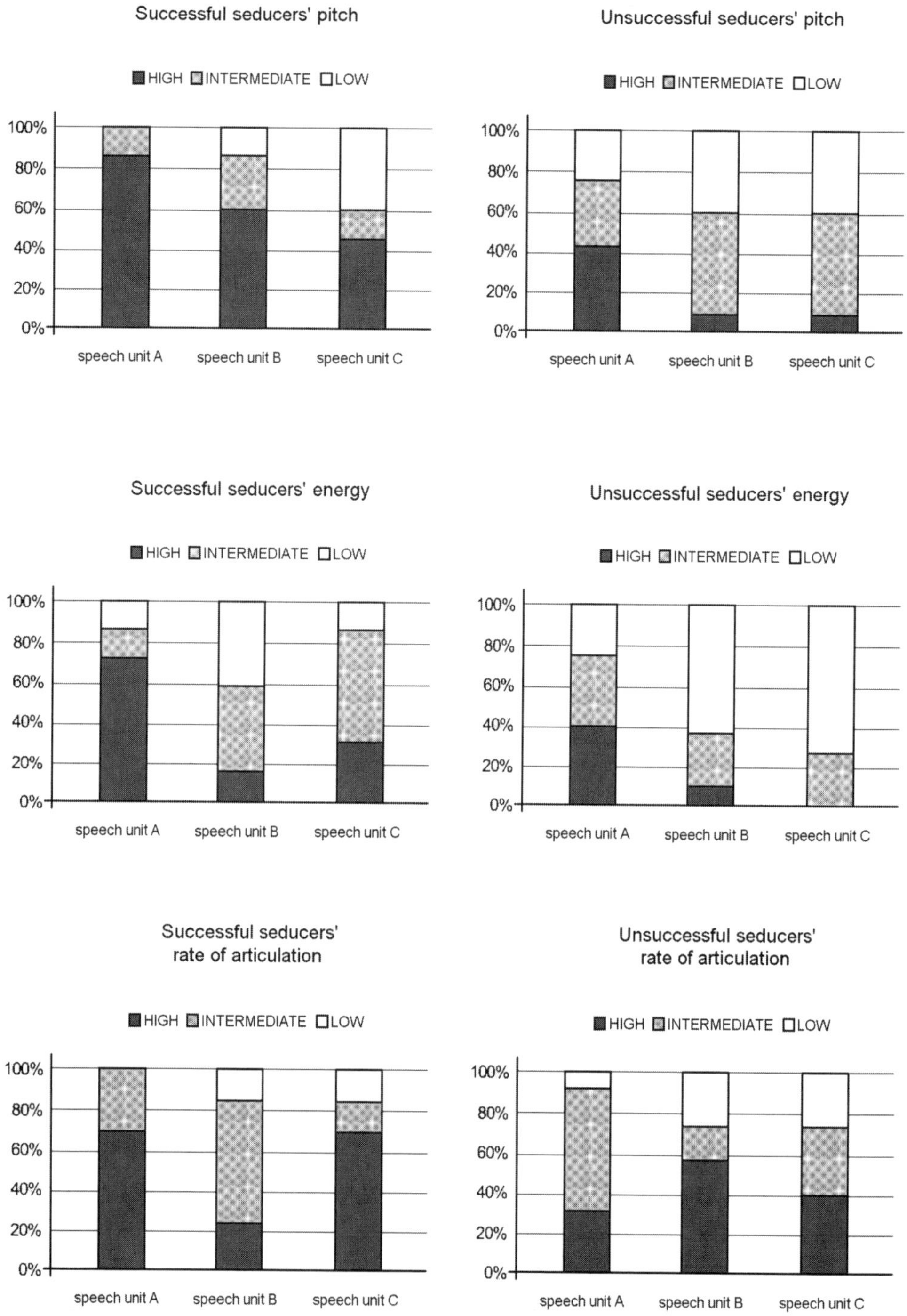

Figure 13–2. Comparison between successful and unsuccessful seducers' vocal patterns.

decreased their rate of articulation (only 28.57% continued speaking quickly), while the unsuccessful ones increased their rate of speech. At the end of the interaction, most of the successful seducers went back to speaking quickly, whereas the unsuccessful ones slowed their speech further.

In a nutshell, the vocal patterns of the successful seducers differed conspicuously from those of the unsuccessful ones, in pitch, intensity, and rate of articulation during the whole seductive interaction. The successful seducers displayed greater variability in their vocal patterns than did the unsuccessful ones.

Conclusions

Voice seems to be a basic device in communicating interest and attraction during the seductive interaction. The increase in mean pitch is reminiscent of childlike speech (so-called "babyish voice") that is evaluated as warmer and more intriguing, as well as a signal of willingness by the seducer to continue the relationship. Furthermore, the high intensity and the faster rate of speech are typical of a full and tense voice (Scherer, 1989), which is connected with a bright and interesting personality—someone who is strong and vital and emotionally involved in, and committed to, the task he is carrying out (Addington, 1968).

However, the voice of seduction is not a stereotypical pattern, as if there were a fixed and unchangeable vocal profile. Seducers use their voices in a flexible and suitable way through a wide range of vocal features. At the start, the potential seducer speaks mainly in a high-pitched voice with frequent modulations. Such an *orotund* voice may be effective in impressing the potential partner, as it suggests strength, vitality, virility, sociability, and confidence (Addington, 1968; Pittam, 1987; Scherer, 1978).

The *vocal orotundity* stresses the vocal exhibition, in order to create a favorable and attractive image of the seducer. This kind of voice is effective in the process of establishing contact with the potential partner. The aspiring seducer has to be noticed in order to be chosen. However, he or she must quickly change the vocal pattern. Should he persist in speaking at a high pitch and loud intensity, he or she could become boring or irritating, since his or her behavior may be interpreted as arrogant and domineering, or, on the contrary, as a manifestation of insecurity and weakness.

This quick and noticeable change requires the skill to switch to a different vocal register, by lowering pitch and weakening volume. This new vocal pattern, by displaying warmth, tenderness, and affability, reassures the potential partner as well as encouraging his or her feedback. The encounter may become more relaxed and cozy in an atmosphere of mutual intimacy.

In consequence, the voice of seduction undergoes many changes throughout the seductive process. This modularity and changeability enable the male partner to adjust his behavior moment by moment during the ongoing interaction with the potential partner. Given this contingent condition, some individuals are better than others at managing the different vocal registers in order to reach their goal.

Essentially, successful seducers display greater flexibility and variability in balancing their vocal patterns compared to unsuccessful ones. The former show more competence in local management of communication (O'Keefe & Lambert, 1995). They are able to choose the most effective vocal profile at a given moment, to optimize the emotional, cognitive, and relational resources available at that time, to process the hints offered by the partner, and turn them into opportunities. Conversely, the unsuccessful seducers show less variability during the seductive interaction. They speak in a flat voice, with a more limited range of oscillations and variations and typically characterized by a low pitch and weak intensity. This kind of voice tends to be associated with shy and depressed individuals, or with people who prefer to be ignored.

In sum, voice is a key manifestation of the self, able to reveal self-identity in a holographic way. It possesses not only structural features (like gender, age, health condition, and so on) but also functional ones associated with the individual's ideas, emotions, desires, and intentions. In seductive interactions, the voice seems to dance in a phantasmagorical way, swinging on the wave of feelings, ranging from high to low, strong to weak, harsh to smooth, in order to bring about disclosure of both self and the other.

References

Abbey, A., Cozzarelli, K., McLaughlin, K., & Harnish, R. (1987). The effects of clothing and dyad sex composition on perceptions of sexual intent: Do women and men evaluate these cues differently? *Journal of Applied Social Psychology, 17*, 108-126.

Addington, D. W. (1968). The relationship of selected vocal characteristics to personality perception. *Speech Monographs, 35*, 492-503.

Andersen, P. A. (1985). Nonverbal immediacy in interpersonal communication. In A. W. Siegman & S. Feldstein (Eds.), *Multichannel integrations of nonverbal behavior* (pp. 1-36). Hillsdale, NJ: Erlbaum.

Anolli, L., & Ciceri, R. (2002). Analysis of the vocal profiles of male seduction: From exhibition to self-disclosure. *The Journal of General Psychology, 129*, 149-169.

Argyle, M. (1988). *Bodily communication* (2nd ed.). London: Methuen.

Baudrillard, J. (1979). *De la seduction [About seduction]*. Paris: Colette.

Berry, D. S. (1990). Vocal attractiveness and vocal babyishness: Effects on stranger, self, and friend impression. *Journal of Nonverbal Behavior, 14*, 141-153.

Bruch, M. A., Giordano, S., & Pearl, L. (1986). Differences between fearful and self-conscious shy subtypes in background and adjustment. *Journal of Research in Personality, 20*, 172-186.

Buss, D. M. (1992). Mate preference mechanism: Consequences for partner choice and intrasexual competition. In L. Cosmides, J. Tooby, & J. Barkow (Eds.), *The adapted mind* (pp. 249-266). Oxford, UK: Oxford University Press.

Buss, D. M., & Schmitt, D. P. (1993). Sexual strategies theory: An evolutionary perspective on human mating. *Psychological Review, 100*(2), 204-232.

Coker, D. A., & Burgoon, J. K. (1987). The nature of conversational involvement and nonverbal encoding patterns. *Human Communication Research, 13*, 463-494.

Cupach, W., & Metts, S. (1994). *Facework*. Thousand Oaks, CA: Sage.

Derlega, V. J., Metts, S., Petronio, S., & Margulis, S. T. (1993). *Self-disclosure*. Thousand Oaks, CA: Sage.

Dindia, K. (1994). The intrapersonal-interpersonal dialectical process of self-disclosure. In S. Duck (Ed.), *Understanding relationship processes. IV: The dynamics of relationships* (pp. 27-57). Newbury Park, CA: Sage.

Dindia, K. (2000). Sex differences in self-disclosure, reciprocity of self-disclosure, and self-disclosure and liking: Three meta-analyses reviewed. In S. Petronio (Ed.), *Balancing the secrets of private disclosures* (pp. 21-35). Mahwah, NJ: Erlbaum.

Duck, S. (1998). *Human relationships*. Thousand Oaks, CA: Sage.

Edmonson, C., & Conger, J. (1985). The impact of mode of presentation on gender differences in social perception. *Sex Roles, 32*, 169-183.

Eibl-Eibesfeldt, I. (1995). *Die Biologie des menschlichen Verhaltens. [The biology of human behaviour]*. München, Germany: Piper.

Ekman, P., O'Sullivan, M., Friesen, W. V., & Scherer, K. R. (1991). Face, voice, and body in detecting deceit. *Journal of Nonverbal Behavior, 15*, 25-135.

Fehr, B. J., & Exline, R. V. (1987). Social visual interaction: A conceptual and literature review. In A. W. Siegman & S. Feldstein (Eds.), *Nonverbal behavior and communication* (pp. 225-326). Hillsdale, NJ: Erlbaum.

Givens, G. (1978). The non-verbal basis of sexual attraction: Flirtation, courtship, and seduction. *Psychiatry, 41*, 346-359.

Grammer, K. (1990). Strangers meet: Laughter and non-verbal signs of interest in opposite-sex encounters. *Journal of Nonverbal Behavior, 14*, 209-236.

Grammer, K. (1992). Human courtship behavior: Biological basis and cognitive processing. In A. E. Rasa, C. Vogel, & E. Voland (Eds.), *The socio-biology of sexual reproductive strategies* (pp. 147-169). London: Chapman & Hall.

Grammer, K., Honda, M., Juette, A., & Schmitt, A. (1999). Fuzziness of nonverbal courtship communication unblurred by motion energy detection. *Journal of Personality and Social Psychology, 77*, 487-508.

Grammer, K., Kruck, K., Juette, A., & Fink, B. (2000). Non-verbal behavior as courtship signals: The role of control and choice in selecting partners. *Evolution and Human Behavior, 21*, 371-390.

Grammer, K., Kruck, K., & Magnusson, M. (1998). The courtship dance: Patterns of non-verbal synchronization in opposite-sex encounters. *Journal of Nonverbal Behavior, 22*, 3-29.

Grammer, K., Renninger, L. A., & Fischer, B. (2004). Disco clothing, female sexual motivation, and relationship status: Is she dressed to impress? *Journal of Sex Research, 41*, 66-74.

Hass, H. (1970). *The human animal*. New York: Putnam's Sons.

Kendrick, D. T., & Trost M. R. (1987). A biosocial theory of heterosexual relationships. In K. Kelley (Ed.), *Females, males, and sexuality: Theories and research* (pp. 59-100). Albany, NY: State University of New York Press.

Kleck, R. E., & Rubinstein, S. (1975). Physical attractiveness, perceived attitude similarity, and interpersonal attraction in an opposite-sex encounter. *Journal of Personality and Social Psychology, 31*, 107-114.

Kleinke, C. L., Bustos, A. A., Meeker, F. B., & Staneski, R. A. (1973). Effects of self-attributed gaze in interpersonal evaluations between males and females. *Journal of Experimental Social Psychology, 9*, 154-163.

Köppel, L. B., Montagne-Miller, Y., O'Hair, D., & Cody, M. J. (1993). Friendly? Flirting? Wrong? In P. J. Kalbfleisch (Ed.), *Interpersonal communication: Evolving interpersonal relationships* (pp. 13-32). Hillsdale, NJ: Erlbaum.

Montepare, J. M., & Zebrowitz-McArthur, L. (1987). Perception of adults with childlike voices in two cultures. *Journal of Experimental Social Psychology, 23*, 331-349.

Moore, M. M. (1985). Non-verbal courtship patterns in women: Context and consequences. *Ethology and Sociobiology, 6*, 237-247.

Morris, D. (1971). *Intimate behaviour*. London: Cape.

Morris, D. (1997). *The human sexes: A natural history of man and woman*. London: Network Books.

O'Keefe, B. J., & Lambert, B. L. (1995). Managing the flow of ideas: A local management approach to message design. In B. R. Burleson (Ed.), *Communication year-*

book 18 (pp. 54-82). Thousand Oaks, CA: Sage.

Pittam, J. (1987). The long-term special measurement of voice quality as a social marker: A review. *Language and Speech, 30*, 1-12.

Renninger, L. A., Wade, T. J., & Grammer, K. (2004). Getting that female glance: Patterns and consequences of male nonverbal behavior in courtship contexts. *Evolution and Human Behavior, 25*, 416-431.

Scherer, K. R. (1978). Inference rules in personality attribution from voice quality: The loud voice of extroversion. *European Journal of Social Psychology, 8*, 467-487.

Scherer, K. R. (1989). Vocal correlates of emotional arousal and effective disturbance. In H. Wagner & A. Manstead (Eds.), *Handbook of social psychophysiology* (pp. 165-197). Chichester, UK: Wiley.

Taylor, R. E., Hoy, M. G., & Haley, E. (1996). How French advertising professionals develop creative strategy. *Journal of Advertising, 25*, 1-14.

Trivers, R. L. (1972). Parental investment and sexual selection. In B. Campbell (Ed.), *Sexual selection and the descent of man 1871-1971* (pp. 136-179). Chicago: Aldine.

Walbott, H. G. (1984). Audiovisual recording: Procedures, equipment and troubleshooting. In K. R. Scherer & P. Ekman (Eds.), *Approaches to emotion* (pp. 542-579). Hillsdale, NJ: Erlbaum.

Zuckerman, M., Hodgins, H. S., & Miyake, K. (1990). The vocal attractiveness stereotype: Replication and elaboration. *Journal of Nonverbal Behavior, 14*, 97-112.

CHAPTER 14

Vocal Indicators of Coping Style in Patients with Breast Cancer: A Pilot Study

Branka Zei Pollermann and Jürg Bernhard

Abstract

Coping styles are thought to be largely determined by the patient's emotional reactions to illness. Assessing such reactions is usually done via self-report questionnaires or by semistructured interviews evaluating the patients' mental adjustment to the disease (adaptive vs. maladaptive). As an alternative, more direct approach, a pilot study was conducted to assess the patients' coping styles as reflected in their oral communication. Voices of 10 breast cancer patients speaking spontaneously were analyzed acoustically. Their coping reactions were previously rated as adaptive versus maladaptive. Four samples of each patient's speech were acoustically analyzed and an index of vocally expressed emotional arousal was calculated for each voice sample. For three samples, the vocal arousal index (VAI) was consistently higher in cases with active/adaptive as opposed to passive/maladaptive coping style. In addition, a vocal differential index (VDI) representing the difference between the VAI of the highest and that of the lowest vocal arousal condition was calculated. With one exception, cases with adaptive coping style (median VDI = 53.8) had higher VDI scores than those with passive/maladaptive coping (median VDI = 21.3). In conclusion, the results show a strong tendency for the vocal arousal to be associated with the patients' coping style.

Theoretical Framework for Measuring Vocal Indicators of Coping Styles

The patient's way of coping with illness is of major importance for both psychosocial (e.g., well-being) and biomedical (e.g., compliance with treatment) aspects of the disease. Obrist (1981) described *passive coping* as a state of enduring a stressor without expending effort to act upon it, while *active coping* was defined as tonic readiness to act upon an event. This corresponds to the action readiness dimension of Cannon's emergency response (Cannon, 1929). Generally speaking, active coping styles are thought to be more appropriate for dealing with stressful events, while avoidant coping appears to be a psychological risk factor from a long-term perspective (Holahan & Moos, 1987).

An important determinant of coping reactions is the *feeling* of potency or control over the illness. The feeling of control, or lack of control, can induce cognitive-affective states of hopefulness or hopelessness (Ortony, Clore, & Collins, 1988, p. 132) and thus significantly influence the patients' coping reactions, which include both somatic and autonomic reactions. The latter can be induced by anticipated activity (Obrist, Webb, Sutterer, & Howard, 1970). ß-adrenergic sympathetic effects on the heart have been found to predominate during active rather than passive coping, particularly when environmental uncertainty and behavioral uncertainty are high (Bongard, 1995; Brener, 1987; Kelsey, 1991; Kelsey et al., 1999; Light & Obrist, 1980; Sherwood, Allen, Obrist, & Langer, 1986). Obrist (1981) also provided evidence regarding the role of parasympathetic physiological reactions in subjects with passive coping style.

As voice and speech production mechanisms (respiration, phonation, and articulation) are strongly influenced by the subjects' autonomic reactions, studying the patients' vocal expression appeared to be a more direct method of assessing the emotional factors associated with coping styles.

What Is Measured: The Voice of Full-Blown Emotions or the Voice of Affective Dimensions?

Research on vocal indicators of affective states has been dominated by designs based on the relations between acoustic features and semantic tasks of emotion labeling. Psychologists and speech scientists rely on the subjects' intuitive labeling of the states called "emotions," often in forced choice recognition tasks (Cowie & Douglas-Cowie, 1996; Kienast & Sendlmeier, 2000; Mozziconacci & Hermes, 1999; Pereira, 2000; Schröder, 2001; Yuan,

Shen, & Chen, 2002). This kind of research can be "contaminated" inherently as the word *emotion* is semantically treacherous, because its meaning shifts according to context. This point has often been made by scholars such as Mandler (1981; 1990; 1992), Ortony and Turner (1990), and Russell & Barrett (1999). As recently pointed out by Roddy Cowie, the word *emotion* has only too often been taken "to refer to entities—natural units that have distinct boundaries, and that can be counted" (Cowie & Cornelius, 2003).

In addition to the ambiguities inherent to intuitive categorizations of emotions, states of arousal often overlap with emotions proper. Research has studied various states involving arousal such as excitement, agitation, lethargy, or stress. The latter has become a subtopic in its own right (Murray, Baber, & South, 1996). Yet, it is not clear whether the arousal associated with what is commonly known as "stress" can be distinguished from the arousal associated with an emotional state such as fear or happiness.

Other conceptions of emotions are based on broad elementary affective dimensions. The latter approach dates back to Wilhelm Wundt (1874/1905). Subsequently, Osgood, Suci, and Tannenbaum's theory (1957) as well as other authors (Davitz, 1964; Mehrabian & Russel, 1974) suggested that affective reactions could be described in terms of two or three major bipolar dimensions (Bachorowski, 1999; Bachorowski & Owren, 1995; Davidson, 2000; Laukka, Juslin, & Bresin, 2005; Russell & Barrett, 1999), such as:

1. valence (displeasure—pleasure), i.e., how positively or negatively the situation is appraised,
2. arousal (sleepy—hyperactivated), i.e., the degree of physiological activation, and
3. potency/control (powerful—powerless), i.e., the degree of power or sense of control over the situation (Argyle & Crossland, 1987; Fecteau, Armony, Joanette, & Belin, 2005; Mehrabian & Russel, 1974; Osgood, May, & Miron, 1975).

In such an approach, emotion categories emerge as specific configurations in a two- or three-dimensional space. Intercultural research in emotion recognition from voice has shown that confusions are often made between emotions sharing the same degree of arousal (van Bezooijen, Otto, & Heenan, 1983). This led critics to suggest that judges' ability to infer emotion from the voice might be limited to basing inference systematically on perceived arousal (Pittam & Scherer, 1993; Scherer, 1979; 1986). It thus appears that vocal indicators of affective states are more closely tied with basic emotional dimensions than with an emotion per se. In Schröder's study of vocal outbursts (2000), an analysis of confusions among inferred emotions suggests two main dimensions: valence and arousal/activation. A vocal signature for a specific emotion thus remains elusive and the activation dimension often seems to dominate (Pittam, Gallois, & Callan, 1990). Activation dimension is of particular interest as it is related to the preparation for instrumental action (Frijda & Tcherkassof, 1997). In Frijda's model of emotion, action readiness (or action tendency) plays a central role. As we considered the "feeling" of potency as one of cognitive prerequisites for action readiness, our approach to studying emotional factors associated with coping styles was based on dimensional theories of affect (e.g., Lang, Greenwald, Bradley, & Hamm, 1993; Russell, 1980).

Vocal Indicators of Coping Style

While coping styles are usually assessed via self-report scales (Carver, 1997; Carver, Scheier, & Weintraub, 1989), we tried to use a more direct way of measuring, that is, via the acoustic indicators of emotional dimensions associated with the patients' coping style. Our focus was on vocal indicators of the potency and arousal dimensions of emotions. Based on evidence about the link between the coping style and autonomic reactions (Waldstein, Bachen, & Manuck, 1997), we then investigated their relation to voice production mechanisms. The impact of the autonomic component of emotional arousal on voice was first modeled by Williams and Stevens (1972) in terms of direct causal relationships between high (dominantly sympathetic) or low (dominantly parasympathetic) arousal states on the one hand, and voice intensity, vocal cord vibration, and timing of speech on the other.

We hypothesized that the degree of vocal expressiveness would be higher in subjects using active/adaptive coping style than in those with passive/maladaptive style. This hypothesis was rooted in the chain of links:

1. the cognitive state of confidence in one's own control (the potency dimension of emotion) of the situation induces
2. a certain degree of cortical and physiological arousal (both autonomic and somatic), which influence
3. the three systems involved in speech production: respiration, phonation, and articulation (Scherer & Zei, 1988), which in turn influence the
4. vocal characteristics of the person's verbal expression.

Design of the Pilot Study

Study Sample

This study included a sample of 10 patients with operable breast cancer who were randomized within 6 weeks after primary surgery into different adjuvant therapy trials conducted by the International Breast Cancer Study Group (IBCSG). The data reported here were collected within two psychosocial substudies. The patients came from three main language areas of Switzerland (Swiss German, Italian, and French) and were interviewed in their primary language. Their ages ranged between 34 and 68 years. All patients were informed about the studies and agreed to participate.

Interview Rating

The patients were interviewed in the hospital about 2 to 3 months after randomization. At that time, patients had to cope with their disease, surgery sequelae, and side effects of adjuvant therapy (Hürny et al., 1996). The interview was semistructured and it was adapted from an interview evaluating mental adjustment in patients with early breast cancer (Morris, Blake, & Buckley, 1985). It covered disease- and treatment-related topics ranging from the discovery of the node in the breast to the thoughts regarding the patient's future. The interviews lasted 40 to 60 minutes, and were conducted by trained interviewers.

The audio-taped interviews were "blindly" rated by two female psychologists with experience in caring for breast cancer patients. The rating consisted of predefined categories in a binary response format (e.g., hopefulness versus hopelessness) as listed in Table 14-1.

These categories were applied to all topics. At the end, the raters estimated the overall mental adjustment as "adaptive" or "maladaptive" based on the ratings of each of the five criteria (Table 14-1). The raters were trained on other cases and reached a moderate agreement on the overall mental adjustment with kappa = 0.47 (N = 32). The test-retest agreement within each rater over several months was kappa = 0.55 and 1, respectively. For this pilot study, we selected five cases with adaptive and five cases with maladaptive adjustment on which the two raters had complete agreement.

Voice Analyses

In experimental settings, voice analyses are typically done by computing the deviation of emotional speech patterns from a neutral or a baseline reference level (Schröder, Cowie, Douglas-Cowie, Westerdijk, & Gielen, (2001); Amir & Ron, 1998; Simonov, Frolov, & Ivanov, 1980). As we measured vocal expression in a natural setting, the baseline level was not available. We therefore established for each subject her own range of vocal reactions by screening the interview for a passage of perceptually high vocal and one of perceptually low vocal arousal. The semantic content of the verbal passages was not predefined, although it was more likely to find low vocal arousal in "footnote-type" of statements or descriptions of sad events. Vocal characteristics of these passages were used to outline the range of vocal reactions for each subject.

The final parts of the interview, where patients talked about coping with illness and about their future prospects, were excluded from the screening for perceptually high vs. low vocal arousal. We assumed that these parts would be closely related to the potency dimension of the patient's emotional reactions and to her mental adjustment. These passages were analyzed separately for their degree of vocal arousal. The duration of

Table 14–1. Rating criteria for adaptive versus maladaptive mental adjustment*

Tendencies toward	
Adaptive adjustment	**Maladaptive adjustment**
1. Hopefulness	Hopelessness
2. Active attitude toward disease and treatment	Passive attitude toward disease and treatment
3. Flexible coping style toward different problems of disease and treatment	Rigid coping style toward different problems of disease and treatment
4. Perceived good social support	No perceived social support
5. Conscious dealing with the malignancy and its implications	No conscious dealing with the malignancy and its implications

*Global summary rating based on ratings of each of the five criteria.

each voice sample varied between 30 and 60 seconds.

The screening and the analysis of vocal parameters were performed by two voice analysts independently. Neither had information on the results of the clinical ratings or on the patient characteristics.

Three categories of vocal parameters were measured:

1. fundamental frequency (mean F_0, F_0 range, F_0 sd);
2. acoustic energy expressed in pseudodecibel units computed from the raw signal (mean and voiced energy range);
3. speed of delivery expressed as the number of syllables uttered per second.

The acoustic variables were normalized by external reference values obtained from emotionally neutral speech samples Zei (1999). Each vocal parameter was thus expressed as a percentage of the respective reference value. All the acoustical analyses were done by means of Signalyze (Keller, 1994), a Macintosh platform software.

Data Transformations

Vocal Arousal Index (VAI)

Because of the trading relationships between vocal intensity, fundamental frequency, and timing (Lieberman, 1960), a *vocal arousal*[1] index (VAI) was created. It was computed as the averaged sum of normalized values of the parameters significantly related to vocal differentiation between low-arousal and high-arousal emotions (mean F_0, F_0max/min ratio, F_0 coefficient of variation, voiced energy range, rate of delivery) (Zei & Archinard, 2002). The *vocal arousal* index thus reflected an overall degree of vocally expressed emotional arousal. The VAI was calculated for each condition.

Vocal Differential Index

VAI was expected to be higher in samples of high emotional arousal compared with those of low emotional arousal. To measure such differentiation, we computed a vocal differential index (VDI), which represented the difference between the VAI of the perceptually highest and that of the perceptually lowest arousal condition. Our assumption was that vocal differential index would reflect the width of what we termed the subject's *emotional space*.

The Concept of Emotional Space

Based on evidence from research in normal vocal expression (Kaiser & Scherer, 1998) and that of affective disturbances (Porges, Doussard-Roosevelt, & Maiti, 1994), we hypothesized that high vs. low level of vocal variation could be related to high vs. low level of affective involvement. Andreasen and colleagues (Andreasen, Alpert, & Martz, 1981) demonstrated that affective flattening was reflected in speech in a diminished variance in both amplitude and fundamental frequency. Similar findings (Zei & Archinard, 2001) support the link between affective flat-

[1]By analogy to the concept of emotional arousal, the term *vocal arousal* is used to signify the amount of vocal activation resulting from emotional arousal.

tening and poor vocal expressiveness. We thus expected a narrow emotional space (low VDI) to be related to passive coping, that is, maladaptive mental adjustment, and a wide emotional space (high VDI) to be related to active coping, or adaptive mental adjustment.

Statistical Analysis

The exact Wilcoxon test was used to compare the VDI in the cases rated as adaptive with the VDI in the cases rated as maladaptive (two-sided test; StatXact, version 4). To check for consistency, the association between mental adjustment, vocal parameters, and the VAI was explored separately for each condition and illustrated by confidence intervals of the medians (Hodges & Lehmann, 1963).

Results

As shown in Figure 14–1, the (VAI) was consistently higher in cases with adaptive than in those with maladaptive adjustment. This was found for the following conditions: high arousal (90% CI of median = 108.3–129.6 vs. 91.6–119.4), topics of coping (90% CI of median = 85.6–129.6 vs. 84.5–104.9), and the topic of future (90% CI of median = 93.8–110.1 vs. 80.0–111.6). In four cases (Table 14–2: A, C, E, F), the perceptually high arousal condition was identical to that in the topics of *coping* or *future*.

The associations between the pitch parameters and mental adjustment were mostly consistent. Of particular interest is a bigger difference in pitch range between high and low arousal conditions

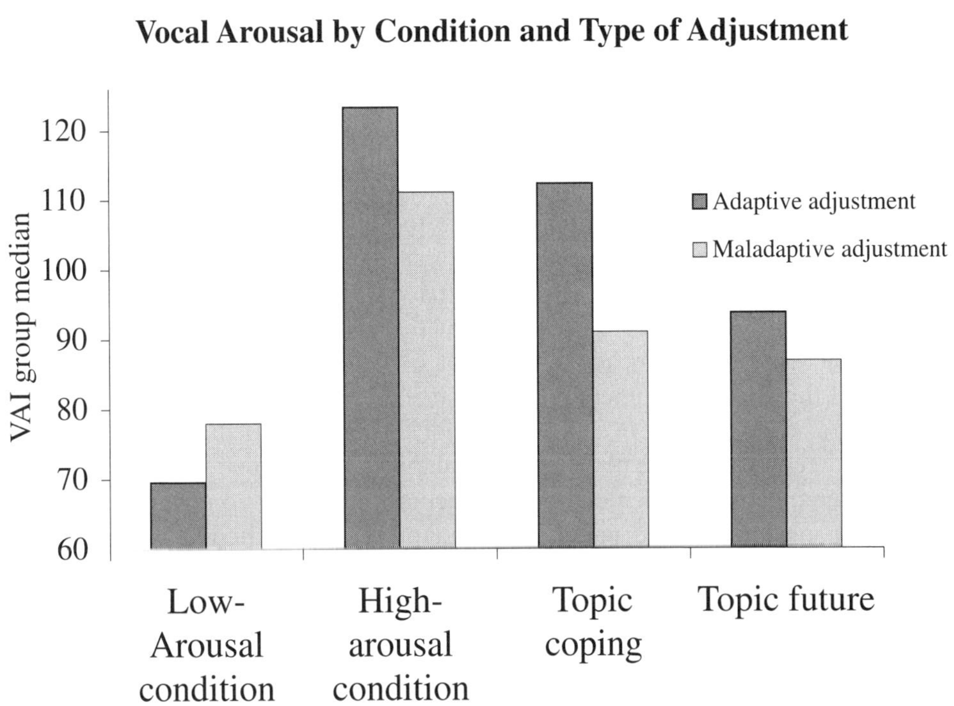

Figure 14–1. Median values of vocal arousal index per type of topic.

Table 14–2. Differential index according to adaptive versus maladaptive mental adjustment

Cases	Vocal differential index	Mean (SD)	Wilcoxon rank-sum test P
Adaptive mental adjustment			
A	64.5		
B	54.3		
C	53.8	49.7 (11.7)	
D	40.0		
E	35.7		0.095 (0.05)*
Maladaptive mental adjustment			
F	58.5 (42.6)*		
G	28.6		
H	24.3	28.5 (17.7)	
I	16.1		
K	15.2		

*Value obtained after correcting subsequent to unblinding the data.

in cases with adaptive (median = 55.2, 90% CI = 46.0–60.4) versus those with maladaptive adjustment (median = 35.2, 90% CI = 8.0–42.4).

Figures 14–2(a) and 14–2(b) illustrate the differences in emotional space and the position of the vocal parameters related to the topic of future.

One notices that the adaptive group is characterized by a wider emotional space. The position of the parameters related to the topic of future was considered as indicative of mental adjustment. It was hypothesized that a mid-position (reflecting a medium level of vocal arousal for this topic) would be associated with adaptive coping, while too low or too high arousal levels would reflect a maladaptive coping style. This hypothesis was conceptually linked to overestimation of threat and/or underestimation of own resources—states liable to produce underaroused or overaroused reactions. The graphs below show that in the adaptive group most of the parameters occupy a mid-position, while in the nonadaptive group their position is very close to either low or high limits of the *emotional space*. Figure 14–3 illustrates the group differences regarding the values for each vocal parameter across all topics.

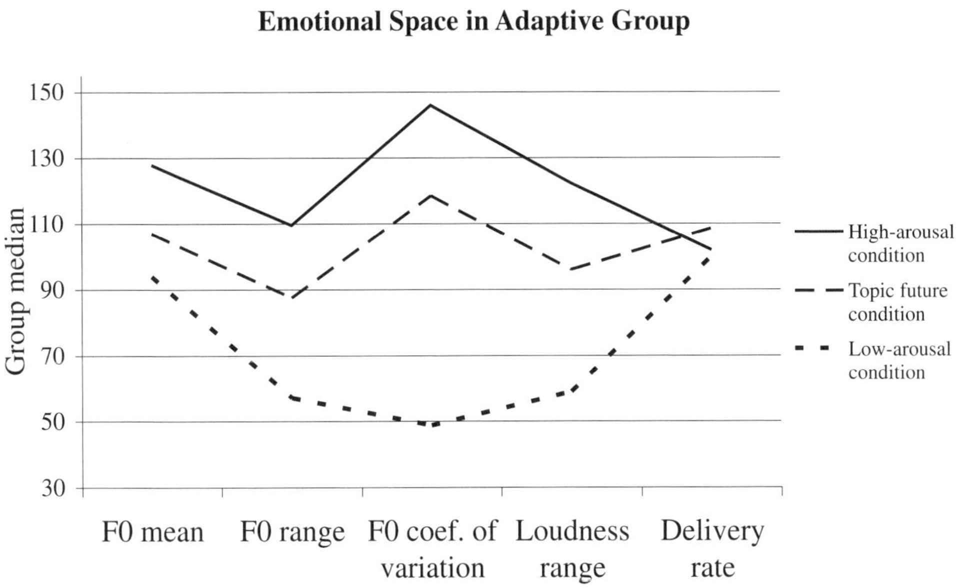

Figure 14–2(a). Emotional space delimited by the values related to low and high arousal conditions and the position of those related to the topic *future* for the group of adaptive cases.

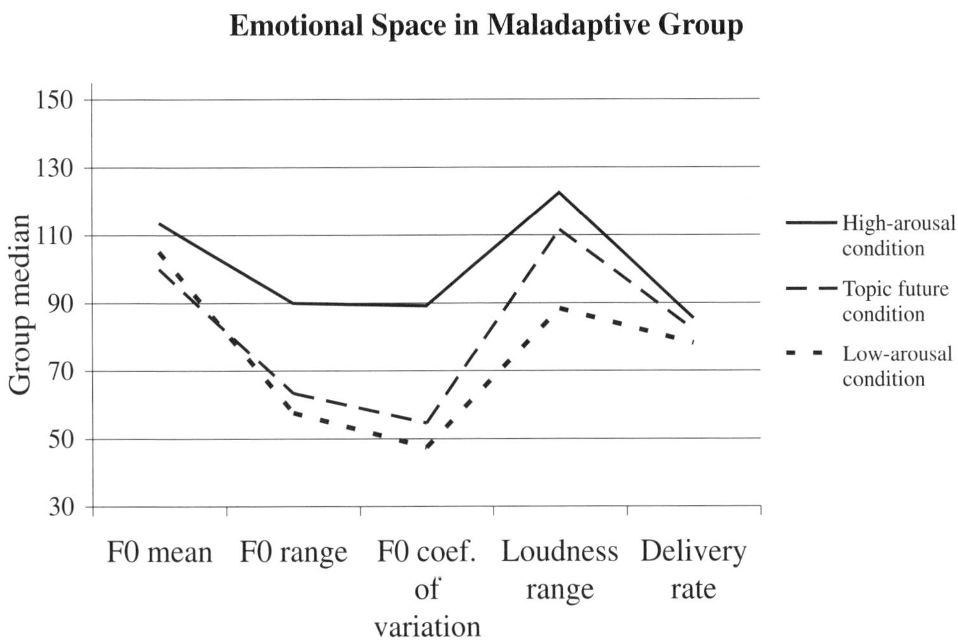

Figure 14–2(b). Emotional space delimited by the values related to low and high arousal conditions and the position of those related to the topic *future* for the group of maladaptive cases.

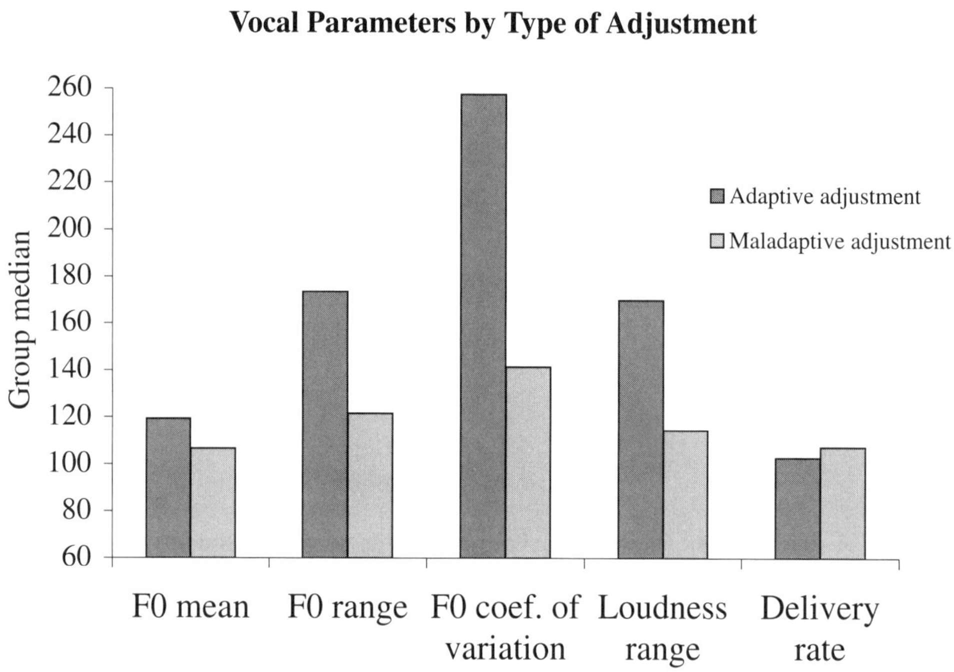

Figure 14–3. Vocal parameters pooled across all topics and displayed by condition (adaptive and maladaptive).

The ranking of the differential index scores is shown in Table 14–2. As expected, the cases whose mental adjustment was rated as adaptive had a higher score (median VDI = 53.8) than those with maladaptive adjustment (median VDI = 24.3; $p = .09$). The only exception was case F whose VDI was high. After unblinding the ratings of adjustment, this case was reinvestigated. We found an incorrect notification of the low arousal passage. A revised analysis resulted in a considerably lower differential index score for this case (VDI = 42.6) and significant result on the Wilcoxon test ($p < .05$).

Discussion

In this pilot study we investigated mental adjustment via vocal indicators of emotional reactions. We hypothesized that patients rated as having an adaptive mental adjustment would display active emotional involvement in their communicative behavior, which in turn would be reflected in a wider VDI. The vocal differential index represented a cumulative mean score of differences between the values of five vocal parameters (mean F_0, F_0 max/min, F_0 coefficient of variation, voiced energy range, rate of delivery) measured in the low arousal condition and those found in the high arousal condition. Prior to the creation of the VDI, each value was normalized by its respective external (emotionally neutral) reference value and expressed on a percentage scale. In our model, the VDI represented the subject's individual *emotional space*. A high VDI score was expected to reflect a wide *emotional space* with adaptive mental adjustment.

We hypothesized that a narrow space would be related to maladaptive mental adjustment.

We found that adaptive versus maladaptive adjustment to breast cancer as rated by clinicians was associated with both *vocal arousal* index and vocal differential index in the expected direction. We used dichotomous categories of adjustment to reduce variability and reach a sufficient agreement between the raters. Thus, the resulting judgment did not provide a grading as it is to be expected clinically. The vocal indices scores showed a plausible pattern, suggesting that this measure may reflect such grading.

The VDI as related to the *emotional space* is a concept with links to theories on emotions, mental adjustment, and mind-body interaction. Adaptive adjustment and the corresponding action are usually linked to higher and more dynamic emotional involvement and consequently to higher *vocal arousal* in speech communication. In patients with advanced breast cancer, self-reported emotional expression was associated with better adjustment (Classen, Koopman, Angell, & Spiegel, 1996). Indirect support for our hypothesis is given by two consistent findings in various chronic diseases. Patients with a generalized high appraisal of threat and those with a response of helplessness or hopelessness are particularly vulnerable, as shown for cancer patients in a longitudinal design (Parle, Jones, & Maguire, 1996). Both an overestimation of threat and an underestimation of own resources are characterized by generalizing the focus of concern and consequently by a poor differentiation between low and high arousal topics.

In our data, this differentiation was particularly reflected in pitch range. The substantially greater difference in this parameter between low and high arousal condition in cases with adaptive adjustment may be taken as an indication of "normal" emotional functioning (Zei & Archinard, 1998; Scherer & Zei, (1988).

Individuals characterized by active coping and internal locus of control usually exhibit higher cardiovascular arousal as compared to those with passive coping (Chevrie-Muller, Dodart, Seguir-Dermier, & Salomon, 1978), thus creating the conditions for sympathetically driven *vocal arousal*. In subjects with passive coping, Obrist (1981) provided evidence of cardiovascular reactions resulting from parasympathetic vagal activity. Scherer (1985) proposed a model relating sympathetic and parasympathetic autonomic reactions to mental adjustment potential and in turn to well-defined vocal characteristics.

We developed the vocal differential index as an indicator of mental adjustment in general and not for specific disorders such as depression for which vocal parameters have been established (Hargreaves, Starkweather, & Blacker, 1965; Helfrich, Standke, & Scherer, 1984; Scherer, 1979; 1987; 1989; Siegman & Boyle, 1993). This concept of a broad "bandwidth" is similar to that of the distress thermometer as proposed for the care of cancer patients (Holland, 2000; Roth et al., 1998). Capturing this vocal information may be a method to identify patients with poor adjustment, for example in monitoring psychiatric morbidity induced by experimental drugs or burdensome situations (e.g., bone marrow transplantation).

We used interviews taped for clinical ratings and not for voice analysis. The quality and standardization of the recordings were suboptimal. Our method is distinct from self- and observer-reported measures. In clinical settings, vocal information may be less influenced by interfering factors such as social desirability.

In a standardized setup a high reliability and responsiveness could be assumed. Given these features, the differential index may be an alternative measure of emotional functioning for studying mind-body interactions, for example with the immune or endocrine systems. Finally, in teaching clinicians on how to recognize psychological distress, nonverbal cues usually do not receive the attention deserved. Our method may be used to sensitize clinicians for the immense richness of vocal information.

Acknowledgments. We thank the patients, the interviewers (E. Lustenberger, M. Rabeus, I. Rousselle, U. Spek, H. Egli, G. Bianchi, and M. Tomamichel), and the raters (S. Fenyoe and S. Herzig) as well as R. Maître for acoustic analysis and M. Bacchi and S.-F. Hsu Schmitz for statistical advice. This study was funded by a grant provided by the Bernese Cancer League and Swiss Cancer Research.

We extend special thanks to Professor Krzysztof Izdebski for his constructive remarks in the elaboration of the manuscript.

References

Amir, N. & Ron, S. (1998): Towards an automatic classification of emotions in speech. Paper No 0199 presented at *ICSLP-98 (International Conference on Spoken Language Processing)*, November 30-December 4, Sidney, Australia

Andreasen, N. C., Alpert, M., & Martz, M. J. (1981). Acoustic analysis. *Archives of General Psychiatry, 38*, 281-285.

Argyle, M., & Crossland, J. (1987). The dimensions of positive emotions. *Journal of Social Psychology, 26*(Pt. 2), 127-137.

Bachorowski, J. A. (1999). Vocal expression and perception of emotion. *Current Directions in Psychological Science, 8*(2), 53-57.

Bachorowski, J. A., & Owren, M. J. (1995). Vocal expression of emotion: Acoustic properties of speech are associated with emotional intensity and context. *Psychological Science, 6*(4), 219-224.

Bongard, S. (1995). Mental effort during active and passive coping: A dual-task analysis. *Psychophysiology, 32*, 242-248.

Brener, J. (1987). Behavioural energetics: Some effects of uncertainty on the mobilization and distribution of energy. *Psychophysiology, 24*, 499-512.

Cannon, W. B. (1929). *Bodily changes in pain, hunger, fear and rage*. New York: Appelton.

Carver, C. S. (1997). You want to measure coping but your protocol's too long: Consider the Brief COPE. *International Journal of Behavioral Medicine, 4*(1), 92-100.

Carver, C. S., Scheier, M. F., & Weintraub, J. K. (1989). Assessing coping strategies: A theoretically based approach. *Journal of Personality and Social Psychology, 56*(2), 267-283.

Chevrie-Muller, C., Dodart, F., Seguir-Dermier, N., & Salomon, D. (1978). Étude des paramètres acoustiques de la parole au cours de la schizophrénie de l'adolescent. *Folia Phoniatrica, 23*, 401-428.

Classen, C., Koopman, C., Angell, K., & Spiegel, D. (1996). Coping styles associated with psychological adjustment to advanced breast cancer. *Health Psychology, 15*, 434-437.

Cowie, R., & Cornelius, R. R. (2003). Describing the emotional states that are expressed in speech. Special issue on speech and emotion [Special issue]. *Speech Communication, 40*(1-2), 5-32.

Cowie, R., & Douglas-Cowie, E. (1996, October). *Automatic statistical analysis of the signal and prosodic signs of emotion in speech.* Paper presented at the International Conference on Spoken Language Processing, Philadelphia.

Davidson, R. J. (2000). Affective style, psychopathology, and resilience: Brain mechanisms and plasticity. *American Psychologist, 55*, 1196-1214.

Davitz, J. R. (1964). Auditory correlates of vocal expression of emotional feeling. In J. R. Davitz (Ed.), *The communication of emotional meaning* (pp. 101-112). New York: McGraw-Hill.

Fecteau, S., Armony, J. L., Joanette, Y., & Belin, P. (2005). Judgment of emotional nonlinguistic vocalizations: Age-related difference. *Applied Neuropsychology, 12*(1), 40-48.

Frijda, N., & Tcherkassof, A. (1997). Facial expressions as modes of action readiness. In J. Russell & J. M. Fernandez-Dols (Eds.), *The psychology of facial expression* (pp. 78-102). Cambridge, UK: Cambridge University Press.

Hargreaves, W. A., Starkweather, J. A., & Blacker, K. H. (1965). Voice quality in depression. *Journal of Abnormal Psychology, 70*, 218-220.

Helfrich, H. R., Standke, R. & Scherer, K. R. (1984). Vocal indicators of psychoactive drug effects. *Speech Communication, 3*, 245-252.

Hodges, J. L., & Lehman, E. L. (1963). Estimates of location based on rank tests. *The Annals of Mathematical Statistics, 34*, 598-611.

Holahan, C. J., & Moos, R. H. (1987). Risk, resistance, and psychological distress: A longitudinal analysis with adults and children. *Journal of Abnormal Psychology, 96*, 3-13.

Holland, J. (2000). Psychosocial distress in the patient with cancer. Standards of care and treatment guidelines. *Oncology, 15*, 19-24.

Hürny, C., Bernhard, J., Coates, A. S., Castiglione Gertsch, M., Peterson, H. F., Gelber, R. D., et al. (1996). Impact of adjuvant therapy on quality of life in women with node- positive operable breast cancer. International Breast Cancer Study Group. *Lancet, 347*, 1279-1284.

Kaiser, S., & Scherer, K. (1998). Models of "normal" emotions applied to facial and vocal expressions in clinical disorders. In W. F. J. Flack & J. D. Laird (Eds.), *Emotions in psychopathology* (pp. 81-98). New York: Oxford University Press.

Keller, E. (1994). *Signal analysis for speech and sound*. Lausanne, Switzerland: Info Signal.

Kelsey, R. M. (1991). Electrodermal lability and myocardial reactivity to stress. *Psychophysiology, 28*(6), 619-631.

Kelsey, R. M., Blascovich, J., Tomaka, J., Leitten, C. L., Schneider, T. R., & Wiens, S. (1999). Cardiovascular reactivity and adaptation to recurrent psychological stress: Effects of prior task exposure. *Psychophysiology, 36*(6), 818-831.

Kienast, M., & Sendlmeier, W. F. (2000). Acoustical analysis of spectral and temporal changes in emotional speech. In R. Cowie, E. Douglas-Cowie, & M. Schröder (Eds.), *Proceedings of the ISCA workshop on speech and emotion* (pp. 92-98) [CD-ROM]. Belfast, Ireland: International Speech Communication Association.

Lang, P. J., Greenwald, M. K., Bradley, M. M., & Hamm, A. O. (1993). Looking at pictures: Affective, facial, visceral, and behavioral reactions. *Psychophysiology, 30*, 261-273.

Laukka, P., Juslin, P. N., & Bresin, R. (2005). A dimensional approach to vocal expression of emotion. *Cognition and Emotion, 19*(5), 633-653.

Lieberman, P. (1960). Some acoustic correlates of word stress in American English. *Journal of the Acoustical Society of America, 32*, 451-454.

Light, K. C., & Obrist, P. A. (1980). Cardiovascular response to stress: Effects of opportunity to avoid, shock experience, and performance feedback. *Psychophysiology, 17*(3), 243-252.

Mandler, G. (1981, August). *Affect, emotion, and other cognitive curiosities*. Paper presented at the Third Annual Meeting of the Cognitive Science Society, Berkley, CA.

Mandler, G. (1990). A constructivist theory of emotion. In N. S. Stein, B. L. Leventhal, & T. Trabasso (Eds.), *Psychological and biological approaches to emotion* (pp 21-43). Hillsdale, NJ: Lawrence Erlbaum Associates.

Mandler, G. (1992). Cognition and emotion: Extensions and clinical applications. In D. J. Stein & J. E. Young (Eds.), *Cognitive science and clinical disorders* (pp. 61-78). San Diego, CA: Academic Press.

Mehrabian, A., & Russel, J. (1974). *An approach to environmental psychology*. Cambridge, MA: MIT Press.

Morris, T., Blake, S., & Buckley, M. (1985). Development of a method for rating cognitive responses to a diagnosis of cancer. *Social Science & Medicine.*, *20*, 795-802.

Mozziconacci, S. J. L., & Hermes, D. J. (1999, August). *Role of intonation patterns in conveying emotion in speech*. Paper presented at the ICPhS 99, San Francisco.

Murray, I., Baber, C., & South, A. (1996). Towards a definition and working model of stress and its effects on speech. *Speech Communication*, *20*, 1-12.

Obrist, P. A. (1981). *Cardiovascular psychophysiology: A perspective*. New York: Plenum.

Obrist, P. A., Webb, R. A., Sutterer, J. R., & Howard, J. L. (1970). The cardiac somatic relationship: Some reformulations. *Psychophysiology*, *6*, 569-587.

Ortony, A., Clore, G. L., & Collins, A. (1988). *The cognitive structure of emotions.* New York: Cambridge University Press.

Ortony, A., & Turner, T. J. (1990). What's basic about basic emotions? *Psychological Review*, *97*, 315-331.

Osgood, C. H., May, W. H., & Miron, M. S. (1975). *Cross-cultural universals of affective meaning*. Urbana: University of Illinois Press.

Osgood, C. E., Suci, G. J., & Tannenbaum, P. H. (1957). *The measurement of meaning*. Urbana: University of Illinois Press.

Parle, M., Jones, B., & Maguire, P. (1996). Maladaptive coping and affective disorders among cancer patients. *Psychological Medicine 26*, 735-744.

Pereira, C. (2000). Dimensions of emotional meaning in speech. In *Proceedings of the ISCA workshop on Speech and Emotion*, September 5-7 (pp. 25-28). Newcastle, Northern Ireland.

Pittam, J., Gallois, C., & Callan, V. (1990). The long-term spectrum and perceived emotion. *Speech Communication*, *9*, 177-187.

Pittam, J., & Scherer, K. R. (1993). Vocal expression and communication of emotion. In M. Lewis & J. M. Haviland (Eds.), *Handbook of emotions* (pp. 185-197). New York: Guilford.

Porges, S. W., Doussard-Roosevelt, J. A., & Maiti, A. K. (1994). Vagal tone and the physiological regulation of emotion. *Monographs of the Society for Research in Child Development*, *59*, 167-186.

Roth, A. J., Kornblith, A. B., Batel, Copel, L., Peabody, E., Scher, H. I., et al. (1998). Rapid screening for psychologic distress in men with prostate carcinoma: A pilot study. *Cancer*, *82*, 1904-1908.

Russell, J. A. (1980). A circumplex model of affect. *Journal of Personality and Social Psychology*, *39*, 1161-1178.

Russell, J. A., & Barrett, L. F. (1999). Core affect, prototypical emotional episodes, and other things called emotion: Dissecting the elephant. *Journal of Personality and Social Psychology*, *76*, 805-819.

Scherer, K. R. (1979). Nonlinguistic vocal indicators of emotion and psychopathology. In C. E. Izard (Ed.), *Emotions in personality and psychopathology* (pp. 495-529). New York: Plenum Press.

Scherer, K. R. (1985). Vocal affect signaling: A comparative approach. In J. S. Rosenblatt, C. Beer, M. C. Busnel, & P. J. B. Slater (Eds.), *Advances in the study of behavior* (Vol. 15, pp. 189-244). New York: Academic Press.

Scherer, K. R. (1986). Vocal affect expression: A review and a model for future research. *Psychological Bulletin*, *99*(2), 143-165.

Scherer, K. R. (1987). Vocal assessment of affective disorder. In J. D. Maser (Ed.), *Depression and expressive behaviour* (pp. 57-83). Hillsdale NJ: Erlbaum.

Scherer, K. R. (1989). Vocal correlates of emotional arousal and affective disturbance. In H. Wagner & A. Manstead (Eds.), *Handbook of social psychophysiology* (pp. 165-197). New York: Wiley.

Scherer, K. R., & Zei, B. (1988). Vocal indicators of affective disorders. *Psychotherapy and Psychosomatics, 49*, 179-186.

Schröder, M. (2000). Experimental study of affect bursts. In R. Cowie, E. Douglas-Cowie, & M. Schröder (Eds.), *Proceedings of the ISCA workshop on speech and emotion* (pp. 132-135) [CD-ROM]. Belfast, Ireland: International Speech Communication Association.

Schröder, M., Cowie, R., Douglas-Cowie, E., Westerdijk, M. & Gielen, S. (2001). Acoustic correlates of emotion dimensions in view of speech synthesis. *Proceedings of Eurospeech 2001*, September 3-7 (Vol. 1, pp. 87-90). Aalborg, Denmark: International Speech Communication Association.

Sherwood, A., Allen, M. T., Obrist, P. A., & Langer, A. W. (1986). Evaluation of beta-adrenergic influences on cardiovascular and metabolic adjustments to physical and psychological stress. *Psychophysiology, 23*(1), 89-104.

Siegman, A. W., & Boyle, S. (1993). Voices of fear and anxiety and sadness and depression: The effects of speech rate and loudness on fear and anxiety and sadness and depression. *Journal of Abnormal Psychology, 102*, 430-437.

Simonov, P. V., Frolov, M. V., & Ivanov, E. A. (1980). Psychophysiological monitoring of operator's emotional stress in aviation and astronautics. *Aviation, Space, and Environmental Medicine, 51*, 46-49.

van Bezooijen, R., Otto, S. A., & Heenan, T. A. (1983). Recognition of vocal expressions of emotion: A three-nation study to identify universal characteristics. *Journal of Cross-Cultural Psychology, 14*, 387-406.

Waldstein, S. R., Bachen, E. A., & Manuck, S. B. (1997). Active coping and cardiovascular reactivity: A multiplicity of influences. *Psychosomatic Medicine, 59*(6), 620-625.

Williams, C. E., & Stevens, K. N. (1972). Emotions and speech: Some acoustical correlates. *Journal of the Acoustical Society of America, 52*, 1238-1250.

Wundt, W. (1905). *Grundzüge der physiologischen psychologie* [Fundamentals of physiological psychology, originally published 1874] (5th ed.). Leipzig, Germany: Engelmann.

Yuan, J., L. Shen, & F. Chen (2002). The acoustic realization of anger, fear, joy and sadness in Chinese. *Proceedings of ICSLP* (pp. 2025-2028). Denver, CO.

Zei, B., & M. Archinard (1998). La variabilité du rythme cardiaque et la différentiation prosodique des émotions, Actes des XXIèmes Journées d'Etudes sur la Parole. Martigny-Switzerland, IDIAP, 167-170.

Zei, B. (1999, April). *Acoustic patterns of emotions.* Paper presented at COST 258 (European Cooperation in the field of Scientific and Technical Research) Meeting on Improving the naturalness of synthetic speech, Morges, Switzerland.

Zei, B., & M.Archinard (2001). The role of autonomic balance in experiencing emotions. In A. Kaszniak (Ed.), *Emotions, qualia, and consciousness* (pp. 278-284). Singapore: World Scientific.

Zei, B., & Archinard, M. (2002). Acoustic patterns of emotions. In E. Keller, G. Bailly, A. Monagham, J. Terken & M. Huckvale (Eds.), *Improvements in speech synthesis* (pp. 237-245). Chichester: Wiley.

CHAPTER 15

Why Are We Attracted to Certain Voices?

Voice as an Evolved Medium for the Transmission of Psychological and Biological Information

Susan M. Hughes and Gordon G. Gallup, Jr.

Abstract

Our research has demonstrated that the sound of an individual's voice correlates with information that bears on his or her reproductive value (e.g., age, sex, bilateral symmetry, body configuration, sexual behavior). The research hence suggests that there appears to be neurological mechanisms in the human brain that evolved to decipher and distinguish between individual differences in voice attractiveness. The possible reason for our apparent ability to attend to these subtle affective/emotional features of the human voice, which serve as a medium for the transmission of such information, is explored here. Our work shows that people are enabled to distinguish and respond differentially to others based on the sound of their voice.

Introduction

Quite independent of the content of speech, the tonal features of the human voice convey a rich array of nonverbal information about the speaker. Consider, for instance, answering the telephone as a case in point. Even though you may not know or have ever met the person who is calling, as soon as he or she starts to talk, you can immediately tell if you are speaking to a male or a female, or to an adult or a child.

Voices contain much more embedded information than just gender and developmental status. Studies have shown that listeners who hear voice samples can accurately infer the speaker's race (Lass, Tecca, Mancuso, & Black, 1979), gender (Lass, Hughes, Bowyer, Waters, & Bourne, 1976), socioeconomic status (Ellis, 1967; Harms, 1963), personality traits (Addington, 1968; Allport & Cantril, 1934; Zuckerman & Driver, 1989), and emotional and mental state attributes related to deception (Ekman, Friesen, & Scherer, 1976; Streeter, Krauss, Geller, Olson, & Apple, 1977). Listeners are also capable of estimating the age, height, and weight of speakers with the same degree of accuracy achieved by examining photographs (Krauss, Freyberg, & Morsella, 2002; Lass & Colt, 1980; Lass & Davis, 1976). Independent raters are capable of matching a speaker's voice with the person's photograph over 75% of the time (Krauss et al., 2002). Furthermore, there is evidence that the sound of an individual's voice is an external attribute that is used as a cue for assessing potential mates and plays an important role in interpersonal attraction (Miyake & Zuckerman, 1993; Oguchi & Kikuchi, 1997).

Voice Attractiveness

What makes some voices sound more attractive than others? There have been a variety of investigations on this matter using acoustic and sound spectrographic analyses, but, as yet, no one has been able to identify or agree on all of the physical properties that distinguish attractive from unattractive voices. For instance, with regards to pitch, Daniel and McCabe (1992) found that both sexes rate mid-pitch voices as being the "most sexy," whereas Oguchi and Kikuchi (1997) found that both sexes evaluated a low-toned voice with a small pitch range as attractive, but the exact opposite was shown by Oksenberg, Coleman, and Cannell (1986), where a higher pitch with greater variation was associated with voice attractiveness.

Whatever the underlying tonal/acoustic features may be that constitute attractive voices, there is high inter-rater reliability (i.e., consensus) with regards to which voices sound attractive (Hughes, Dispenza, & Gallup, 2004; Hughes, Harrison, & Gallup, 2002; Zuckerman & Driver, 1989; Zuckerman, Hodgins, & Miyake, 1990). Not only do people tend to agree about which voices are attractive, they are usually capable of making this decision as soon as they hear a person begin to talk. In addition, individuals rate the attractiveness of same-sex and opposite-sex voices with the same degree of consensus (Addington, 1968; Hughes et al., 2002).

Vocal attractiveness appears to exert an influence on mate selection, and individuals with voices that sound attractive are perceived as having more desirable personality characteristics (Zuckerman & Driver, 1989). Individuals with attractive voices are thought to be warmer, more likable, honest, dominant, and more likely to achieve (Berry, 1990; Zuckerman & Driver, 1989). Thus, a "vocal attractiveness stereotype" appears to exist (Zuckerman & Driver, 1989; Zuckerman et al., 1990). Furthermore, the higher the rating of vocal attractiveness, the more similar the speaker is judged to be to like the listener and the more the listener would like to affiliate with the speaker (Miyake & Zuckerman, 1993). Favorable impressions of speakers with attractive voices have been obtained under conditions where observers only heard the speaker's voice, as well as when they both saw and heard the speaker (Miyake & Zuckerman, 1993).

There is evidence suggesting that reliable impressions of other personality attributes can also be inferred on the basis of the sound of a person's voice (Allport & Cantril, 1934; Berry, 1990; Zuckerman & Driver, 1989). Addington (1968) found that when making inferences about personality based upon vocal samples, the average inter-rater reliability coefficient was a .81 across 40 measured personality traits. When listeners form an impression of the speaker's personality traits, they are influenced more by the speaker's tone of voice than by the content of the speech (Yogo, Ando, Hashi, Tsutsui, & Yamada, 2000). Furthermore, the effects of manipulating a single vocal sample by changing the rate, mean, and variance of fundamental frequency all showed a corresponding change in personality ratings (Brown, Strong, & Rencher, 1974).

Most studies that investigate vocal attractiveness use voice samples that are neutral (such as a standardized sentence, word count, or vowel recitation) and attempt to control for such things as content, speech patterns, dialect, accents, visual information, intonations, and inflections (Collins & Missing, 2003; Daniel & McCabe, 1992; Hughes et al., 2002; Hughes et al., 2004; Zuckerman, et al., 1990; Zuckerman & Miyake, 1993). But in certain contexts, it can be argued that it is possible that individuals modify their vocal patterns in order to persuade, seduce, or influence potential mates. For example, there is evidence showing that males' vocal style in seductive speech produces a profile that differs significantly from the one used in normal speech (Anolli & Ciceri, 2002). On the other hand, the sound of a person's voice can only be manipulated within limits, and much of the variance in vocal quality is undoubtedly influenced by one's biology and genetic makeup. (To learn more about vocal attractiveness, see Chapter 2 in Volume 1: Editor.)

Voice and Physical Features

A person's voice not only conveys psychological information about that person, but it can also reveal information about one's basic biological features. For instance, both height and weight can be inferred from a person's voice with the same degree of accuracy as viewing a photograph (Krauss et al., 2002; Lass & Colt, 1980; Lass & Davis, 1976).

There are also several studies showing that ratings of voice attractiveness predict certain physical features. For instance, we have shown that voice attractiveness is related to bilateral symmetry. Individuals who possess symmetrical bilateral traits (such features as length of the fingers, hand widths, etc.) tend to have voices that are rated as more attractive (Hughes et al., 2002). Bilateral symmetry is a feature that reflects heritable fitness and is an indicator of genetic quality (Thornhill & Møller, 1997). Measures of symmetry across several morphological traits can be used to quantify deviations (that occur during ontogeny) from our genetic blueprint of having perfectly symmetrical bilateral traits. Therefore, symmetry is considered a measure of developmental stability. Moreover, these particular findings that relate voice and symmetry in humans are consistent with the animal literature in showing that, in some species (e.g., jungle fowl, *Gallus gallus*), symmetric males tend to have more attractive mating calls (Furlow, Kimball, & Marshall, 1998).

Another marker of prenatal development, the ratio of the length of the second digit (the index finger) to the fourth digit (the ring finger), also known as the 2D:4D ratio, appears to be related to certain vocal features. Research has shown that digit ratios are influenced by prenatal exposure to sex steroids. The 2D:4D ratio is negatively correlated with exposure to prenatal testosterone and positively correlated to prenatal estrogen (Manning, Scutt, Wilson, & Lewis-Jones, 1998; Manning et al., 2000). Although 2D:4D is not directly related to voice attractiveness, females with low 2D:4D, who therefore have had a greater exposure to prenatal androgen, have voices that are rated as more dominant and mature (Hughes, Pastizzo, & Gallup, 2008). Therefore, voice appears to be influenced by organizational effects of hormones during prenatal development. Indeed, the development of the voice box and larynx and the exposure to sex hormones, which shape the brain and genital anatomy, both occur during the first trimester of pregnancy (Moore, 1977).

Voices are not only subject to the organizational effect of hormones, but they appear to be even more influenced by short-term, activational effects of hormones seen during puberty. For instance, it is well known that voices are shaped and modified by testosterone for males and estrogen and progesterone for females at puberty (J. Abitbol, P. Abitbol, & B. Abitbol, 1999). It has been shown that tonal features of women's voices change during menarche/puberty (Abitbol et al., 1999; Hagg & Taranger, 2003), across the menstrual cycle, especially at ovulation (Amir & Biron-Shental, 2004; Higgins & Saxman, 1989), in women experiencing menopause (Amir & Biron-Shental, 2004; Schneider, van Trotsenburg, Hanke, Bigenzahn, & Huber, 2004), during pregnancy (Seemann, 1930), and in women taking oral contraceptives (Amir, Kishon-Rabin, & Muchnik, 2002). In addition, female preferences for male voices also appear to change across the menstrual cycle. Women who are in their fertile phase, prefer males with lower pitched voices as short-term mates (Puts, 2005).

The same sex hormones that modify vocal development during adolescence also contribute to the differences seen between males and females with regards to changes in body configurations that occur at puberty (Abitbol et al., 1999; Dijkstra & Buunk, 2001; Hughes et al., 2004; Singh, 1993). For instance, female waist-to-hip ratio (WHR) becomes more accentuated (lower) during puberty, and WHR is an indicator of a female's hormonal profile (increased estrogen) and reproductive status (Singh, 1993). Women with a low (WHR), whereby the waist is noticeably narrower than their hips (what is commonly referred to as an hourglass figure), are typically perceived as being more physically and sexually attractive (Singh, 1993). From an evolutionary perspective, a narrow waist and broad hips signal two things to a potential mate: (a) the female is not currently pregnant and (b) her hip morphology may provide for relatively unencumbered childbirth (Hughes et al., 2004).

For males, broad shoulders and narrow hips seem to be an important corollary body configuration that signals high levels of testosterone (Kasperk, et al., 1997) and is seen as an attractive male trait (Dijkstra & Buunk, 2001). During puberty the male's shoulders broaden, increasing his shoulder-to-hip ratio (SHR). SHR correlates positively with beta-lipoproteins, hormones that are related to testosterone and muscle development (Evans, 1972), and higher androgen levels in males contribute to the development of sex-related differences in skeletal morphology and muscle mass at puberty (Kasperk et al., 1997). Consistent with evolutionary theory, both WHR and SHR appear to have an impact on mate selection. We found that females with attractive, low waist-to-hip ratios and males with high shoulder-to-hip ratios had significantly more sexual experience and began having sex at an earlier age (Hughes & Gallup, 2003; Hughes et al., 2004).

Voice attractiveness is related to both of these sex-specific differences in the body configuration of men and women (Hughes et al., 2004). Females with attractive voices tended to have a more accentuated/attractive hourglass figure, whereas males with attractive voices tended to have broad shoulders and narrow hips (Hughes et al., 2004). The reason voice attractiveness and body configuration are related may be due to the fact that both are being influenced by sex hormones at the advent of puberty; there may be a fairly direct hormonal link between these features.

Another explanation as to why voice and physical features (such as digit ratios and bilateral symmetry) are related involves sexual selection pressure. The tonal features of voice may be a medium for the transmission of cues that signal biologically important information. In other words, one might expect to find selection for mate preferences based on traits that correlate with fitness (Thornhill & Gangestad, 1999) and voice may have been a salient marker of underlying genetic quality and viability as it relates to mate choice (Hughes et al., 2002; Hughes et al., 2004). Vocal cues are especially important because they can provide information about potential mates when visual cues are ambiguous or not available, such as during the night before the advent of artificial illumination.

Voice and Sexual Behavior

Individual differences in voice attractiveness are also related to sexual behavior. We discovered that both men and women with voices rated as attractive experienced first sexual intercourse at an earlier age, had more sexual partners, and were more likely to commit infidelity (Hughes et al., 2004). Indeed, we found a particularly striking relationship between voice attractiveness and promiscuity among females. The correlation between opposite sex ratings of voice attractiveness and number of sex partners for women was +.49, which means that individual variation in the perceived attractiveness of women's voices accounts for almost 25% of the variation in their overall level of promiscuity. The same effect holds for males, but it is not as robust. The ratings of male voices by females account for about 13% of the individual differences in male promiscuity.

The fact that favorable psychological attributes are associated with attractive voices (the vocal attractiveness stereotype) may promote sexual opportunities. In addition, Collins and Missing (2003) found that vocal and visual attractiveness are related in women, while Hughes et al. (2004) showed that voice attractiveness is related to attractive, sex-specific body configurations. Therefore, individuals with attractive voices may also appear physically attractive, and this may promote more sexual opportunities, as well. Similarly, the sex hormones that influence the voice at puberty may also exert an influence on sexual drive/libido and may lead to a greater motivation to access sexual partners. (More on voice and sexual behavior can be found in Chapter 1, Volume 1)

Conclusion

Because the sound of an individual's voice is correlated with important information that bears on their reproductive value (e.g., age, sex, bilateral symmetry, body configuration, sexual behavior), there appear to be neurological mechanisms in the human brain that evolved to decipher and distinguish between individual differences in voice attractiveness. These subtle affective/emotional features of voice, which serve as a medium for the transmission of such information, may have been especially important prior to the invention of sources of artificial illumination, thus enabling people at night to distinguish and respond differentially to others based on the sound of their voices.

References

Abitbol, J., Abitbol, P., & Abitbol, B. (1999). Sex hormones and the female voice. *Journal of Voice*, *13*, 424-446.

Addington, D. (1968). The relationship of selected vocal characteristics to personality perception. *Speech Monographs*, *35*, 492-503.

Allport, G. W., & Cantril, H. (1934). Judging personality from voice. *Journal of Social Psychology*, *5*, 37-55.

Amir, O., & Biron-Shental, T. (2004). The impact of hormonal fluctuations on female vocal folds. *Current Otolaryngological Head and Neck Surgery*, *12*, 180-184.

Amir, O., Kishon-Rabin, L., & Muchnik, C. (2002). The effect of oral contraceptives on voice: Preliminary observations. *Journal of Voice*, *16*, 267-273.

Anolli, L., & Ciceri, R. (2002). Analysis of the vocal profiles of male seduction: From exhibition to self-disclosure. *Journal of General Psychology*, *129*, 149-169.

Berry, D. (1990). Vocal attractiveness and vocal babyishness: Effects on stranger, self and friend impressions. *Journal of Nonverbal Behavior*, *14*, 141-153.

Brown, B., Strong, W., & Rencher, A. (1974). Fifty-four voices from two: The effects of simultaneous manipulations of rate, mean fundamental frequency, and variance of fundamental frequency on ratings of personality from speech. *Journal of the Acoustical Society of America*, *55*, 313-318.

Collins, S. A., & Missing, C. (2003). Vocal and visual attractiveness are related in women. *Animal Behaviour*, *65*, 997-1004.

Daniel, H. J., & McCabe, R. B. (1992). Gender differences in the perception of vocal sexiness. In J. M. G. van der Dennen (Ed.), *The nature of the sexes: The sociobiology of sex differences and the "battle of the sexes"* (pp. 55-62). Groningen, Netherlands: Origin Press.

Dijkstra, P., & Buunk, B. P. (2001). Sex differences in the jealousy-evoking nature of a rival's body build. *Evolution and Human Behavior, 22*, 335-341.

Ekman, P., Friesen, W. V., & Scherer, K. (1976). Body movements and voice pitch in deceptive interaction. *Semiotica, 16*, 23-27.

Ellis, D. S. (1967). Speech and social status in America. *Social Forces, 45*, 431-437.

Evans, R. B. (1972). Physical and biochemical characteristics of homosexual men. *Journal of Consulting and Clinical Psychology, 39*, 140-147.

Furlow, B. F., Kimball, R. T., & Marshall, M. C. (1998). Are rooster crows honest signals of fighting ability? *Auk, 115*, 763-766.

Hagg, U., & Taranger, J. (2003). Menarche and voice change indicators as indicators of the pubertal growth spurt. *Biological Reviews of the Cambridge Philosophical Society, 78*, 385-407.

Harms, L. S. (1963). Listener comprehension of speakers of three status groups. *Language Speech, 4*, 109-112.

Higgins, M. B., & Saxman, J. H. (1989). Variations in vocal frequency perturbation across the menstrual cycle. *Journal of Voice, 3*, 233-243.

Hughes, S. M., Dispenza, F., & Gallup, G. G., Jr. (2004). Ratings of voice attractiveness predict sexual behavior and body configuration. *Evolution and Human Behavior, 25*, 295-304.

Hughes, S. M., & Gallup, G. G., Jr. (2003). Sex differences in morphological predictors of sexual behavior: Shoulder to hip and waist to hip ratios. *Evolution and Human Behavior, 24*, 173-178.

Hughes, S. M., Harrison, M. A., & Gallup, G. G., Jr. (2002). The sound of symmetry: Voice as a marker of developmental instability. *Evolution and Human Behavior, 23*, 173-180.

Hughes, S. M., Pastizzo, M. J., & Gallup, G. G., Jr. (2008, in press). The sound of symmetry revisited: Subjective and objective analyses of voice. *Journal of Nonverbal Behavior.*

Kasperk, C., Helmboldt, A., Borcsok, I., Heuthe, S., Cloos, O., Niethard, F., et al. (1997). Skeletal site-dependent expression of the androgen receptor in human osteoblastic cell populations. *Calcified Tissue, 61*, 464-473.

Krauss, R. M., Freyberg, R., & Morsella, E. (2002). Inferring speakers' physical attributes from their voices. *Journal of Experimental Social Psychology, 38*, 618-625.

Lass, N. J., & Colt, E. G. (1980). A comparative study of the effect of visual and auditory cues on speaker height and weight identification. *Journal of Phonetics, 8*, 277-285.

Lass, N., & Davis, M. (1976). An investigation of speaker height and weight identification. *Journal of the Acoustical Society of America, 60*, 700-704.

Lass, N., Hughes, K., Bowyer, M., Waters, L., & Bourne, V. (1976). Speaker sex identification from voiced, whispered and filtered isolated vowels. *Journal of the Acoustical Society of America, 59*, 675-678.

Lass, N., Tecca, J., Mancuso, R., & Black, W. (1979). The effect of phonetic complexity on speaker race and sex identification. *Journal of Phonetics, 7*, 105-118.

Manning, J. T., Barley, L., Walton, J., Lewis-Jones, D. I., Trivers, R. L., Singh, D., et al. (2000). The 2nd:4th digit ratio, sexual dimorphism, population differences, and reproductive success: Evidence for sexually antagonistic genes? *Evolution and Human Behavior, 21*, 163-183.

Manning, J. T., Scutt, D., Wilson, J., & Lewis-Jones, D. I. (1998). The ratio of 2nd to 4th digit length: A predictor of sperm numbers and concentrations of testosterone, luteinizing hormone and oestrogen. *Human Reproduction, 13*, 3000-3004.

Miyake, K., & Zuckerman, M. (1993). Beyond personality impressions: Effects of physical and vocal attractiveness on false consensus, social comparison, affiliation, and assumed and perceived similarity. *Journal of Personality*, *61*, 411-437.

Moore, K. L. (1977). *The developing human: Clinically orientated embryology.* Philadelphia: W.N. Saunders.

Oguchi, T., & Kikuchi, H. (1997). Voice and interpersonal attraction. *Japanese Psychological Research*, *39*, 56-61.

Oksenberg, L., Coleman, L., & Cannell, C. F. (1986). Interviewers' voice and refusal rates in telephone surveys. *Public Opinion Quarterly*, *50*, 97-111.

Puts, D. (2005). Mating context and menstrual phase affect women's preferences for male voice pitch. *Evolution and Human Behavior*, *26*, 388-397.

Schneider, B., van Trotsenburg, M., Hanke, G., Bigenzahn, W., & Huber, J. (2004). Voice impairment and menopause. *Menopause*, *11*, 151-158.

Seemann, M. (1930). Sexual function and voice. Abstract from Časopis lékařů českých, 112-115.

Singh, D. (1993). Adaptive significance of female physical attractiveness: Role of waist-to-hip ratio. *Journal of Personality and Social Psychology*, *65*, 293-307.

Streeter, L. A., Krauss, R. M., Geller, V. J., Olson, C. T., & Apple, W. (1977). Pitch changes during attempted deception. *Journal of Personality and Social Psychology*, *35*, 345-350.

Thornhill, R., & Gangestad, S. W. (1999). The scent of symmetry: A human sex pheromone that signals fitness? *Evolution and Human Behavior*, *20*, 175-201.

Thornhill, R., & Møller, A. P. (1997). Developmental stability, disease and medicine. *Biological Reviews*, *72*, 497-548.

Yogo, Y., Ando, M., Hashi, A., Tsutsui, S., & Yamada N. (2000). Judgments of emotion by nurses and students given double-blind information on a patient's tone of voice and message content. *Perception Motor Skills*, *9*, 855-863.

Zuckerman, M., & Driver, R. (1989). What sounds beautiful is good: The vocal attractiveness stereotype. *Journal of Nonverbal Behavior*, *13*, 67-82.

Zuckerman, M., Hodgins, H., & Miyake, K. (1990). The vocal attractiveness stereotype: Replication and elaboration. *Journal of Nonverbal Behavior*, *14*, 97-112.

CHAPTER 16

From Perception to Communication: Sensolinguistic Therapy to Restore Voice and Vocal Emotions

Lilla-Teresa Sadowski, Alois Mauerhofer, Sabine Hoffman, and Krzysztof Izdebski

Abstract

Patients with severe emotional disturbances may be subject to communicative withdrawal and to severely altered vocalization, and may even be electively silent, rendering their vocalization both pathologic and, when present, subject to the internal and the external emotional load.

In this chapter, we present our global therapy concept, which uses both perception and motor coordination, including an innovative instrumental approach capable of providing thermal stimulation, vibration, voice, music, and speech feedback to both the patient and the therapist. This feedback can be integrated with filters or special effects so that the patient may hear herself in the way she may be perceived by others, including effects of different acoustic environments.

Application of this therapy with patients presenting with a variety of psychiatric disorders (depression, anxiety, panic attacks, or schizophrenia) is reviewed here, but in general, the technique is also applicable to other voice/speech/communication disorders. The basic concept behind this multistage treatment program is the exploration of the connection between vocal, emotional, and social development, with each therapy stage aimed at addressing the various developmental stages (i.e., the awareness phase, the instrumental phase, and the communicational phase).

Introduction

It is well established that the various psychiatric conditions can severely affect all aspects of human communication including the voice (Andersson & Schalen, 1998; Aronson, 1990; Baker, 1998; 2002; 2003; Baker & Lane, 2006; Friedl, Friedrich, & Egger, 1990; Friedl, Friedrich, Egger, & Fitzek, 1993; White, Deary, & Wilson, 1997). Severe restrictions to voice production, including both the effect upon the voice and restoration of the "normal" voice in these cases, may be difficult, lengthy, and at times very protracted (Schlömicher-Thier, Weikert, B. Kirchner, & B. Kirchner, 2006).

Therapy

To aid the recovery process, a unique therapy method supported by psychotherapy and instrumentation was developed (Sadowski & Mauerhofer, 1998; Sadowski & Taucher, 1995a; 1995b). The efficacy of this therapy was the object of research studies between 1995 and 1998 (Sadowski & Mauerhofer, 1998; Sadowski & Taucher, 1995a; 1995b; 1997), and the technique has since been put into practice at the Psychiatric Department, University Clinic, University of Graz, Graz, Austria.

The therapy is divided into three steps or phases, in which implementation is spaced sequentially. These stages are: (a) perception-awareness phase, (b) respiration and voice phase, and (c) instrumental-communicational phase.

This first therapy stage, the *perception-awareness stage*, is crucial to all patients, but more so to the severely inhibited patients, specifically those showing stupor. The goal of therapy at this stage is to make the patient deduce the concept of "I feel, therefore I am," which describes the fundamental relationship between an individual and his or her environment. In other terms, at this initial therapy stage, we focus on patient reintegration, namely the capacity of the patient to relate or to be in contact with self and with surroundings (the world around) and to remove any possible distortions in perception.

In the second stage, the *respiration and voice stage*, both vocalization and breathing are addressed to allow integration of self perception, emotions, and environment with the motor actions needed to produce and restore normal or near normal vocalization patterns for declarative and the primary emotional voice types.

Concerning respiration, attention is paid to the expiratory air flow and to the ventilatory pauses. Voice must be produced only during expiration, and inspiratory (ingressive) phonation is eliminated. At this time cathartic like reactions may be observed in some patients.

Another focus is placed at this stage on the perception of one's own voice and speech output and quality. Objectification of perception allows the patient to effectively make immediate adjustments concerning posture and respiratory and articulatory musculature and to immediately perceive the changes being implemented.

The third stage, the *instrumental-communicational stage*, is indicated for all of the patients who completed the first two stages. The therapy in this phase is for those patients who completed the two previous stages, for those patients who desire to continue therapy after being released from the inpatient **hospital** setting, and for those for whom the social aspects of communication are severely compromised.

When group therapy is initiated at this stage, the participants are asked to accomplish group tasks together, that is, to prepare and to perform a theater play or to organize a fancy-dress ball or a social event requiring engagement of social and creative capacities, but performed in a protected and psychologically safe environment.

Working Hypothesis

The working hypothesis behind this approach incorporates some basic concepts that include the cognitive, social, and emotional aspects, all to be integrated into corresponding developmental stages for which each primary deficit area must be identified. Healing and catharsis are possible through partial reproduction of early developmental stages in accordance with their developmental sequence. Each phase of the developmental stage is compared to the degree of subconsciousness or unconsciousness of the behavioral patterns exhibited by each patient.

Partial reproduction of the developmental blocks is intended in each stage. It is crucial that the therapist and the setting are both capable of relating positively to the patient. Simple, positive stimuli are thus used to evoke, to correct, and to integrate perception of reality into a more concrete environment, as a form of operative conditioning to reach appropriate social relatedness.

The voice therapy portion plays a special function as the integrator between the subconscious emotional states and conscious perception, and it (the voice) may catalyze cathartic effects. On the other hand, using the sensations of touch, heat, and external sound, patients are invited to passively perceive simple, basic, and positive inputs. This therapy setting is repeated for several days, but for no longer than 10 minutes of stimulation at one time.

The Instrument

To support the concept of integration of the external stimuli with the patient's needs, the sensolinguistic therapy instrument has been developed and tested since its introduction at the Graz International Spring Congress for Medicine in 1997. The instrument has three basic setting modes: (a) Warmth and Music, (b) Sound Recording and Playback, and (c) Mixture of Rhythm, Sound, and Voice (Moshammer, Gross St. Florian, Austria).

One of the reasons for developing this instrumental aid was the fact that for some patients direct hands-on, physical contact with the clinician might not be desired. Contacting (relating) to the patient with the instrument via two hand-sized warmth pillows was thought to offer a patient a less stressful transmission mode and thus facilitate a more neutral interaction. In addition, the thermal pillows regulate the body temperature of the breathing zones and increase blood flow, which results in respiratory muscle relaxation and improved patient control, enabling better expansion of the breathing apparatus.

The other advantage of using this **instrument** is that it provides an objective acoustical feedback to both the patient and the therapist, therefore increasing the opportunity for the patient to critically listen to him- or herself.

Research Results

The efficacy of this approach has been studied (Sadowski & Mauerhofer, 1998; Sadowski & Taucher, 1995a; 1995b; 1997), demonstrating excellent acceptance of the technique by the patients and the clinicians, and a significant improvement in therapy outcomes. The percentage of amelioration was best in patients affected by depressive syndrome. In a test on the effectiveness of the Sensotherm instrument, 98% of the patients tested showed positive responses using questionnaire methodology (Van der Ploeg, 1989).

The Concept of the Development

The concept of the developmental stages in the acquisition of human sound and speech is crucial to the basis of the therapy proposed here. Going back to the "original" experience permits the patient in stupor to relate to the antecedent primary knowledge and to transfer this experience to the therapy requirements. We use the following language developmental stages to convey our therapy goals to the patient. These stages are based on the building blocks of a child's normal voice-speech-language acquisition, and are incorporated into the therapy protocol we are describing next. The actual therapy tasks are grouped as outlined below:

1. Passive exercises for respiration—hand contact (thermal pillows) on different respiratory muscles
2. Exercises for respiration—from breathing to vocalization
3. Exercises for respiration—body posture, breathing, and voice
4. Humming exercises produced on expiration and supported by abdominal appoggio

5. Transfer of vocalization to tentative text
6. Texts with appoggio and interpretation (1. through 6. and 8. are individual exercises with the Sensotherm instrument)
7. Group work involving reading and interpreting of known or unfamiliar texts/scripts; stress on accentuation
8. Preparation of new texts for the audience (acoustic self-awareness exercises)
9. Presenting (emotional expression) of texts
10. Adding mood effects via light, texture, colors—costumes
11. Communication between actor and audience

Summary

The therapy protocol described here has been tested over the years with a wide variety of patients with emotional disturbances affecting voice, speech, emotional expressions, and global aspects of human-to-human communication, varying from mild to extremely severe cases. The approach has been very successful in ameliorating deficits in vocalization in these clinical subgroups. The three-stage consecutive therapy technique we describe here is supported by the use of an instrument that provides an improved access to the patient's inner self via application of heat, touch, sound, and feedback. The patient, in turn, learns again to feel him-self, recognizes his own feelings and emotions, articulates them and hears them, and thus regains access to himself and his surroundings.

For purely the voice patients the instrument can be used to provide acoustical self-help in voice therapy and voice monitoring. This combined operative-instrumental approach has been successful in restoring both declarative and emotionally loaded vocalization.

References

Andersson, K., & Schalen, L. (1998). Etiology and treatment of psychogenic voice disorder: Results of a follow-up study of thirty patients. *Journal of Voice*, *12*(1), 96–106.

Aronson, A. E. (1990). Psychogenic voice disorders. In A. E. Aronson, (Ed.), *Clinical voice disorders: An interdisciplinary approach* (3rd ed., pp. 116–159). New York: Thieme.

Baker, J. (1998). Psychogenic dysphonia: Peeling back the layers. *Journal of Voice*, *12*(4), 527–535.

Baker, J. (2002). Psychogenic voice disorders —Heroes or hysterics? A brief overview with questions and discussion. *Logopedics, Phoniatrics, Vocology*, *27*, 84–91.

Baker, J. (2003). Psychogenic voice disorders and traumatic stress experience: A discussion paper with two case reports. *Journal of Voice*, *17*(3), 308–318.

Baker, J., & Lane, R. (2008). Psychogenic voice disorders. In K. Izdebski (Ed.), *The emotions in the human voice.* San Diego, CA: Plural.

Friedl, W., Friedrich, G., & Egger, J. (1990). Personality and coping with stress in patients suffering from functional dysphonia. *Folia Phoniatrica*, *42*, 13–20.

Friedl, W., Friedrich, G., Egger, J., & Fitzek, T. (1993). Zur psychogenese funktioneller dysphonia. *Folia Phoniatrica*, *45*, 10–13.

Lytwyn, H. Sadowski, L.-T., & Tschetsch, V. (2002). Das wahrnehmungstraingsgerät. *Sensotherm* (Vol. 3, pp. 26–27). Logopädie, Wein: Verband der Depl. Logopadinna.

Sadowski, L.-T., Kenner, B., Mauerhofer, A., & Kenner, T. (1998). Eine sensolinguistische evolutionäre therapie-methode zur behandlung der recurrensparese. *Sprache und Sprachen* (pp. 2-15). München, Germany: Zeitschriftder Geselschaft für Sprache und Sprachen, E. V.

Sadowski, L.-T., & Taucher, J., Steinbauer, M., & Zapotoczky, H. G. (1995). *Elisabeth: Psycholinguistische therapii bei einer patintin mit major depression, menschmacht-maschine* (pp. 160-171). Insbruck, Wein: Integrative Psychiatrie-Verlag.

Sadowski, L.-T., Taucher, J., Steinbauer, M., & Zapotoczky, H. G. (1995). Stimme-stimmung: Psycholinguistische therapie mit psychiatrischen patienten. *Wiener Medizinische Wochenschrift, 145*, Heft 9, 201-206.

Schlömicher-Their, J., Weikert, M., Kirchner, B., & Kirchner, B. (2006). Diagnostics and treatment of psychogenic dysphonia. In K. Izdebski (Ed.), *The emotions in the human voice.* San Diego, CA: Plural.

Taucher, J., Sadowski, L.-T., Taucher, J., Steinbauer, M., & Zapotoczky, H. G. (1997). Wärme und Atemtherapie im Therapiekonzept der Stimmungstherapie nach Sadowski für psychiatrische patienten. *Klinische Psychotherapie* (pp. 97-103). Wien/New York: Springer Verlag.

van der Ploeg, H. M. (1989). *Self-assessment questionnaire-Nijmegen (SAQ-N).* Nijimegen, Netherlands: Swets and Zeitlinger.

White, A., Deary, I. J., & Wilson, J. A. (1997). Psychiatric disturbance and personality traits in dysphonic patients. *European Journal of Disorders of Communication, 32*, 307-314.

CHAPTER 17

Restoration of Vocal and Facial Emotive Production in Tardive Dyskinesia, Cerebral Palsy, and Closed Head Injury Using Selective Chemical Denervation

Krzysztof Izdebski and Raul M. Cruz

Abstract

A variety of neurologic conditions can leave patients with spastic-like dysphonias and abnormal facial contractions. For example, tardive dyskinesia (TD) is an iatrogenic syndrome that may rob patients' normal communicative production, rendering voice, speech, and associated facial expressions severely disrupted. Similarly, patients with cerebral palsy (CP) or closed head injury (CHI) presenting with dysphonia and dysarthria can manifest a variety of phonatory and facial disturbances. Using selective botulinum toxin type-A, (Allergan, Inc. Irvine, CA) EMG guided sequential injections into laryngeal and facial musculature, we were able to improve significantly vocal and facial functions resulting in improved emotive expressions in these patients.

Introduction

The purpose of this chapter is to describe the blunting of vocal emotive expression in select examples of patients with TD, CP, and CHI. All of these patients were plagued with spasmodic-like dysphonias and abnormal facial contractions. Restoration of improved vocal and facial function resulting in greater ability to express vocal emotions was obtained using a technique of targeting specific muscle groups for chemical denervation with EMG guided botulinum toxin injections.

Tardive Dyskinesia

TD belongs to the group of so-called movement disorders (MD) and is considered a neurological syndrome of iatrogenic origin. A wide variety of drugs can cause this condition: anticholinergics, antidepressants, antiemetics, antiepileptics, antimalarials, antihistamines, anxiolytics, stimulants, mood stabilizers, and even oral contraceptives. However, the prototypic form of TD is caused by the long-term use of neuroleptic drugs, which are dopamine receptor blockers. (Neuroleptic drugs may also be categorized as antipsychotic or psychotropic drugs.) These agents are prescribed for patients suffering various psychiatric conditions that include schizophrenia, schizoaffective disorder, and bipolar disorder.

Typical antipsychotic drugs include: haloperidol (Haldol), chloropromazine (Thorazine), trifluoperazine (Stelazine), molindone (Moban), and thiothixene (Navane). The newer atypical antipsychotic agents are believed to have a lower incidence of TD and one of them, clozapine (Clozaril), is often prescribed in refractory schizophrenia cases with TD (Keck, McElroy, Strakowski, & Soutullo, 2006).

The long-term side effects of using any of these agents may result in repetitive, involuntary, and apparently purposeless muscular movements affecting various motor activities including: respiration, posturing, deglutition, articulation, phonation, and facial expression. Hence, these patients may present with profound problems in the control of musculature associated with voice production. Altered speech production is characterized by reduced fluency, intelligibility, and intonation. Facial grimacing and contortions, repetitive eye blinking, tongue protrusion, and lip smacking, puckering, and pursing may be present during speech. Abnormal facial appearance often results in mismatching or camouflaging of the intended emotional content of speech. (To learn more about this phenomenon, consult Chapter 8 in this volume: Editor.)

In addition to bizarre speech production and facial contortions, atypical movements of the trunk, neck, arms, and even fingers may be observed (Gharabawi et al., 2005). These movements can be exacerbated when speaking in the declarative mode, even more so when expressing emotions. These distortions affect respiratory support and worsen speech production. Extraneous body movements may also distract the listener from the nuances of emotional content in patients' speech.

In all, patients with TD may exhibit bizarre speech patterns, and akin to severe adductor spasmodic dysphonia (ADDSD) patients (Izdebski, Dedo, & Boles, 1984), this may render them functional vocal cripples. This often results in complete social isolation and reclusive behavior, as their appearance during speech (but not at rest) is so bizarre that these patients do not want to communicate in public.

Currently, there is no standard treatment for TD. It remains highly individualized and includes reducing dosage, stopping drugs, or changing to the newer atypical neuroleptics; yet the symptoms of TD may remain long after drug discontinuation or change.

Our successful experience in treating another MD, namely ADDSD (Aminoff, Izdebski, & Dedo, 1978; Izdebski, 1990), using techniques aimed at denervation either through RLN nerve resection (Dedo, 1976: Dedo & Izdebski, 1981; 1983a; 1983b; 1984) or botulinum toxin injections (Izdebski & Ward, 1997) encouraged us to treat "an extreme case of TD," labeled such by the referring clinician. We pursued this avenue, because many of the symptoms present in TD are similar to the successfully treated symptoms of ADDSD, and Botox injections in severe dystonic posturing have been recently reported (Arikan, Tan, Kendi, & Koc, 2006; Rapaport et al., 2000; Schneider et al., 2006; Suskind & Tilton, 2002; Tarsy et al., 1997).

Tardive Dyskinesia (TD) Case

A 51-year-old woman was referred for evaluation of her dysphonia associated with TD. She had begun psychiatric treatment 30 years previously for paranoid schizophrenia that eventually evolved into a bipolar condition over several years. She was treated with thiothixene (Navane) at varying doses for more than 20 years, and subsequently lithium and carbamazepine (Tegretol) were added to her regimen. For the last 8 years, she has been treated with a newer atypical neuroleptic agent, clozapine (Clozaril). This drug is thought useful in reducing the TD symptoms in patients requiring psychiatric medication.

After 17 years of drug usage, she began to notice a movement disorder. Her initial symptoms affected speech. Employed as an executive secretary, she began mispronouncing words on the phone and eventually people had difficulty understanding her speech. Six years later, facial grimacing began. Her psychiatrist referred her as "one of the most severe cases of TD ever seen" in 20 years with a large HMO practice. She quit her job 8 years ago because she experienced a psychotic break, which she claimed was caused primarily by being treated "funny" at work because of her voice and facial appearance. Her marked facial grimacing also led to the development of a TMJ problem during her last 6 months of employment. The consequences of her condition rendered her a complete social recluse for at least the prior 5 years.

Pretreatment Symptoms

Symptoms were subdivided into vocal (speech) and facial. Vocal symptoms include severely overpressured speech accompanied by a mild dysarthria and worsened by facial contortions. This rendered speech intelligibility severely distorted. The facial expression muscles contracted abnormally, particularly in the perioral and glabellar regions. Overall, her appearance during speech created the painful perception of a suffering woman. However, at rest, a completely normal facial appearance was noted. Figure 17-1 shows facial contortions during reading of a random text.

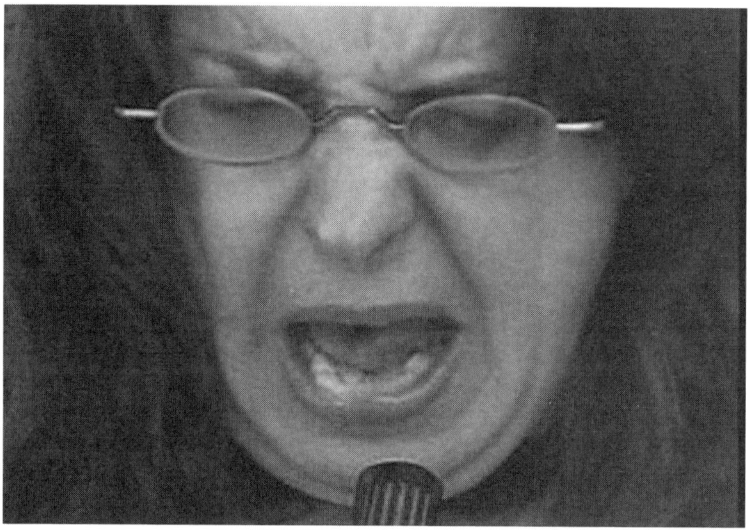

Figure 17–1. Facial contortions in a TD patient while reading a standard text before botulinum toxin treatment.

Treatment

Botulinum toxin type A injection therapy was initiated in a stepped fashion. Initially, treatment was directed at selected intrinsic laryngeal musculature, and later the muscles of facial expression were treated using previously described techniques (Izdebski & Ward, 1997). During the initial injection session the left thyroarytenoid muscle was unilaterally injected to reduce vocal spasticity and to observe its effect on facial expression. This resulted in an increase in breathiness, less pressured speech, and some reduction of facial contortions. Upon symptom recurrence three months later, the muscles of facial expression were included in the injection treatment. Facial muscles injected included the bilateral risorius, depressor anguli oris, and procerus/corrugators. Figure 17-2 shows the dramatic reduction of facial contortions during reading. Since this second session, combined laryngeal and facial muscle injections have been performed and supported with speech therapy. The gratifying outcome has allowed this patient to reenter social life. She is now looking for employment for the first time in eight years.

Cerebral Palsy Case

A 41-year-old male pediatric nurse with the diagnosis of CP self-referred himself complaining of distorted speech making communication at work with patients and families difficult. The quality of his speech was pressed, high pitched, dysfluent, and dysarthric. There was a tendency to drool during speech. Marked facial, cervical, truncal, and extremity spasticity was present. This contorted his body positioning and gait. He noted all of these symptoms, especially vocal symptoms, were worse when experiencing strong

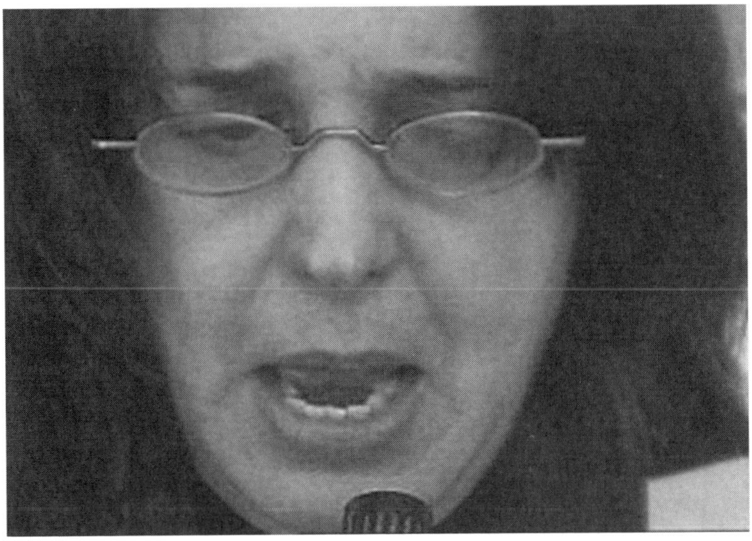

Figure 17–2. The same TD patient reading the same text after botulinum toxin treatment.

emotions. The overall impression created was of a person suffering and whining. However, in reality, this individual had a positive life attitude and has overcome his severe handicaps.

We elected to perform laryngeal and facial musculature botulinum toxin injections in this patient. The left thyroarytenoid and bilateral cricothyroid muscles were injected. This reduced pressed phonation and dysfluency. It also lowered his pitch to a more gender-appropriate level. Injected facial muscles included the bilateral risorius, levator/depressor anguli oris, and procerus/corrugator muscles. This moderately improved his drooling and unwanted facial contractions. Overall, treatment has improved his speech and given him a more presentable appearance. He continues his employment and has recently been promoted to an administrative position within the same HMO system. He continues to return for periodic injections.

Closed Head Injury Case

A 52-year-old woman, a veterinarian, was referred almost 4 years after a motor vehicle accident for her chronic dysphonia. She had suffered a CHI with the subsequent development of an organic brain syndrome. A MRI 2 years before had revealed changes consistent with ischemia/gliosis of her left frontal lobe and deep white matter. She had undergone an extensive period of physical and combined voice/speech therapy. She was maintained on gabapentin (Neurontin) medical therapy. Although she manifested a generalized spasticity, her examination was remarkable for her pressed, dysfluent speech and unwanted facial contractions. She was noted to be emotionally labile, with a tendency for inappropriate laughter or crying. Again we began combined injection therapy of her laryngeal and facial muscles. Her left thyroarytenoid, bilateral depressor anguli oris, procerus/corrugators, and frontalis muscles were injected. This has resulted in moderate improvement in her dysphonia and reduction in unwanted facial contortions. She is pleased with the results and continues to return for periodic injections.

Summary and Conclusions

Several clinical conditions can cause significant disruptions of voice, speech, and associated facial expression that are difficult to correct purely through behavioral or speech therapy. These conditions can also affect emotive expression in these patients either by introducing unwanted representation of emotion, especially during declarative speech, or by magnifying intended emotions. The idea for using botulinum toxin type A injections was based on our long history of treating ADDSD using these techniques. The use of these injections in MD patients has been described before (Arikan et al., 2006; Rapaport et al., 2000; Schneider et al., 2006; Suskind & Tilton, 2002; Tarsy et al., 1997). Botulinum treatment of drooling in CP patients has been reported (Arikan et al., 2006), but not for vocal or facial problems. Finally, we were not able to locate any reports of the use of this therapy for these indications in CHI patients (http://www.ncbi.nlm.nih.gov/PubMed), May, 2007. Our results have been encouraging to date. In select patients manifesting these problems, botulinum toxin injection therapy may prove useful. All three of our patients feel they have benefited and have continued periodic treatment for over a year. Specifically, patients with spasmodic-like dysphonias and facial grimacing and in particular who experience difficulty with emotional expression may benefit from this therapy.

References

Aminoff, M., Izdebski K., & Dedo, H. H. (1978). Clinical aspects of spasmodic dysphonia. *Journal of Neurology, Neurosurgery, and Psychiatry*, *41*(4), 361-365.

Arikan, O. K., Tan, F. U., Kendi, T., & Koc, C. (2006). Use of botulinum toxin type A for the treatment of masseteric muscle hypertrophy. *Journal of Otolaryngology*, *35*(1), 40-43.

Dedo, H. H. (1976) Recurrent laryngeal nerve section for spastic dysphonia. *Annals of Otology, Rhinology, and Laryngology*, *85*, 451-459.

Dedo, H. H., & Izdebski, K. (1981). Surgical treatment of spastic dysphonia. *Contemporary Surgery*, *19*, 75-90.

Dedo, H. H., & Izdebski, K. (1983). Intermediate results of 306 recurrent laryngeal nerve sections for spastic dysphonia. *Laryngoscope*, *93*(1), 9-16.

Dedo, H. H., & Izdebski, K. (1983). Problems with surgical (RLN section) treatment of spastic dysphonia. *Laryngoscope*, *93*(3), 268-271.

Dedo, H. H., & Izdebski, K. (1984). Evaluation and treatment of recurrent spasticity after recurrent laryngeal nerve section. A preliminary report. *Annals of Otology, Rhinology, and Laryngology*, *93*(4, Pt. 1), 343-345.

Gharabawi, G. M., Bossie, C. A., Lasser, R. A., Turkoz, I., Rodriguez, S., & Chouinard, G. (2005). Abnormal Involuntary Movement Scale (AIMS) and Extrapyramidal Symptom Rating Scale (ESRS): Cross-scale comparison in assessing tardive dyskinesia. *Schizophrenia Research*, *77*(2-3), 119-128.

Izdebski, K. (1992). Symptomatology of adductor spasmodic dysphonia: A physiologic model. *Journal of Voice*, *6*, 306-319.

Izdebski, K., Dedo, H. H., & Boles, L. (1984). Spastic dysphonia: A patient profile of 200 cases. *American Journal of Otolaryngology*, *5*(1), 7-14.

Izdebski, K., & Ward, R. (1997). Glottic physiology after Botox treatment of ADDuctor spasmodic dysphonia, ABDuctor spasmodic dysphonia and vocal tremor. In M. Pais Clemente (Ed.), *Voice Update, International Congress Series 1997*, 131-146. Amsterdam: Elsevier.

Keck, P. E., Jr., McElroy, S. L., Strakowski, S. M., & Soutullo, C. A. (2000). Antipsychotics in the treatment of mood disorders and risk of tardive dyskinesia. *Journal of Clinical Psychiatry*, *61*(Suppl. 4), 33-38.

Rapaport, A., Sadeh, M., Stein, D., Levine, J., Sirota, P., Mosheva, T., et al. (2000). Botulinum toxin for the treatment of oro-facial-lingual-masticatory tardive dyskinesia. *Movement Disorders*, *15*(2), 352-355.

Schneider, S. A., Aggarwal, A., Bhatt, M., Dupont, E., Tisch, S., Limousin, P., et al. (2006). Severe tongue protrusion dystonia: Clinical syndromes and possible treatment. *Neurology*, *67*(6), 940-943.

Suskind, D. L., & Tilton, A. (2002). Clinical study of botulinum—A toxin in the treatment of sialorrhea in children with cerebral palsy. *Laryngoscope*, *112*(1), 73-81.

Tarsy, D., Kaufman, D., Sethi, K. D., Rivner, M. H., Molho, E., & Factor, S. (1997). An open-label study of botulinum toxin A for treatment of tardive dystonia. *Clinical Neuropharmacology*, *20*(1), 90-93.

CHAPTER 18

A Comprehensive Model of How the Stress Chain Affects Voice

W. A. R. Wellens and M. J. M. C. Van Opstal

Abstract

Stress (Latin: *stringere*) is a global term that is used broadly in daily communication. It is the nonspecific effect of any demand upon the body and mind. It is the nonspecific biological and mental excitement caused by everyday life. The authors present a comprehensive behavior model of stress in voice users. Stress is a circular process of a dynamic behavior chain that includes different elements: stimuli or signals, biological and mental arousal, emotions, coping behavior, and short- and long-term effects. The stress level is postulated to be on a continuum, from complete rest to intensive hyper-excitement. Voice users are at risk of being exposed to high stress. Physiological effects of the stress response may directly interfere with the delicate mechanism of vocal tract and body, impeding the quality of the vocal performance. Cognitive aspects of the stress chain may have a disrupting effect on the skills of the performance of speaker and singer. Stress is not always detrimental to verbal performance: a certain level of stress, known as *eustress*, is necessary in order to perform well. Voice users have to keep stress in balance in order to perform without endangering their basic needs of safety, security, and creativity. It is obvious that constant, too high stress, known as *distress*, can be detrimental to the quality of the voice. Distress may result in physical problems, voice and articulation disorders, and even psychological dysfunction. Moreover, disturbed vocal performance and dysphonia may become a stress-inducing stimulus resulting in different types of anxiety states. Stress factors should be recognized in the etiology of voice complaints and symptoms, and addressed in the voice therapy management.

Introduction

Verbal communication makes human beings different from other living species. We use our voice for communication and to express our meaning and emotions (Aronson, 1990; Brockway, 1979; Freidl, 1989; Hollien, 1980; Izard, 1991; Kenny, 2004; Schutte, 1980; Seifert, 2005, Simovov, 1977; Smith, 1977; Stemple, 1993).

It is commonplace to state the obvious relationship between emotion and voicing, between stress and voicing (Freidl, 1989; Kenny, 2004). Most of the so-called "non-organic" or "functional" voice disorders are primarily caused by stress (Hollien, 1980). Punt (1979) stated, "The vocal mechanism may be healthy and undamaged, but the precision with which it responds to the subtle and intricate demands made upon it is so often affected by the state of mind and emotions of the performer." House and Andrews (1988) found that voice disorders frequently occurred as a response to a specific sort of stress.

Over the years there has been a wide range of publications on how emotions are conveyed acoustically (Cosmides, 1983; Engstrand, 1988; Fuller, 1992; Hollien, 1980; Mendoza, 1998; Seidner, 1981; Simovov, 1977; Smith, 1977; Williams, 1972). However, only rarely is there specific reference to what the stated relationship between emotion and voicing consists of, and what the consequences of it are for diagnostics, therapy management, and training (Fresnel, 1999; Rosen, 1997; Wellens, 2001; Butcher, 1993).

The term *professional voice user* applies to any person whose profession or livelihood relies on the use of his voice. They all experience high vocal loading (Rubin, 1995; Sataloff, 1991).

Professional voice users have many attributes that make their work and lifestyle particularly vulnerable to stress. Being a professional voice user is a particular risk factor for exposure to high stress levels. Stress is a main cause of disturbed acting, voice and articulation disorders, or even psychological and physical problems.

Behavioral Analysis of Stress in Professional Voice Users

In order to analyze stress in relationship with vocal performance we conceptualize stress in terms of a dynamic circle of functional entities interacting with the structural and functional aspects of the organs of vocal communication, singing, and acting (Wellens, 2001).

This clinical model is mainly based upon:

1. The behavioral model for functional analysis of Kanfer and Philips (1970);
2. Selye's concept of stress (1950; 1974);
3. Lindsley's activation theory (1951; 1957); and
4. The principles of behavior modification.

In this conceptual model, stress is considered to be a circular process, which constitutes a dynamic behavior chain including:

- Stressors;
- Arousal, both biological and mental;
- Emotions;
- Coping behavior; and
- Effects of the behavior on the internal and external environment.

We will systematically extend on these functional entities within the stress process. For each of these links in the stress chain we will reflect on its involvement in the different aspects of vocal performance.

Stressors

A stressor is an external or internal event, which elects a biological and mental alarm reaction. All kinds of stimuli (signals, invaders) can become stressors. Stimuli are more or less consciously perceived as signals for needs, either for danger or needs at different levels of human well-being. Basic needs are motivational systems necessary for survival. Maslow (1971) categorized three main types of basic needs:

- Safety: physical well-being resulting in health;
- Security: personal well-being by personal and social appraisal; and
- Creativity: spiritual well-being or fulfillment.

The different levels of well-being are involved in a specific way in professional voice users before, during, and after the public performance. Some examples:

- Safety: the constant concern not to harm the vocal instrument, staying sane in the art, in teaching;
- Security: earning a living as a professional voice user, appreciation by the audience or pupils or customers, having rewarding relationships;
- Creativity: the concerns of performing at a high artistic level, delivering a convincing oral presentation, to teach or preach well, to provide an excellent service. Only the performer who has achieved a sense of physical and mental quietude gains creativity.

Artists (Maisel, 1992) and teachers (de Jong, 2004; Knothe, 1990) represent a specific subgroup in stress management because they are the most obvious and demanding professional voice users. In addition to the stress of simply being human, they are also confronted by strong performance-related stressors (Maisel, 1992). Most of the artistic people are driven, ambitious, perfectionist, and tightly controlled (Rosen, 1997). They are used to working hard and long, are under excessive pressure, and often have to race against the clock.

Artistic performance necessitates a wider than usual vocal quality, vocal range, intensity dynamics, and prosody (Bunch, 1995). Most of the time, artists lead a very hectic lifestyle, experience a lot of competition, and sometimes have to perform in far from ideal circumstances.

It's obvious that a broad range of stressors is inherent to vocal performance. Professional voice users represent a group of high-risk individuals for external and internal stressors (Rubin, 1995; Sataloff, 1991; Seidner, 1997). Biological noxious stimuli are quite common and may invade from the external environment, for example: dry atmosphere, space acoustics, noise, medication, alcohol, tobacco, stimulants, tranquilizers, narcotics, microorganisms, allergens, and dust. Biological invaders can harm their body or larynx, especially if the voice user is predisposed to either hereditary or acquired vulnerability. Stimuli generated by the internal environment play an important role in the stress response. Numerous proprioceptive stimuli from sensory receptors located in the larynx, skin, joints, ligaments, postural muscles, and other tissues of the body constantly relay information to the brain for processing. Such information is important in order to coordinate the mental and physical factors involved in vocal performance. Among other things, disturbed biorhythm, jet lag, exhaustion, discomfort from spotlights, vocal abuse, misuse, vocal discomfort, overloaded muscles, and inability of a teacher to instill and maintain discipline may fire a salvo of internal stimuli.

Task demands are high on the professional stage and professional voice presupposes a high degree of awareness and self-control. This can easily disappear when confronted with intensive stress. Stressors may accumulate. The overall performance-related stress experienced is built up by the cumulative effects of the biological and mental stress triggered by the different external and internal stressors involved in a particular vocal performance situation.

Arousal

Arousal is a cluster of biological and psychological excitement, which prepares the individual to cope with the perceived needs, especially with endangered needs. It is primarily a survival mechanism preparing the organism for fight and/or flight in order to defend the physical, personal, and spiritual values endangered by the stressors.

Biological Arousal in the General and Local Adaptation Syndromes of Selye

The endocrinologist Hans Selye paved the way for the concept of the stress chain (1950; 1976). As he mentioned in *The Stress of Life* (1976), already in the early 1930s he described a general response of the organism to stressors in his experiments with animals. He analyzed their responses to biological stressors and postulated that the physiology of the animals was attempting to counteract the noxious invaders. He termed the whole process the General Adaptation Syndrome or GAS. He described three consecutive stages of biological reactions: the general alarm reaction, the stage of resistance, and the stage of exhaustion.

Each of these stages has its specific physiological changes. Stressors activate the hypothalamus. The result is a widespread mass reaction through the nervous and endocrine systems in the target organs throughout the body by the activity of the autonomic nervous system (ANS). This massive alarm response prepares the *organism for coping with the perceived needs.*

Two mechanisms, a neuronal and a hormonal one, are involved in the stress response. The mediator of the sympathetic or adrenergic system is the neuroeffector cellular secretion of norepinephrine (norarenaline).

The arousal level is on a continuum from rest to maximal activation. It can be general or local. In the GAS, a general arousal reaction is evoked in different organs in order to maintain or to restore adaptation. This is the common denominator of illness. An anaphylactic shock can be defined as a state of exhaustion, the third stage of GAS.

In the Local Adaptation Syndrome (LAS), a local arousal reaction is evoked in an organ in order to develop local adaptation. Contact allergy, local inflammation, and vocal cord edema are examples of LAS.

GAS and LAS Interact

The mediators of the hormonal system are the adrenocorticotropic hormone (ACTH) and the antidiuretic hormone vasopressin (ADH). ACTH releases two types of corticosteroids in the bloodstream: glucocorticoids and mineralocorticoids.

The role of the alarm reaction is primarily a stimulative one providing extra activation of the bodily functions to prepare the organism for coping with the perceived needs. Among others it decreases the blood flow and function of those organ systems that are not critical for the fight or flight reaction, and it excites those organ functions that are necessary in order to cope with the perceived need.

The role of the parasympathetic or cholinergic system, mediated by the neuroeffector secretion of acetylcholine, is primarily a restorative system. It tends to repair the body's physiological functions and to restore the energy levels after the fight or flight reactions.

Mental Arousal in the Activation Syndrome of Lindsley

In the 1950s, Lindsley (1951; 1957) developed the activation theory of emotions and behavior. He states that the arousal is not only biological, but also it has a cognitive pendent of mental activation. Either external or internal stimuli evoke responses in the ANS and endocrine functions. Such stimuli also activate the brainstem, which in turn sends impulses to the thalamus and cortex. The activation mechanism transforms these impulses into behavior characterized by "emotional excitement." Increased mental activity is reflected in heightened vigilance and awareness and activated memory and concentration. Cognitive processing selects and reduces the number of dimensions in a threatening situation in order to focus better on the danger or challenge.

The cognitive interpretation of the stimuli and arousal results in an emotional state and the performer has a feeling of being mentally prepared for the vocal performance. In the vocal performer, biological and mental arousal can reach very high levels.

The psychological makeup of the performer is complex. Performing at a constant high artistic level is very demanding. Already during the pre-stage period the biological and mental stress may rise to very high levels. Business aspects (Will I get the contract?) tend to provoke heightened stress. Critics, dependence of the audience and fans, and responsibility for a company, clients, or pupils can make them very vulnerable.

During the performance the already built-up prestage biological and mental stress level is likely to increase due to the high physical, social, and creative demands of putting on a good performance, delivering a good speech, giving a good lesson, or having a fruitful meeting.

Emotions

A selection from Izard's publication (1972, pp. 41-54) and considerations highlight some aspects of emotion that illustrate its relevance as an element in the stress chain.

For Arnold (1960a, 1960b), emotion results from a sequence of events described by the concepts of perception and appraisal. He used the term *perception* to mean simple apprehension of an object; *appraisal* is the evaluation what effect it has on the perceiver. Appraisal itself is characterized as direct, immediate, and intuitive, not the result of reflection or deliberation. It immediately follows and completes perception. Schachter and Singer (1962) proposed that emotion results from the physiological arousal and the cognitive appraisal or evaluation of the stimuli-context that elicited the arousal. Plutchnik (1962) defines emotion as a patterned bodily reaction corresponding to an underlying adaptive biological process.

The perception of stressors and the elicited excitement give the feeling of pleasure or displeasure, depending on the interpretation of the signals, and is labeled along a gradient of indifference, basic interest, surprise, and fear (Charlesworth, 1969; Darwin, 1965; Plutchnik, 1962).

Emotions play an important role in human behavior. Izard (1971; 1972) and Tomkins (1962; 1963) maintain that the emotions constitute the primary motivational system in humans. Some scientists have argued that for the most part emotions disrupt and disorganize behavior, and are a primary source of human problems (Lazarus, 1968; Young, 1961). Others state that the emotions play an important role in organizing, motivating, and sustaining behavior (Charlesworth, 1969; Izard, 1971; 1972; Tomkins, 1962; Young, 1961). Some experts maintain that emotions are primarily a matter of visceral functions and activities by the ANS (Gasanov, 1974; Wenger, 1950). Mowrer (1960) states that "the emotions play a central role, indeed an indispensable role, in those changes in behavior or performance which are said to represent 'learning'" (1960, p. 307) and "If the present analysis is sound, the emotions are of quite extraordinary importance in the total economy of living organisms and do not at all deserve being put into opposition with 'intelligence'" (1960, p. 30).

According to Izard (1991), emotions organize and motivate significant aspects of individual behavior, personality development, and social relationships (1991, p. 3). An emotion is experienced as a feeling that motivates, organizes, and guides perception, thought, and action (1991, p. 12). Emotions constitute the primary motivational system of human beings, which activates neural, cognitive, and motor processes, mobilizes and channels energy, and motivates and guides mental and physical activity. According to Selye (1976) stress is neutral. He introduced the term *eustress* and contrasted it with *distress* to reinforce his theory, namely, it is what each individual does with personal stressors that makes the difference in physiological stress response and the short- and long-term effects (1954; 1974). The emotions play an important role in the self-awareness and self-identity and hence in shaping a person's personality and functioning.

Fundamental or basic emotions can be distinguished, each of which has distinct properties. Izard (1991) lists interest, enjoyment, surprise, sadness, anger, disgust, contempt, fear, shame, shyness, and guilt as fundamental emotions.

At the expressive or neuromuscular level, emotion is primarily facial activity and facial patterning. Secondarily, it is expressed bodily by postural, gestural, and vocal behavior. Each of the basic emotions has an expressive component with distinctive facial, vocal, gestural, and bodily expression (Izard, 1991). Being skilled in these distinctive expressive components is, of course, extremely important in performing and vocal communication (Kramer, 1963).

There is widespread confusion about the terms stress and emotion. Although they have their roots in the approach and avoidance system, emotions are in no way synonymous for stress. They only represent one link within the stress chain: the cognitive labeling of the stimuli and/or arousal and activation state. Anxiety can be defined as the conscious concern regarding a person's functioning and abilities.

Seifert and Kollbrunner (2005) put forward that psychosocial conflicts seem less often to be deep-rooted psychopathological problems but rather daily anxieties, failures, injuries, annoyances, disappointments regarding the sufferer him- or herself and others, the nonfulfillment of desires, and feelings of inadequacy and of lack of self-confidence (Pruett, 1991). Patients may find it difficult to speak about conflicts and feelings, and they follow social conventions to an excessive extent.

Anxiety can function as a state and as a trait. Trait anxiety is the degree of susceptibility to anxiety in stressful conditions, whereas state anxiety is transient experienced anxiety.

An occupational voice user as any human being experiences the common anxiety related to ego threat. And, more over, singers and actors have been told to be very sensitive. Self-esteem and pride, social esteem and success, and drive to achieve treasured goals may provoke performance-disturbing emotions.

In a group of elite chorus artists employed full-time by a national opera company, Kenny, Davis, and Oates (2004) found higher trait anxiety, higher occupational role concerns, and higher occupational personal strain than in normative samples. Trait anxiety and musical performance were closely related. Higher scores on personal resources were associated with the higher scores on trait anxiety. It appears that these resources were used adaptively to manage anxiety (Kenny et al., 2004).

Freidl et al. (1989) found that, compared to a control group, functional dysphonic patients show a higher level of state anxiety in situations causing stress.

Coping or Adaptive Reactions

Reflex is a specific unlearned/inborn adaptive response to particular stimuli; it is the simplest form of behavior. Reflexes are automatic responses that require no evaluation and appraisal of the stimulus; no decision about how to behave is involved. Human beings are born with only a few reflexes. Moreover, reflexes are rigid, standard responses and stimulus dependent. When decision-making and flexibility in strategy or performance are required, these are not enough (Fuller, 1992). This is why humans have to learn a great variety and complexity of coping or adaptive behaviors.

Coping is the process of managing the demands that are appraised as taxing or exceeding the resources of a person (Lazarus, 1984). It's similar to the stress response, a homeostatic mechanism, with its main effect to counteract or to eliminate the source of stress.

Coping behaviors are the constant cognitive and behavioral strategies to manage the biological and mental arousal, and to develop skills to meet the basic needs of human well-being. Every individual develops his own coping style, his favorite ways of coping (Dantzer, 1993).

A comparative study by McHugh-Munier et al. (1997) concluded that emotional strategies are used more and cognitive coping strategies are used less by female patients diagnosed with vocal nodules and polyps in comparison to controls with no history of voice pathology.

A person's emotional appraisal and the self-evaluation of his competence lead to coping or adaptive reactions, either to meet the perceived need, or to counteract the perceived danger. Coping behaviors can be differentiated in two main types:

- An approach or fight reaction, in the case of a decision to stay and to gain control over the situation;
- Or a flight reaction, in the sense of an avoidance or an escape reaction, in the case of a decision to flee rather than to face the situation.

Facing the problem and taking up the challenge are examples of approach and fight reactions; not showing up at an audition, canceling the performance, or pretending sickness are typical flight reactions. In behavior terms voicing, acting, and speaking can be defined as either adapted or maladapted coping behavior. In professional voice users the approach has to result in a consciously directed and efficient action, using arousal energy appropriately, in order to sing or speak or teach well. They must be able to stand long-term and intensive arousal and be able to manage stress, keeping it at an efficient and nondisturbing level.

Effects

Effective coping behaviors meet in the short or long term, at least partially, the needs of safety, security, and creativity. As a consequence the arousal level is reduced and adaptation is reached.

Maladaptive coping behavior however doesn't lead to the desired positive effects. The effect may be positive or negative, short- or long-term.

For the occupational voice user, the positive effects of adapted coping behavior can be:

- On a physical level: performing without harming the vocal tract; in the long term
- developing a healthy technique of voicing, speaking, singing, acting;
- On a personal and social level: passing an audition, signing a contract, self-esteem and appraisal by the audi-

ence; in the long term being estimated as an excellent singer, actor, lawyer, teacher; earning a living as a professional voice user;

- On a creative level: the intrinsic pleasure of mastering a technique, putting on a vocal performance that transcends the ordinary; in the long term spiritual well-being or fulfillment.

The negative effects of maladaptive behavior are:

- On a physical level: vocal fatigue, vocal discomfort, and edema of the vocal fold can be defined as short-term, and vocal nodules as a long-term effect of vocal misuse and abuse;
- On a personal level: doubts about one's social position, occupational incapacity; in the long term work incapacity;
- On a creative level: suffering from burnout.

To summarize: the dynamic stress chain consists of: stressors; neuroendocrinocrine reactions; physical signs and organic changes; cognitive aspects, feelings, and emotions; instrumental behaviors; short- and long-term effects, which meet to some extent the needs of safety, security, and creativity.

Figure 18-1 and Figure 18-2 summarize the biological and mental stress chain.

Interaction of Biological and Mental Activation

The interaction of primarily biological and mental excitement and the most common types of secondary kinesthetic emotional excitement are listed in Table 18-1.

Interference of Stress with Vocal Performance

The obvious relationship between vocal communication and stress is commonly stated (Brockway, 1979). Even in the field of aviation and space medicine there exist data about the correlation of voice pitch with emotional excitation (Johannes, 1994; 1995; Ruiz, 1990).

Stress affects the physiological and motor mechanism of vocal performance (Sundberg, 1987). This is reflected in several acoustic parameters such as pitch and intensity variations, vocal range (Seidner, 1981), timbre and prosodic changes, jitter, shimmer, (Fuller, 1992; Mendoza, 1998), duration of the syllables, and other speech aspects (Engstrand, 1988; Fuller, 1992). Moreover, voice and speech modulations are the vehicles to communicate, for adequately expressing the broad spectrum of human feelings and emotions. The listener can easily detect the emotional state of a speaker and singer just by listening and watching the mimic (Sundberg, 1987). Voice, posture, and mimic are very precise emotion indicators. The emotional state of a speaker and singer has a considerable effect on the way the vocal tract is used (Cosmides, 1983; Sundberg, 1987).

Changes of fundamental frequency (F_0), in particular, have significant relationship with emotional load. The maximum F_0 constitutes the primary indicator of the perception of emotional stress (Cosmides, 1983; Protopapas, 1997; Wittels, 2002).

The influence of life events has been shown to have an important effect on the etiopathogenesis of functional dysphonias (Butcher, 1993; Freidl, 1990; 1993; House, 1988). Voice pitch mode

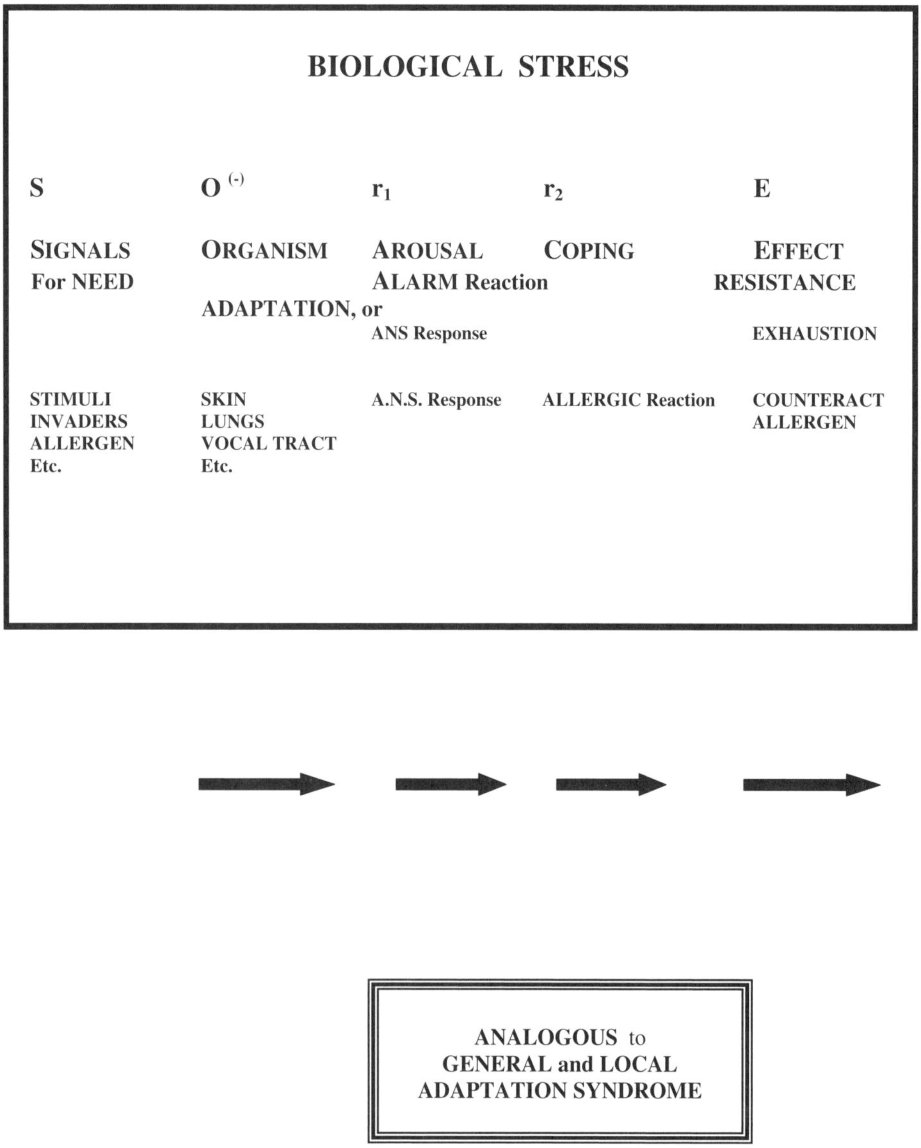

Figure 18–1. Biological stress. *Note.* From by H. Selye (1976). This scheme is an application to voice by the authors Wellens & Van Opstal of the more general scheme of biological stress. Reprinted courtesy of Phoniatrics ENT Department, University Clinics KULeuven, Kapucijnenover, 35 B 300 Belgium.

(F_{om}) is less related to physical than to psychological load. The reactivity of F_{om} to mental load depends on psychological personality traits (Johannes, 1995).

Actors and singers have not only to deal with their personal emotions; they also have to be very skilled on the stage in conveying various feelings and emo-

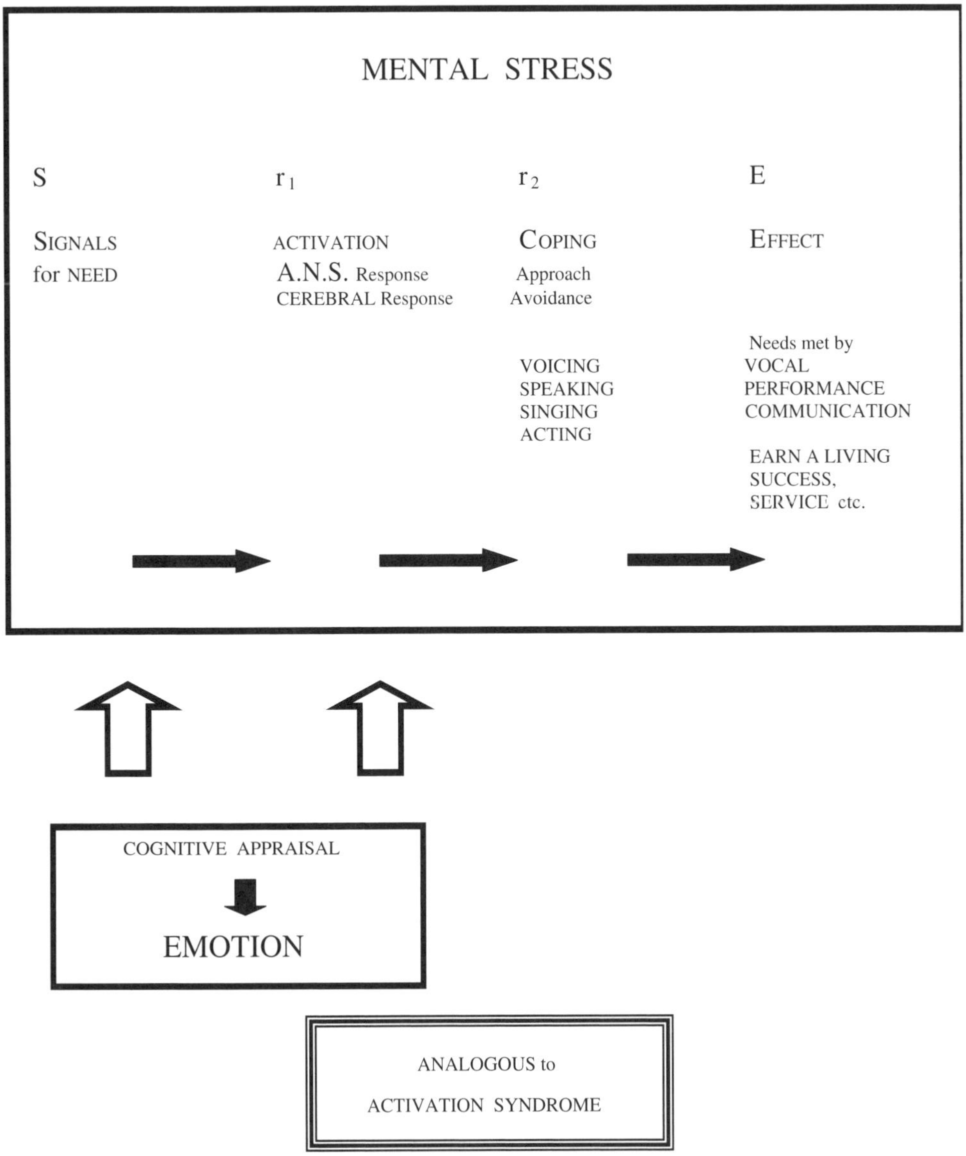

Figure 19–2. Mental stress. *Note.* From by D. B. Lindsley (1951; 1957). This scheme is an application to voice by the authors Wellens & Van Opstal of the more general scheme of biological stress. Reprinted courtesy of Phoniatrics ENT Department, University Clinics KULeuven, Kapucijnenover, 35 B 300 Belgium.

tions of the roles they perform (Bunch, 1995).

Whatever are the technical skills the individual has developed, the final level of his performance depends on to what extent he manages to perform within the functional circle of stress (Misterek, 1989; Wellens, 2001).

The stress response has numerous physical consequences as listed in Table 18–1.

Table 18–1. Interaction of the biological and mental activation

PRIMARY EXCITEMENT (Biological and Mental)	SECONDARY EXCITEMENT (Kinesthetic and Emotional)
PHYSIOLOGICAL ASPECTS	
Muscular strength increases	Headache, neck and shoulder pain
Heart and respiration rate increases	Heart palpitation Changes in rate and depth of respiration Hyperventilation
Reduced range of perception, tunnel vision Pupils change size, field of vision narrows	Attention sharply and narrowly focused on stressor
Mucus / saliva production decreases	Swallowing feels difficult Dry mouth and throat Throat is getting tight Throat clearing
Visceral reflexes	Nausea, diarrhea, gastric acid production Urinary urgency
Sweating increases	Palms feel cold and sweaty
Vasoconstriction	Complexion becomes pale Syncope High blood pressure
Metabolic, endocrine functions increase: Catecholamines, ACTH, Cortisone	Positive feeling of "Being pumped up Negative feeling of "Being exhausted"
MOTOR ASPECTS	
Increased muscle strength, tone	Alteration in voicing, singing
Motor (dys)co-ordination, trembling	Hoarseness Tremor Restricted frequency range, prosody, intensity dynamics Resonance: poor harmonics Articulation problems Phonofatigue, phonodiscomfort Poor relaxation, posture, breath support Psychomotor agitation Musculoskeletal tension Affected acting, etc.
COGNITIVE ASPECTS	
Mental activity increases	Heightened vigilance, awareness Sleep pattern changes Impaired memory and concentration
Appraisal of stimuli, arousal & activation Predisposed by: expectancy, perceptual selectivity, concepts, imagination, previous experiences	Pleasure/displeasure Labeling: Indifference Basic interest Surprise Fear Emotions Feeling of being "Mentally prepared Feeling of being "Burned out"

Some physiological manifestations may interfere directly with vocal performance and acting; some may be observed by the vocal performer and recognized as objective signs of stress.

The ANS disturbs respiration rate, pattern, and control. Decrease of lubrication of mouth and throat affects *eu-voicing* and *eu-speaking*. Muscular strength and (dys)coordination directly and indirectly affect the fine motor control of voicing, articulating, mimic (Rusalova, 1975), and acting. Posture, body alignment, and breath support go out of control. The result of severe or sustained stress without appropriate release leads to unnecessarily high muscle tension especially in the face, larynx, neck, and shoulders. The effects are poor vocal performance, mimic, acting, and even complaints of muscle pain, phonofatigue, and phonodiscomfort (Sundberg, 1987).

Cognitive aspects also have a disrupting effect on the performance (Freidl, 1993; McHugh-Munier, 1997; Wellens, 2001). Because attention and concentration are focused on the source of the threat, the cognitive labeling and the concerns, doubts, or worries about one's coping capabilities, attention to other aspects such as vocal technique, artistic interpretation, and contents can be weakened. The effect is a poor vocal performance. Anxiety and negative self-evaluation interfere with the performance and make the performer feel uncertain and unhappy.

Another general aspect of stress is that in modern society we have to learn to inhibit or adapt our physical and mental responses to stress (Maisel, 1992). The immediate expression of adequate coping behaviors to adapt to biological and mental arousal is often not desirable or allowed in society today. There is always some risk when expressing our feelings and coping behaviors (Butcher, 1993). The risk of the negative consequences of expression has to be weighed against the effects of not expressing our feelings and coping behaviors. If adaptation becomes impossible we remain in a constant state of biological and mental hyperexcitement. This can lead to exhaustion and all kinds of dysfunctions and disorders. The irony is that the stress mechanism, which is supposed primarily to save us from life-threatening situations, becomes distress-provoking in some circumstances, contributing to dysfunction, medical and mental health problems, and even to death.

To summarize:

- Only a body and mind that is in eustress results in expressive voice, speech, mimic, and movement;
- The cumulative effects of different external and internal stressors may result in distress;
- Distress has a disrupting effect on vocal performance;
- It is a general clinical observation that distress affects a speaker's voice use, sometimes to the extent that vocal dysfunction and even vocal pathology develops;
- Vocal dysfunction and pathology itself may become a distress-response-inducing stressor.

Different Stress Modalities in Professional Voice Users

Stress is not always a detriment to performance. In general, the amount of energy necessary for artistic or public vocal performance is relatively high. A moderate to high level of arousal is intrinsic to all vocal performance. Selye proposes the term eustress and contrasts this with distress. A certain stress level *"eustress"* (Selye, 1956) is necessary in order to speak well. It's a state of high dynamic energy we need to perform well. Eustress implies the sum of the biological and mental activation, which provides the performer with that extra "buzz" to perform to the best of his or her ability. Eustress is recognized by the individual as the feeling of "Now I'm pumped up; now I'm ready to perform." It is the state of dynamic tension and release that is necessary to the speaker. It prepares one to perform more strenuously than otherwise would be possible.

On the contrary, *"distress"* (Selye, 1974) implies a degree of activation that is inefficient or too high to manage and is detrimental to the performance. It will reduce behavioral efficiency and disturb voicing, speaking, and acting more or less seriously. In particular singing, a sensory-motor phenomenon that requires balanced skills, is easily disturbed. Chronic distress may result in habitual maladaptive vocal behaviors and dysphonias. In the longer term it may even induce organic lesions such as edema, vocal nodules, polyps, granulomas, dysplasias, etc.

Once a dysphonia is installed, it will interfere with daily life and with professional demands. Confronted with the negative impact the patient will respond emotionally to vocal dysfunction, which, together with its consequences, triggers of increased stress (Wellens, 2001).

So Seifert et al. (2005) put forward in making diagnosis an assessment of the degree to which the patient feels him- or herself subjectively affected by the voice disorder.

The emotional reactions to dysphonia are manifold. We list below the most common stress and anxiety states related to vocal dysfunction (Wellens, 2001).

- Stress response induced at the perception of the negative impact of dysphonia on the quality of the performance and the quality of life is almost inevitable in vocal performers (Rosen, 1997; Wellens, 2001).

  Disturbance or loss of voice poses a threat to self-image and identity. What to a nonprofessional speaker or singer may be a minor degree of dysphonia without any negative consequences may have devastating effects on the vocal performance and functioning of a professional voice user. No wonder that, in professional voice users, the perception of a decline in vocal efficiency may become a stress-inducing stimulus. A manageable stress situation may become unmanageable if incapacitating vocal problems have developed.
- Induced anticipatory anxiety is the next step. (My voice will crack again. Will I be able to perform? Will I lose my voice forever?) Actors, singers, teachers, and public speakers, become very anxious if the most important tool of their trade, their vocal tract, is not functioning well. Cognitive anticipation and self-evaluation trigger the anticipatory anxiety. The performer anticipates trouble prior to the vocal performance. The installation of anticipatory anxiety can be the start of a disrupting anxiety-provoking spiral, which has devastating effects on the performance and functioning of the individual (Rosen, 1997).
- Anxiety about disease at the perception of vocal problems (Am I developing nodules?) is very common in this group (Prugh, 1990). Tendency to self-

analysis makes them particularly interested in signals of impairment and vocal dysfunction. Vocal performers with a hypochondriac or psychosomatic personality structure are more likely to develop anxiety for disease.

When talking to the patient and boosting his or her confidence, the anxiety will often disappear.

- Disease phobia (I have vocal nodules. I have cancer.) may be the next anxiety-inducing step in increased sensorial perception and/or imagination of dysfunction of the vocal tract. Disease phobia is a marked and persistent irrational fear, sparked off by the anticipation of a disease. It is highly anxiety provoking and therefore interferes significantly with the patient's personal and occupational functioning (McQuellon, 1997).
- Existential anxiety from conflicting needs (Osterwald, 1991) is very distressing (Should I continue my career?) Several conflicts arise as the voice user attempts to apportion time and energy between the demands of his/her profession and commitments of having a meaningful life. For some artistic performers, their self-esteem is mainly built upon the appraisal by the audience. The artist who became a cult figure is under high pressure to continue to fulfill the expectations of his fans. Fame may be a powerful driving factor, but at the same time can destroy the artist. Moreover, it's also a corrosive condition and lack or decrease of recognition can be even more stress inducing than being a celebrity.

  Perception of growing old is always a potential existential anxiety-inducing stressor. The performer faces the loss of his vocal skills, a decline in success and endurance, and increasing competition from younger colleagues. Existential anxiety is never far away.
- Finally, stage fright is a specific performance-related anxiety state; we will look at in more detail.

Stage Fright

Stage fright is an irrational anxiety state for public speaking, singing, or performing just before starting the task. It blocks the person, who then fails to actualize his ability to perform. Performance anxiety is a condition which has been experienced at one time or another by just about everyone who has to perform in public. Stage fright is not uncommon; it is the number one phobia. We all know the feeling of last minute (hyper) arousal before the dimming of the lights. When its level is mild, it can be helpful for a good performance.

In some performers, however, the anxiety state may rise so high that it becomes a paralyzing condition. Irrational fear of negative evaluation and criticism by the audience is an ego threat (Butcher, 1993). High task demands induce high biological arousal and mental activation (Frederikson, 1992; Fresnel, 1999; Wellens, 2001). Worry about one's vocal and artistic skills and the unpredictability of the events and fear about ability to stand regulate the hyperarousal (fear of losing control, lack of confidence) and anticipation of the negative consequences for the performance task and career emerge. Overwhelming anticipatory anxiety for catastrophic disrupting signals results in ruminations and spooking thoughts (I will miss the high C3). This catastrophic thinking becomes a cue for cognitive anxiety, eliciting even greater levels of anxiety.

The combination of fear and worry results in a high anxiety level. The poor performer gripped by fear, and confronted with an approach/avoidance conflict, will lose control and develop struggling fight and flight reactions. Feelings of helplessness, resulting from previous ineffective efforts to cope with the hyperarousal, and confinement (inability to escape) increase the hyperanxiety already present (Seligman, 1975).

In the end, the vocal performance itself becomes a stimulus of displeasure. Negative task expectancy and negative self-concept intervene with task-oriented activities, which ensures that the anxiety-provoking stimuli remain in an ongoing negative loop. The overwhelmed performer realizes that escaping the anxiety-provoking situation or choosing to avoid the situation (not to perform) offers immediate relief from anxiety; the speaker suddenly falls sick just before the meeting is due to start; the singer becomes dysphonic or complains that he is missing his high notes. The long-term consequences are feelings of helplessness, depression, and apathy ending in feelings of being burned out, and the performer will eventually drop out of the profession.

References

Arnold, M. B. (1960). *Emotion and personality: Vol 1. Psychological aspects*. New York: Columbia University Press.

Arnold, M. B. (1960). *Emotion and personality: Vol. II. Psychological aspects*. New York: Columbia University Press.

Aronson, A. (1990). *Clinical voice disorders* (3rd ed.). New York: Thieme Medical Business.

Brockway, B. F. (1979). Situational stress and temporal changes in self-report and vocal measurements. *Nursing Research, 28*(1), 20-24.

Bunch, M. (1995). *Dynamics of the singing voice* (3rd ed.). Vienna, Austria: Springer-Verlag.

Butcher, P., Elias, A., & Raven, R. (1993). *Psychogenic voice disorders and cognitive behaviour therapy*. San Diego, CA: Singular.

Charlesworth, W. R. (1969). The role of surprise in cognitive development. In D. Elkind & F. Flavell (Eds.), *Studies in cognitive development* (pp. 257-314). London: Oxford University Press.

Cosmides, L. (1983). Invariances in the acoustic expression of emotion during speech. *Journal of Experimental Psycholology: Human Perception and Performance, 9*(6), 864-811.

Dantzer, B. (1993). Coping with stress. In S. C. Standford & P. Salmon (Eds.), *Stress: From synapse to syndrome*. London: Academic Press.

Darwin, C. R. (1965). *The expression of emotions in man and animals*. Chicago: University of Chicago Press. (Original work published in 1872)

de Jong, F. I. C. R. S., Cornelis, B. M., Wuyts, F. L., Kooijman, P. G. C., Schutte, H. K., Oudes, M. J., et al. (2004). A psychological cascade model for persisting voice problems in teachers. *Folia Phoniatrica et Logopedia, 55*, 91-101.

Engstrand, O. (1988). Articulatory correlates of stress and speaking rate in Swedish VCV. *Journal of the Acoustical Society of America, 83*(5), 1863-1875.

Fredrikson, M., & Gunnarsson, R. (1992). Psychobiology of stage fright: The effect of public performance on neuroendocrine, cardiovascular and subjective reactions. *Biological Psychology, 33*(1), 51-61.

Freidl, W., Egger, J., & Friedrich, G. (1989). Personality and coping with stress in patients with functional dysphonia. *Psychotherapy and Psychosomatic Medicine and Psychology, 39*(8), 3000-3005.

Freidl, W., Friedrich, G., & Egger, J. (1990). Personlichkeit und Stressbearbeitung bei Patienten mit functionellen Dysphonia. *Folia Phoniatrica 42*(3), 144-149.

Freidl, W., Friedrich, G., Egger, J., & Fitzek, T. (1993). Zur Pychogenese funktioneller Dysphonien. *Folia Phoniatrica, 45*(1), 3-10.

Fresnel, E. (1999). *Le trac: Trac, stress, anxiété problèmes de communication*. Marseille, France: Solal.

Fuller, B. F., Horii, Y., & Conner, D. A. (1992). Validity and reliability of nonverbal voice measures as indicators of stressor-provoked anxiety. *Research in Nursing and Health, 15*(5), 379-389.

Gasanov, G. G. (1974). Emotions, visceral functions, and limbic system. In G. G. Gasanov (Ed.), *Emotions and visceral functions*. Moscow: Elm Press.

Hollien, H. (1980). Vocal indicators of psychological stress. *Annals of the New York Academy of Sciences, 347* 47-72.

House, A. O. & Andrews, H. B., (1988), Life events and difficulties preceding the onset of functional dysphonia. *Journal of Psychosomatic Research, 32*(3), 311-319.

Izard, C. E. (1971). *The face of emotions*. New York: Springer.

Izard, C. E. (1972). *Patterns of emotions: A new analysis of anxiety and depression*. New York: Academic Press.

Izard, C. E. (1991). *The physiology of emotions*. New York: Plenum Press.

Johannes, B., Eichhorn, C., & Fischer, F. (1994). A complex experimental assessment for objective description of hierarchical psychophysiological behavior as human regulatory phenotype. *Journal of Gravitational Physiology, 1*(1), 73-74.

Johannes, B., Salnitzki, V. P., Haller, H., Wilke, D., Fischer, F., & Schlykova, L. (1995). Comparison of voice stress reactivity under psychological stress test and simulate Mir docking manoeuvre. *Journal of Gravitational Physiology, 2*(1), 107-108.

Kanfer, F. H., & Philips, J. S. (1970). *Learning foundations of behavior therapy*. New York: John Wiley & Sons.

Kenny, D. T., Davis, P., & Oates, J. (2004). Music performance anxiety and occupational stress amongst opera chorus artists and their relationship with state and trait anxiety and perfectionism. *Journal of Anxiety Disorders, 18*(6), 757-777.

Knothe, M., Misterek, M., Meyer, G., & Thummler, D. (1990). Stress in the occupational role of teachers with disabilities and physical disorders. *Zeitschrift fur Gesamte Hygiene 36*(8), 424-427.

Kramer, E. (1963). Judgements of personal characteristics and emotions from nonverbal properties of speech. *Psychological Bulletin, 60*, 408-420.

Lazarus, R. S. (1968). Emotions and adaptation: Conceptual and empirical relations. In W. Arnold (Ed.), *Nebraska Symposium on Motivation* (pp. 175-270). Lincoln: University of Nebraska Press.

Lazarus, R. S., & Folkman, S. (1984). *Stress appraisal in coping*. New York: Springer-Verlag.

Lindsley, D. B. (1951). Emotion. In S. S. Stevens (Ed.), *Handbook of experimental psychology* (pp. 473-516). New York: John Wiley.

Lindsley, D. B. (1957). Psychophysiology and motivation. In M. R. Jones (Ed.), *Nebraska Symposium on Motivation* (pp. 44-103). Lincoln, NE: University of Nebraska Press.

Maisel, E. (1992). *Staying sane in the arts*. New York,: Putnam's Sons.

Maslow, A. (1971). *The further reaches of human nature*. New York: Viking.

McHugh-Munier, C., Scherer, K. R., Lehmann, W., & Scherer, U. (1997). Coping strategies, personality, and voice quality with vocal fold nodules and polyps. *Journal of Voice, 11*(4), 452-461.

McQuellon, R. P., & Hurt, G. J. (1997). The psychosocial impact of the diagnosis and treatment of laryngeal cancer. *Otolaryngologic Clinics of North America, 30*(2), 231-241.

Mendoza, E., & Carballo, G. (1998). Acoustic analysis of induced vocal stress by means of cognitive workload. *Journal of Voice, 12*(3). 263-273.

Misterek, M., Knothe, M., Johannes, E., Heidelbach, J. G., & Scheuch, K. (1989). Beanspruchunguntersuchen bei Lehrterinnen mit functionellen Stimmstorungen in der unterrichtlichen Tatigkeit. *Zeitschrif fur Gesamte Hygiene*, *35*(7), 415-416.

Mowrer, O. H. (1960). *Learning theory and behavior*. New York: John Wiley.

Osterwald, P., & Avery, M. (1991). Psychiatric problems of performing artists. In R. T. Sataloff, A. Brandfonbrenner, & R. Lederman (Eds.), *Textbook of performing arts medicine* (2nd ed., pp. 319-335). New York: Raven Press.

Plutchik, R. (1962). *The emotions: Facts, theories, and a new model*. New York: Random House.

Protopapas, A., & Lieberman, P. (1997). Fundamental frequency of phonation and perceived emotional stress. *Journal of the Acoustical Society of America*, *101*(4), 2267-2277.

Pruett, K. D. (1991). Psychological aspects of the development of exceptional young performers and prodigies. In R. T. Sataloff, A. G. Branfonbrenner, & R. J. Lederman (Eds.), *Textbook for performing arts medicine* (pp. 337-349). New York: Raven Press.

Prugh, D. G., & Thompson, T. L. (1990). Illness as a source of stress: Acute illness, chronic illness, and surgical procedures. In J. Nospitz & R. Coppington (Eds.), *Stressors and the adjustments disorders*. New York: John Wiley and Sons.

Punt, N. (1979). *The singer and the actor's throat*. London: Heineman.

Rosen, D. C., & Sataloff, R. T. (1997). Psychological aspects of voice disorders. In R. T. Sataloff (Ed.), *Professional voice: The science and art of clinical care* (2nd ed., pp. 305-317). New York: Raven Press.

Rosen, D. C., & Sataloff, R. T. (1997). *Psychology of voice disorders*. San Diego, CA: Singular.

Rubin, J., Sataloff, R. T., Korovin, G., & Gould, W. J. (1995). *The diagnosis and treatment of voice disorders*. New York: Igaku-Shoin.

Ruiz, R., Legos, C., & Guell, A. (1990). Voice analysis to predict the physiological or physical state of a speaker. *Aviation, Space, and Environmental Medicine*, *61*(3), 266-271.

Rusalova, M. N., Izard, C. E., & Simonov, A. S. (1975). Comparative analysis of mimical and autonomic components of man's emotional state. *Aviation, Space, and Environmental Medicine*, *46*(9), 1132-1134.

Sataloff, R. T. (1991). Care of the professional voice. In R. T. Sataloff, A. G. Branfonbrenner, & R. J. Lederman (Eds.), *Textbook for performing arts medicine* (pp. 229-286). New York: Raven Press.

Sataloff, R. T. (1997). Patient history. In R. T. Sataloff (Ed.), *Professional voice: The science and art of clinical care* (2nd ed., pp. 193-201). New York: Raven Press.

Schachter, S., & Singer, J. E. (1962). Cognitive, social and physiological determinants of emotional state. *Psychological Review*, *69*, 379-399.

Schutte, H. K. (1980). *The efficiency of voice production*. Groningen, Netherlands: Kemper.

Seidner, W., Sturzebecher, E., & Wagner, H. (1981). Belastungsphonographie. *Folia Phoniatrica*, *33*(2), 100-104.

Seidner, W., & Wendler, J. (1997). Erkrankungen und Gezundhaltung der Stimme. In *Die Sängerstimme* (pp. 228-261). Berlin, Germany: Henschel Verlag.

Seifert, E., & Kollbrunner, J. (2005). Stress and distress in non-organic voice disorders. *Swiss Medical Weekly*, *135*(27-28), 387-397.

Seligman, M. E. P. (1975). *Helplessness: On depression, development and death*. San Francisco: Freeman.

Selye, H. (1950). *The physiology and pathology of exposure to stress*. Montreal, Canada: Acta.

Selye, H. (1954). On the real benefits of eustress. *Psychology Today*, *12*(10), 60-64.

Selye, H. (1974). *Stress without distress*. Philadelphia: Lippencott.

Selye, H. (1976). *The stress of life* (2nd ed.). New York: McGraw Hill.

Simovov, P. V., & Frolov, M. V. (1977). *Aviation, Space, and Environmental Medicine, 48*(1), 23-25.

Smith, G. A. (1977). Voice analysis for the measurements of anxiety. *British Journal of Medical Psychology, 50*(4), 367-373.

Stemple, J. (1993). *Voice therapy: Clinical studies.* St. Louis, MO: Mosby Year Book.

Sundberg, J. (1987). *The science of the singing voice*. Dekalb, IL: Northern Illinois University Press.

Tomkins, S. S. (1962). *Affect, imagery, consciousness: Vol 1. The positive affects.* New York: Springer.

Tomkins, S. S. (1963). *Affect, imagery, consciousness: Vol 2. The negative affects.* New York: Springer.

Wellens, W. A. R., & Van Opstal M. J. C. M. (2001). Performance stress in professional voice users. In P. H. Dejonkere (Ed.), *Occupational voice—Care and cure*. (pp. 81-100). The Hague, Netherlands: Kugler.

Wenger, M. A. (1950). Emotion a visceral action: An extension of Lange's theory. In M. L. Reymert (Ed.), *Feelings and emotions.* The Mooseheart Symposium (pp. 3-10). New York: McGraw-Hill.

Williams, C. E., & Stevens, H. T. (1972). Emotions and speech: Some acoustic correlates. *Journal of the Acoustical Society of America, 52*, 1238-1250.

Wittels, P., Johannes, B., Enne, R., Kirsch, K., & Gunga, H. C. (2002). Voice monitoring to measure emotional load during short-term stress. *European Journal of Applied Physiology, 87*(3), 278-282.

Young, P. T. (1961). *Motivation and emotions: A survey of the determinants of human and animal activity*. New York: Wiley.

CHAPTER 19

Vocal Psychodynamics in the Voice Clinic

Mara Behlau and Gisele Gasparini

Abstract

Here we reinforce the idea that the larynx is an organ of emotions since birth, and then we explain the concept of vocal psychodynamics and the emotional impact of voice on the listener. We propose that any physiological change can affect the main vocal parameters identifying a vocal image of an individual, that is, vocal quality, resonance, loudness, pitch, articulation, rhythm, and breathing. These parameters will produce a psychological response in the listener, and this is specifically crucial in speakers suffering dysphonia. Therefore, we propose the usage of psychodynamic voice evaluation to make the speaker aware of the psychological impact of his or her voice on the listener. To accomplish this task, the verbal message needs to be separated from the vocal expression.

Introduction

In this chapter we discuss the concept of vocal psychodynamics and its role in the clinical approach. We propose here using the Psychodynamic Approach when treating patients presenting with voice disorders, which typically affect the production of emotional prosody; we also propose that the organ of voice, the larynx, is one of the most important organs of emotions.

Voice is present since birth and is a subject of continuous change during the life span. The quality of a specific voice corresponds to the overall development of an individual, both in the physical and in the socio-psychological sense. We postulate that the larynx should be considered an organ of emotions and not merely a motor system reacting to stimuli in a reflexive way to signify changes and as an expression of internal struggle (Connor, 2008; Moses, 1954.

The ongoing process of speech development relies on the voice as a carrier signal for both phonetic and emotional information, with the additional possibility of transferring emotive information (not just through facial and body expressions) but also through vocalization, because vocalization reflects the subtleness of the nervous and somatic systems, and therefore emotion effects would be expected on the voice (Scherer, 1995).

The concept of vocal psychodynamics refers to the psychological impact of one's voice on the listener (Behlau & Ziemer, 1988; Moses, 1954). The relationship between voice, personality, and emotions has been known since antiquity. Aristotle proposed an extensive list of vocal parameters and aspects related to personality, emotion, or social/educational level of speaker, and in more modern times, a scientific summary of these relationships, at least for health practitioners, has been outlined elsewhere (Moses, 1954).

To elaborate on this, cultural, social, gender, and age particularities need to be considered (Behlau, 2001; Behlau & Ziemer, 1988; Bloom, Zajac, & Titus, 1999; Pittam, 1994; Rossit & Behlau, 2006). For example, Brazilian women prefer a low-pitched voice, as low F_0 is a sign of independence and professionalism, while the preferred female voice in Japanese female culture is high-pitched, as it is considered to express femininity and good manners (Behlau, 2001). Moreover, voice characteristics alter significantly according to the personality of the speaker, the context, and the situation. However, there are essential aspects concerning vocal tract configuration, characteristics of personality and the impact of the voice produced on the listeners, which are evident even to the naive listener, regardless of the communication process (Pear, 1931; Scherer, 1979).

Our voice is changing during the life span, even though the basic parameters that determine someone's vocal quality in a broad sense appear to be preserved. The uniqueness of the sound of one's voice arises from the interaction of two main factors, (a) organic (anatomy) and (b) phonetic (usage of a language) (Laver, 2000). Hence, according to a concept proposed by Laver (1968; 1978), someone's voice can be described by both the articulatory settings of the vocal apparatus, including laryngeal, labial, mandibular, lingual tip/blade, body and root, and velar coupling, and by the phonatory modes.

As an example, consider a young adult male who presents with a problem of a long-term adjustment characterized by raised larynx, labiodentalization with lip spread, advanced tip/blade articulation, nasal-velar coupling, and a falsetto voice. This sort of setting can be a result of anatomically determined puberphonia, or due to emotional difficulties encountered in facing adulthood. Well, in true adulthood, such a voice can be a response to an idiopathic vocal fold paralysis (paralytic falsetto) (Izdebski, 2004). Therefore, a young man with such a voice will probably be judged by the listeners as immature or maybe even as representing a sexual conflict, even if his vocal setting represents solely compensation for anatomic reality or is due to an organic problem. On the other hand, the adult male with laryngeal paralysis and so-called paralytic falsetto may be misjudged on the phone as an adolescent (see Chapter 8 in this volume).

People may be categorized and judged by their vocal quality, regardless of the presence of a disorder. It is of importance to consider vocal psychodynamics as a factor when evaluating and treating dysphonic patients. (For more on how vocal pathologies can evoke inappropriate emotional responses, see Chapter 8 in this volume.)

The vocal parameters that typically identify a speaker are: vocal quality, resonance, loudness, pitch, pitch range, articulation, rhythm and speech rate, and breathing pattern. The parameter usage depends on the speaker's anatomy, physiology, and psycho-physiology, as well as on the cultural and social environment. Behlau (2001) recently summarized the main psychodynamic impact of these vocal parameters.

The vocal quality relates to the type of voice and provides the overall vocal impression based on the source and resonance. The vocal quality is fully influenced by the language and culture, and so is the impact caused by it. This parameter provides information about the biological, psychological, and social-educational characteristics of the individual. Any deviation on the vocal quality may impair the real psychodynamic impact, causing communication problems.

The resonance relates to the emotional goal of the speech: a balanced resonance reveals psycho-emotional equilibrium; a laryngo-pharyngeal focus is related to tension and aggressive feelings. For example, an oral focus may be associated with narcissism; a nasal quality (non-tense) is usually used for expressing sensuality and affection, while either hyponasality or hypernasality is typically judged as unpleasant (Behlau, 2001).

Loudness relates to the vocal manifestation of social limits. The use of a balanced loudness shows an awareness of social limits and respect to others. A weak voice, however, displays a lack of social experiences, fear, or shyness. If on one hand a loud voice may demonstrate frankness, on the other its negative facet may transmit aggression and bad manners.

The pitch itself and the range of tones selected by the speaker are going to transmit different information. The pitch alone relates to the intention of the speech and the maturity of the speaker. While a high-pitched voice conveys fragility, femininity, dependence, and immaturity, a low-pitched voice transmits authority, maturity, and masculinity. Higher tones characterize happy and surprising situations, and lower tones, serious and sad circumstances. The pitch range relates to trading attitude and interpersonal flexibility. A rich, controlled range shows happiness, satisfaction, and good feelings. While an excessively wide range shows loss of control and excitation beyond limits, a narrow range shows a variety of characteristics such as character rigidity, excessive emotional control, repressive education, monotone, and boredom.

Articulation refers to the extent by which the information is delivered and to the educational level of the speaker. A well-defined type of articulation conveys an impression of a clear mind, good ideas, education, desire to be understood, and consideration towards the listener. An imprecise articulatory pattern transmits mental confusion, lack of wish to communicate, and lack of education. Over-articulation exhibits narcissism and egocentrism; sometimes overarticulation is needed when comprehension is crucial but it's usually linked to egocentric and vain speakers. Finally, a closed articulatory pattern displays aggression and rage.

Rhythm and speech rate relate to the speaker's mental process. While a slow speech rate conveys emotional equilibrium, a fast rate transmits tension and aggressive feelings; an irregular pattern transmits lack of control, anxiety, and mental confusion; and lastly too regular a rate transmits rigidity, contention, and artificiality. Introduction of tremor to the voice either connotes an illness or can be a vocal sign of deception (Shipp & Izdebski, 1981).

Breathing pattern concerns the rhythms of life and contact with either the situation or the environment. A balanced respiratory mode (inspiration and expiration) transmits clear mind, persistence, and psychological equilibrium. If on one hand a deep pattern gives the impression of an active and energetic person, a shallow pattern shows avoidance of contact and anxiety.

Although the selected options can be the result of anatomic and functional features, psychological traits/state, or laryngeal pathologies, the speaker will be analyzed from an emotional point of view. A spasmodic dysphonia patient with overpressure and phonatory breaks, for instance, may be considered a vocal cripple (Izdebski, 1980) or as being tense and nervous, even when relaxing at the beach. A Parkinson's patient will produce a negative first impact on the listener due to the hypophonia and reduced speech rate (Canuto, Gasparini, & Behlau, 2006). Since several vocal parameters can be severely deviated in dysphonic patients, a psychodynamic evaluation and careful feedback to the speaker is essential in the vocal rehabilitation process.

Vocal Psychodynamics Evaluation

It's a common response to interpret someone's feelings through the voice (Canuto et al., 2006; Rossit & Behlau, 2006). After a single "hello" on the phone a spouse can sense that there is something happening at home. Our voice instantly reacts to inner and outer stimuli, both physical and psychological in nature. As far as the physical nature is concerned, background noise is the main source of vocal quality modification (Södersten, Ternström, & Bohman, 2005), as under noise conditions the voice tends to be higher in pitch and loudness and tenser in quality. During these occasions people can be considered as more aggressive. Considering the psychological nature, basic (or at times referred as modal) emotions, such as happiness, sadness, anger, surprise, disgust, and fear, are easily identified in the voice. Synthesized speech samples can be created and main parameters can be manipulated to explore the limits of certainty or ambiguity in recognition (Cahn, 1990).

Basic emotions have clear acoustic trends (Banse & Scherer, 1996; Pittam & Scherer, 1993); for instance, rage is characterized by high fundamental frequency, large frequency variability with descending contours, higher energy on spectrum, high-frequency energy, and fast speech rate. Fear is characterized by even higher fundamental frequency, large frequency variability, high-frequency energy, and fast speech rate. Sadness is represented by low fundamental frequency, reduced frequency variability, descending contours, reduced energy on all spectra, slow speech rate, and reduced high-frequency energy. Despair is represented by similar parameters as sadness, but with a higher fundamental frequency and higher level of energy on spectrum; happiness is characterized by high fundamental frequency and increased frequency variability, with higher energy level on spectrum, high-frequency energy, and fast speech rate.

In the clinical setting, people may seek voice services for at least three different reasons. The first is to improve the voice for professional usage. Second, people may seek treatment because of a voice problem. A third reason is to maintain a given voice quality, even if pathological, for financial reasons, for example, voice-over artists who require maintaining a specific voice quality at any cost. To perceive voice and to analyze it correctly a clinician must be capable of performing a perceptual assessment. A set of four initial steps is suggested for voice evaluation and for using information in the rehabilitation process (Behlau & Ziemer, 1988):

1. Listen without personal projection.
2. Separate verbal message from vocal expression.
3. Observe any emotional and/or motor reaction triggered by the vocal stimuli.
4. Describe the experience, without personal judgment and interpretation.

The easiest strategy to involve patients in their psychodynamic evaluation is to make them choose 10 words that describe their voice from a given list. An example is Boone's list, 100 Word-Descriptors for voice (Boone, 1991), which contains 100 terms used by patients to describe their own voices, such as abrasive, good, insecure, low, warm, and sexy. Afterwards, patients should classify the terms as positive or negative and then a discussion on the selection should be established. This list can be adapted according to patients' descriptions in each culture.

For Brazilians, a 172-descriptor list was compiled from patients' protocols of the Centro de Estudos da Voz (CEV; Behlau, 2001). For illustration purposes, we show an example of this process with a TV news announcer, 32 years old, who sought voice treatment. The positive terms she selected were brilliant, good, melodic, stable, and rich. The negative terms were sexy, artificial, mellow, and affected. After opening a discussion on the selection made, the patient reported that the main negative issue was related to the sexy component, which is inappropriate for a TV news program.

Another option for involving patients in this process of making them aware of someone's voice impact on the listener is to analyze the information contained in characters' voices in foreign films or soap operas and even news announcers transmitting happy and sad events. More important than identifying the vocal psychodynamics characteristics is to use this information positively to improve communication competence.

Vocal Psychodynamics Approach

The goal of the Psychodynamic Approach (PA) is to offer feedback to let patients recognize the specific impact of their voice on the listener. The patient is guided in identifying the revealed impact, and the clinician makes it clear that vocal parameters are conditioned throughout the life or may be the result of a pathology and do not always represent the patient's emotion or true nature. For this process, examples can provide a great help: a loud voice is common in children that grow up in noisy families; fast speech rate may be due to stressful situations; uncoordinated breathing can be due to a vocal fold paresis and not to anxiety; rough voice can be the result of a distorted mucosal wave from vocal nodules and not due to an abrasive manner. So, it's important to make the patient comprehend that the psychological impact does not always represent the real self; for example, a closed jaw articulation delivers aggression even if the cause is temporomandibular joint dysfunction.

Voice is a primary and automatic instrument for emotional expression, because it has a physiological basis and a communicative function (Scherer, 1995). The voice clinician must be aware that any behavioral change is submitted to the psychological acceptance of the patient. Voice is a strong mirror of one's self. Everybody influences and is influenced by others' vocal patterns. To omit consideration of the vocal psychodynamic of a dysphonic patient can restrict or even impair the vocal rehabilitation outcome.

Table 19–1 summarizes the main naïve interpretations of different types of voice, and Table 19–2 matches frequent vocal problems and common features to their main vocal psychodynamics interpretation.

Table 19–1. Type of voice and main vocal psychodynamic interpretation

Type of Voice	Main Interpretation
Roughness	Aggression, anger, and/or fatigue
Breathiness	Fatigue, sensuality (discrete deviation), lack of power, and/or shyness
Strain	Effort, difficult life, relationship problems, and/or distress
Nasality	Sensuality (discrete deviation), lack of social skills, and/or limited intelligence
Tremulous	Emotional liability, lack of confidence, conflict, and/or fear
Asteny	Lack of energy, shyness, and/or lack of social skills or confidence
Creaky/Basal	Aggression, attempt to control or to express power, villainy

Table 19–2. Vocal problems with common features and their main vocal psychodynamics interpretations

Vocal Problem and Common Features	Main Interpretation
Vocal nodules: Low pitch, high intensity, and roughness	Aggression, anxiety, and invasive personality, with need to control
Reinke's edema: Low pitch, sometimes fry	Virilization, control, and power
Vocal fold paralysis: Breathiness and roughness, pitch instability, and breathing uncoordination	Fatigue, lack of control and power, distress
Parkinson's disease: Hypophonia, slurred articulation, and reduced speech rate	Weakness, sadness, indifference, confusion, depression, and slowness
Amyotrophic lateral sclerosis: Roughness, nasality, and distorted speech	Cognitive impairment and lack of power or energy
Depression: Low pitch, reduced loudness, and monotone	Sadness, lack of interest or energy, low self-esteem, and boredom
Presbyphonia: Unstable vocal quality, reduced loudness, and sometimes high pitch	Weakness, lack of power, and reduced virility (for men)
Spasmodic dysphonia: Overpressure and phonatory breaks	Tension, aggression, stress, despair, and/or the edge of a breakdown
Puberphonia (vocal mutation delay/falsetto): High-pitched voice with limited range	Infantile behavior, immaturity, femininity, crossed gender presentation, sexual conflicts, and/or insecurity
Scar: Roughness, high pitch, and breathing uncoordination	Tension, despair, anxiety, and lack of control
Muscle tension dysphonia: Effortful phonation, usually with low pitch and high intensity	Effort to live, invasive personality, restlessness, anxiety, and tension
Endocrinological virilization: Women with low-pitched voice and reduced range	Masculinity, crossed gender presentation, and/or sexual conflicts
Esophageal/tracheoesophageal speech: Rough/fry voice, low pitch, and loudness	Weirdness, ugliness, rejection, and sickness

Summary

This chapter presented the importance of voice as an expression of emotions. A person with normal voice unconsciously or consciously modifies his or her vocal quality, resonance, loudness, pitch, articulation, rhythm, and breathing to express or reveal feelings, moods, and intentions. In the presence of a vocal pathology this process can be severely impaired. For instance, rough voices can be interpreted as a sign of aggression and a patient with spasmodic dysphonia can be seen as someone tense or on the edge of a breakdown. As indicated, the psychodynamic evaluation requires separation of the verbal message from the vocal expression. The use of the psychodynamic approach offers the opportunity for the patient to recognize the impact of his or her voice on the listener.

References

Banse, R., & Scherer, K. R. (1996). Acoustic profiles in vocal emotion expression. *Journal of Personality and Social Psychology, 70*, 614-636.

Behlau, M. (2001). *Voz. O livro do especialista* (Vol. I). Rio de Janeiro, Brazil: Revinter.

Behlau, M., & Ziemer, R. (1988). Psicodinâmica vocal. In L. P. Ferreira (Eds.), *Trabalhando a voz* (pp. 71-88). São Paulo, Brazil: Summus.

Bloom, K., Zajac, D. J., & Titus, J. (1999). The influence of voice in sex-stereotyped perceptions. *Journal of Nonverbal Behavior, 24*, 271-281.

Boone, D. (1991). *Is your voice telling on you?* San Diego, CA: Singular.

Cahn, J. E. (1990). The generation of affect in synthesized speech. *Journal of American Voice Input/Output Society, 8*, 1-19.

Canuto, V., Gasparini, G., & Behlau, M. (in press). Piscodinâmica vocal de pacientes portadores da Doença de Parkinson. In M. Behlau & I. Gielow (Eds.), *A voz do especialista* (Vol. IV). Rio de Janeiro, Brazil: Revinter.

Connor, S. (2008). In K. Izdebski (Ed.), *The emotions in the human voice*. San Diego, CA: Plural.

Izdebski, K. (1980). Effects of prestimulus interval on phonation initiation reaction times. *Journal of Speech and Hearing Research, 23*(3), 485-489.

Izdebski, K. (2008). Clinical voiceassessment: The role and value of the phonatory function studies. In A. K. Lalwani (Ed.), *Current Diagnosis and Treatment. Otolaryngology Head and Neck Surgery* (pp. 416-429). NY: McGraw Hill Lange.

Laver, J. (1968). Voice quality and indexical information. *British Journal of Disorders of Communication, 3*, 43-54.

Laver, J. (1978). The concept of articulatory settings: A historical survey. *Historiographia Linguistica, 5*, 1-14.

Laver J. (2000) Phonetic evaluation of voice quality. In R. Kent & M. J. Ball (Eds.), *Voice quality measurement.* San Diego, CA: Singular.

Moses, P. (1954). *The voice of neurosis.* New York: Grune & Stratton.

Pear, T. H. (1931). *Voice and personality.* London: Chapman & Hall.

Pittam, J. (1994). *Voice in social interaction: An interdisciplinary approach.* Thousand Oaks, CA: Sage.

Pittam, J., & Scherer, K. R. (1993). Vocal expression and communication of emotion. In M. Lewis & J. M. Haviland (Eds.), *Handbook of emotions* (pp. 185-198). New York: Guilford.

Rossit, L., & Behlau, M. (in press). Opinião leiga quanto à agradabilidade de diferentes vozes. In M. Behlau & I. Gielow (Eds.), *A voz do especialista* (Vol. IV). Rio de Janeiro, Brazil: Revinter.

Scherer, K. R. (1979). Personality markers in speech. In K. R. Scherer & H. Giles

(Eds.), *Social markers in speech* (pp. 147-209). London: Cambridge University Press.

Scherer, K. R. (1995). Expression of emotion in voice and music. *Journal of Voice, 9*, 235-248.

Shipp, T., & Izdebski, K. (1981). Current evidence for the existence of laryngeal macrotremor and microtremor. *Journal of Forensic Science, 26*(3), 501-505.

Södersten, M., Ternström, S., & Bohman, M. (2005). Loud speech in realistic environmental noise: Phonetogram data, perceptual voice quality, subjective ratings and gender differences in healthy speakers. *Journal of Voice, 19*, 29-46.

Index

A

B

C

D

E

F

M

N

O

P

R

S